ABC of Sexually Transmitted Infections

Sixth Edition

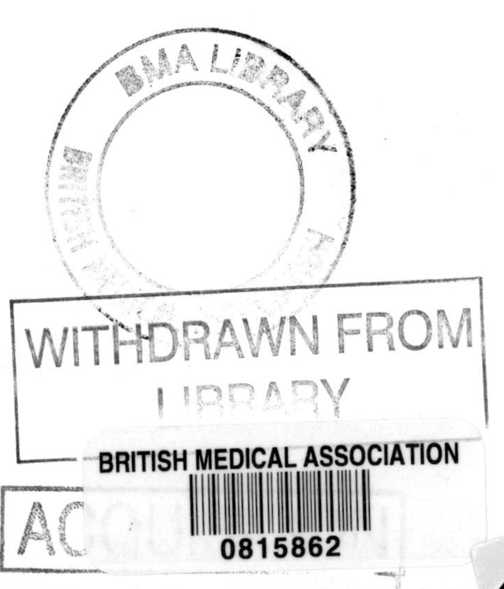

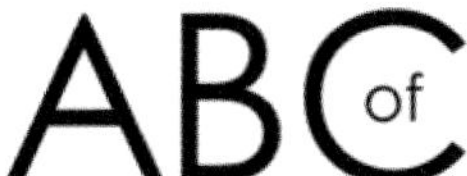

Sexually Transmitted Infections

Sixth Edition

EDITED BY

Karen E Rogstad

Consultant Physician
Sheffield Teaching Hospitals NHS Foundation Trust, Sheffield, UK

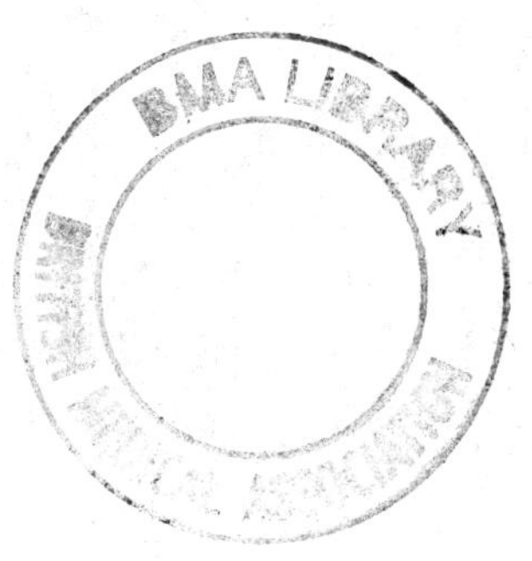

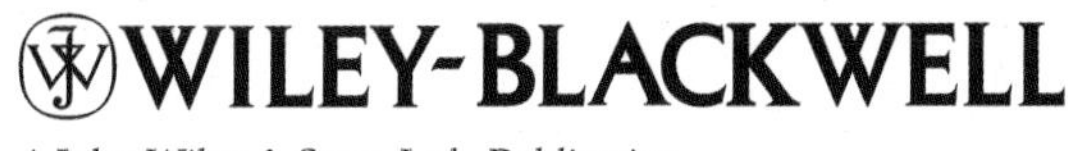

A John Wiley & Sons, Ltd., Publication

BMJ | Books

This edition first published 2011, © Blackwell Publishing Ltd

BMJ Books is an imprint of BMJ Publishing Group Limited, used under licence by Blackwell Publishing which was acquired by John Wiley & Sons in February 2007. Blackwell's publishing programme has been merged with Wiley's global Scientific, Technical and Medical business to form Wiley-Blackwell.

Registered office: John Wiley & Sons Ltd, The Atrium, Southern Gate, Chichester, West Sussex, PO19 8SQ, UK

Editorial offices: 9600 Garsington Road, Oxford, OX4 2DQ, UK
The Atrium, Southern Gate, Chichester, West Sussex, PO19 8SQ, UK
111 River Street, Hoboken, NJ 07030-5774, USA

For details of our global editorial offices, for customer services and for information about how to apply for permission to reuse the copyright material in this book please see our website at www.wiley.com/wiley-blackwell

Library of Congress Cataloging-in-Publication Data
ABC of sexually transmitted infections. – Sixth Edition / edited by Karen Rogstad, Department of Genitourinary Medicine, Royal Hallamshire Hospital, Sheffield, South Yorkshire, UK.
p. ; cm.
Includes bibliographical references and index.
ISBN 978-1-4051-9816-5 (pbk. : alk. paper) 1. Sexually transmitted diseases. 2. Communicable diseases. I. Rogstad, Karen, editor.
[DNLM: 1. Sexually Transmitted Diseases. WC 140]
RA644.V4A24 2011
614.5′47 – dc22

2010047401

A catalogue record for this book is available from the British Library.

Set in 9.25/12 Minion by Laserwords Private Limited, Chennai, India
Printed in Singapore by C.O.S. Printers Pte Ltd

2 2015

To Luke and Annabelle

Contents

Contributors

Sarah Alexander
Clinical Scientist, Sexually Transmitted Bacteria Reference Laboratory, Health Protection Agency, London, UK

Monique Andersson
Specialist Registrar in Virology and Genitourinary Medicine, Health Protection Agency Regional Laboratory South West; Bristol Sexual Health Clinic, Bristol, UK

Gill Bell
Nurse Consultant and Sexual Health Adviser, Genitourinary Medicine, Sheffield Teaching Hospitals NHS Foundation Trust, Sheffield, UK

Alison Bigrigg
Director, The Sandyford Initiative, Glasgow, UK

Aparna Briggs
Specialist Registrar in Genitourinary Medicine, Sheffield Teaching Hospitals NHS Foundation Trust, Sheffield, UK

M Gary Brook
Clinical Lead GUM/HIV, North West London Hospitals NHS Foundation Trust, London, UK

Chris Bunker
Consultant Dermatologist, University College and Chelsea & Westminster Hospital; Professor of Dermatology, University College, London, UK

Elizabeth Carlin
Consultant Physician in Genitourinary Medicine, Sherwood Forest Hospitals NHS Foundation Trust and Nottingham University Hospitals NHS Trust, Nottinghamshire, UK

Frances Cowan
Senior Lecturer and Honorary Consultant, University College London, London, UK

David Daniels
Consultant in Sexual Health and HIV, West Middlesex University Hospital NHS Foundation Trust, Isleworth, UK

Sarah Edwards
Consultant GU Physician, Suffolk Community Health, West Suffolk Hospital, Bury St Edmunds, UK

Claudia Estcourt
Reader in Sexual Health and HIV, Queen Mary University of London, Barts and The London School of Medicine and Dentistry, London, UK

Christopher K Fairley
Chair of Sexual Health Unit, University of Melbourne; Director, Melbourne Sexual Health Centre, The Alfred Hospital, Melbourne, Australia

Kevin A Fenton
Director, National Centers for HIV/AIDS, Viral Hepatitis, STD, and TB Prevention, Coordinating Center for Infectious Diseases, Centers for Disease Control and Prevention, Atlanta, USA

Paul A Fox
Consultant in Sexual Health and HIV, Ealing Hospital; Honorary Senior Lecturer, Imperial College School of Medicine, London, UK

Patrick French
Consultant Physician, Camden Primary Care Trust, London, UK; Honorary Senior Lecturer, University College London, London, UK

Keerti Gedela
Specialist Registrar GUM/HIV, West Middlesex University Hospital NHS Foundation Trust, Isleworth, UK

Nadi Gupta
Specialist Registrar in Genitourinary Medicine, Sheffield Teaching Hospitals NHS Foundation Trust, Sheffield, UK

Phillip Hay
Reader in HIV/GU Medicine, Centre for Infection, St George's, University of London, London, UK

Ashini Jayasuriya
Consultant in Genitourinary Medicine, Nottingham University Hospitals, Nottingham, UK

Vincent Lee
Consultant, Manchester Centre for Sexual Health, Manchester, UK

David A Lewis
Head of the Sexually Transmitted Infections Reference Centre, National Institute for Communicable Diseases, National Health Laboratory Service, Johannesburg, South Africa

Pat Munday
Consultant Genitourinary Physician, Watford Sexual Health Centre; West Herts Hospitals NHS Trust, Watford, UK

Rak Nandwani
Acting Director, The Sandyford Initiative, Glasgow, UK

Raj Patel
Consultant in Genitourinary Medicine, Department of GU Medicine, Royal South Hants Hospital, Southampton, UK

Katrina Perez
Specialist Registrar, Manchester Centre for Sexual Health, Manchester, UK

Anna Pryce
Specialist Registrar in Genitourinary Medicine, Sheffield Teaching Hospitals NHS Foundation Trust, Sheffield, UK

Cecilia Priestley
Consultant in Genitourinary Medicine, Dorset County Hospital NHS Foundation Trust, Dorchester, UK

John Richens
Clinical Lecturer, Centre for Sexual Health and HIV Research, University College London, London, UK

Angela J Robinson
Consultant in Genitourinary Medicine, Mortimer Market Centre, London, UK

Karen E Rogstad
Consultant Physician, Department of Sexual Health and HIV, Sheffield Teaching Hospitals NHS Foundation Trust; Honorary Senior Lecturer, University of Sheffield, Sheffield, UK

Jonathan D C Ross
Professor of Sexual Health and HIV, Whittall Street Clinic; Queen Elizabeth Hospital (Birmingham), Birmingham, UK

John Saunders
Specialist Registrar, Queen Mary University of London, Barts and The London School of Medicine and Dentistry, London, UK

Ian Williams
Senior Lecturer, Centre for Sexual Health & HIV Research, The Royal Free and University College London Medical School; Honorary Consultant Physician, UCL Research Department of Infection and Population Health, London, UK

Janet Wilson
Consultant in Genitourinary Medicine, Department of Genitourinary Medicine, The General Infirmary at Leeds, Leeds, UK

Clare L N Woodward
Specialist Registrar GUM, Department of Genitourinary Medicine, Mortimer Market Centre, London, UK

Preface

It is over a quarter of a century since the first edition of *ABC of Sexually Transmitted Infections* was published. In that time there have been major changes in sexually transmitted infections. AIDS in 1984 was only just being recognised, but then subsequently became a major global epidemic. Initially there was no effective treatment and death was inevitable for most sufferers; now it is treatable, although the infection cannot be eliminated. While there is still no universal access to treatment, significant inroads have been made in treatment provision in resource-poor nations. Syphilis in the western world has shown a decline over the 25 years but there has been a recent resurgence. Lymphogranuloma venereum was a tropical STI but is now endemic in some communities of men who have sex with men. Gonorrhoea continues its relentless progress in developing resistance to antibiotics. STI diagnosis has changed from being labour intensive, requiring laboratory diagnosis by highly trained staff, to more sensitive tests that can be performed by a broader range of providers in the community, including the patient themselves.

The way sexual health care is provided has also shown a dramatic change, with much more community testing and treatment, and the integration of STI and contraceptive care. In addition, there has been an increased awareness of the need to address child protection issues for some sexually active adolescents. Finally, the internet has revolutionised how patients access information and services, and how professionals learn.

This new edition has also evolved over the years to reflect these changes, moving from the excellent 1984 edition written by Professor Michael Adler to a book with international authorship which brings together all the developments listed above to provide a resource for all those providing sexual health services, and those who wish to learn more about the subject. It is hoped that traditional and new sexual health care providers, as well as medical, nursing and pharmacy students, throughout the world will be able to utilise the information in this edition to enhance their own knowledge and thus improve patient care and STI prevention. I would like to acknowledge the expertise and work of the editors of the previous edition, which has formed the basis for this one – Michael Adler, Frances Cowan, Patrick French, Helen Mitchell, and John Richens.

Karen E Rogstad

CHAPTER 1

Sexually Transmitted Infections: Why are they Important?

Kevin A Fenton [1] *and Karen E Rogstad* [2]

[1]Centers for Disease Control and Prevention, Atlanta, USA
[2]Department of Sexual Health and HIV, Sheffield Teaching Hospitals NHS Foundation Trust, Sheffield, UK

OVERVIEW

- There are more than 30 different sexually transmissible bacteria, viruses and parasites
- A million people acquire HIV or another STI every day
- There are 33.4 million people with HIV worldwide, with 2.7 million new HIV infections and 2 million HIV-related deaths annually (1998 data)
- STIs (excluding HIV) are the second most common cause of healthy life lost in 15- to 44-year-old women
- STIs cost $16 billion annually to the health care system
- Preventing a single HIV transmission would save £0.5–1 million in health benefits and costs

What are sexually transmitted infections?

Sexually transmitted infections (STIs) are infections that are spread primarily through person-to-person sexual contact. There are more than 30 different sexually transmissible bacteria, viruses, and parasites (Table 1.1). Several, in particular HIV and syphilis, can also be transmitted from mother to child during pregnancy and childbirth, and through blood products and tissue transfer.

In general, the viral STIs (including sexually transmitted HIV and hepatitis A, B, and C) are more prevalent, often causing lifelong infections, frequently asymptomatic in their early phases, and may result in serious long-term sequelae including chronic morbidity or even mortality. In contrast, the bacterial and protozoal STIs are generally curable, and often asymptomatic. The causative organisms may cause a spectrum of genitourinary symptoms, including urethral discharge, genital ulceration, and vaginal discharge with or without vulval irritation.

STIs are among the most commonly diagnosed infectious diseases in many parts of the world. More than a million people acquire HIV or another STI every day, and there are 450 million new cases of curable STIs occurring in adults each year. There is marked variation in the prevalence and incidence of infections throughout the world, and even within countries (Figure 1.1 and Table 1.2).

ABC of Sexually Transmitted Infections, Sixth Edition.
Edited by Karen E. Rogstad.

Why are STIs important?

Being diagnosed with an STI can have a tremendous physical, emotional, and psychological toll on individuals. Symptoms are unpleasant and may cause considerable pain, and have systemic complications. HIV and hepatitis B and C may have an aggressive course leading to lifelong morbidity and death. Some human papillomavirus (HPV) types are a cause of cervical, penile, anal, and oropharyngeal cancer (Table 1.3). Chlamydia and gonorrhoea are both the most serious, and also most preventable, threats to women's fertility worldwide. The World Bank estimated that STIs (excluding HIV) were the second most common cause of healthy life lost after maternal morbidity in 15- to 44-year-old women (Figure 1.2).

Effects on pregnancy, neonates, and children

STIs can lead to miscarriage, intrauterine growth retardation, and *in utero* death. They can also cause neonatal illness and death, and long-term sequelae. The consequences of congenital herpes and HIV are well recognised in developed nations. However, the magnitude of the congenital syphilis burden, globally, rivals that of HIV infection in neonates yet receives little attention. Congenital syphilis results in serious adverse outcomes in up to 80% of cases and is estimated to affect over 1 million pregnancies annually.

Effects on partners

STIs are also important to sexual partners, who may have asymptomatic infection. Partner notification is a key strategy for identifying and treating sexual partners for most STIs (see Chapter 2). The diagnosis of an acute STI may indicate that a partnership is non-monogamous, with negative impacts on relationships. For some couples who are discordant for infections such as HIV or herpes, there are long-term implications such as whether to have unprotected sex and psychological issues.

Stigma

The stigma and fear of STIs cannot be over-emphasised. There is significant psychological morbidity associated with being diagnosed with an STI which ranges from mild distress to severe anxiety and depression. Stigma can result in people living with HIV and other STIs being rejected, shunned, and discriminated against by partners,

Table 1.1 Main sexually transmitted pathogens and the diseases they cause.

Pathogen	Clinical manifestations and other associated diseases
	Bacterial infections
Neisseria gonorrhoea	GONORRHOEA *Men:* urethral discharge (urethritis), epididymitis, orchitis, infertility. *Women:* cervicitis, endometritis, salpingitis, pelvic inflammatory disease, infertility, preterm rupture of membranes, peri-hepatitis. *Both sexes:* proctitis, pharyngitis, disseminated gonococcal infection. *Neonates:* conjunctivitis, corneal scarring and blindness
Chlamydia trachomatis	CHLAMYDIAL INFECTION *Men:* urethral discharge (urethritis), epididymitis, orchitis, infertility. *Women:* cervicitis, endometritis, salpingitis, pelvic inflammatory disease, infertility, preterm rupture of membranes, peri-hepatitis; commonly asymptomatic. *Both sexes:* proctitis, pharyngitis, Reiter's syndrome. *Neonates:* conjunctivitis, pneumonia
Chlamydia trachomatis (strains L1–L3)	LYMPHOGRANULOMA VENEREUM *Both sexes:* ulcer, inguinal swelling (bubo), proctitis
Treponema pallidum	SYPHILIS *Both sexes:* primary ulcer (chancre) with local adenopathy, skin rashes, condylomata lata; bone, cardiovascular, and neurological damage. *Women:* pregnancy wastage (abortion, stillbirth), premature delivery. *Neonates:* stillbirth, congenital syphilis
Haemophilus ducreyi	CHANCROID *Both sexes:* painful genital ulcers; may be accompanied by bubo
Klebsiella (Calymmatobacterium) granulomatis	GRANULOMA INGUINALE (DONOVANOSIS) *Both sexes:* nodular swellings and ulcerative lesions of the inguinal and anogenital areas
Mycoplasma genitalium	*Men:* urethral discharge (nongonococcal urethritis). *Women:* bacterial vaginosis, probably pelvic inflammatory disease
Ureaplasma urealyticum	*Men:* urethral discharge (nongonococcal urethritis). *Women:* bacterial vaginosis, probably pelvic inflammatory disease
	Viral infections
Human immunodeficiency virus	ACQUIRED IMMUNODEFICIENCY SYNDROME (AIDS) *Both sexes:* HIV-related disease, AIDS
Herpes simplex virus type 2 Herpes simplex virus type 1 (less commonly)	GENITAL HERPES *Both sexes:* anogenital vesicular lesions and ulcerations. *Neonates:* neonatal herpes (often fatal)
Human papillomavirus	GENITAL WARTS *Men:* penile and anal warts; carcinoma of the penis. *Women:* vulval, anal and cervical warts, cervical carcinoma, vulval carcinoma, anal carcinoma. *Neonates:* laryngeal papilloma
Hepatitis B virus	VIRAL HEPATITIS *Both sexes:* acute hepatitis, liver cirrhosis, liver cancer
Cytomegalovirus	CYTOMEGALOVIRUS INFECTION *Both sexes:* subclinical or nonspecific fever, diffuse lymph node swelling, liver disease, etc.
Molluscum contagiosum virus	MOLLUSCUM CONTAGIOSUM *Both sexes:* genital or generalized umbilicated, firm skin nodules
Kaposi's sarcoma associated herpes virus (human herpes virus type 8)	KAPOSI'S SARCOMA *Both sexes:* aggressive type of cancer in immunosuppressed persons
	Protozoal infections
Trichomonas vaginalis	TRICHOMONIASIS *Men:* urethral discharge (nongonococcal urethritis); often asymptomatic. *Women:* vaginosis with profuse, frothy vaginal discharge; preterm birth, low birth weight babies. *Neonates:* low birth weight
	Fungal infections
Candida albicans	CANDIDIASIS *Men:* superficial infection of the glans penis. *Women:* vulvo-vaginitis with thick curd-like vaginal discharge, vulval itching or burning
	Parasitic infections
Phthirus pubis	PUBIC LICE INFESTATION
Sarcoptes scabiei	SCABIES

Source: World Health Organization, 2007.

family, and community, and being victims of physical violence. Stigma not only makes it more difficult for people trying to come to terms with and manage their illness, but it also interferes with attempts to fight the disease more generally. On a national level, stigma can deter governments from taking fast, effective action against STI epidemics.

Economic burden

STIs can have significant economic impacts on the individual and community. Even where treatment for STIs is free or low cost, individuals may pay for care in the private sector, or access traditional healers, because of stigma. Aditionally, there are opportunity costs incurred through missing work, travelling to the clinic, or purchasing treatment and returning for follow-up.

The global economic impact of STIs is staggering. However, treatment costs for STIs vary tremendously between countries and are influenced a range of factors. Reproductive ill-health (death and disability related to pregnancy, childbirth, STIs, HIV, and reproductive cancers) is thought to account for 5–15% of global disease burden. In developing countries they account for 17%

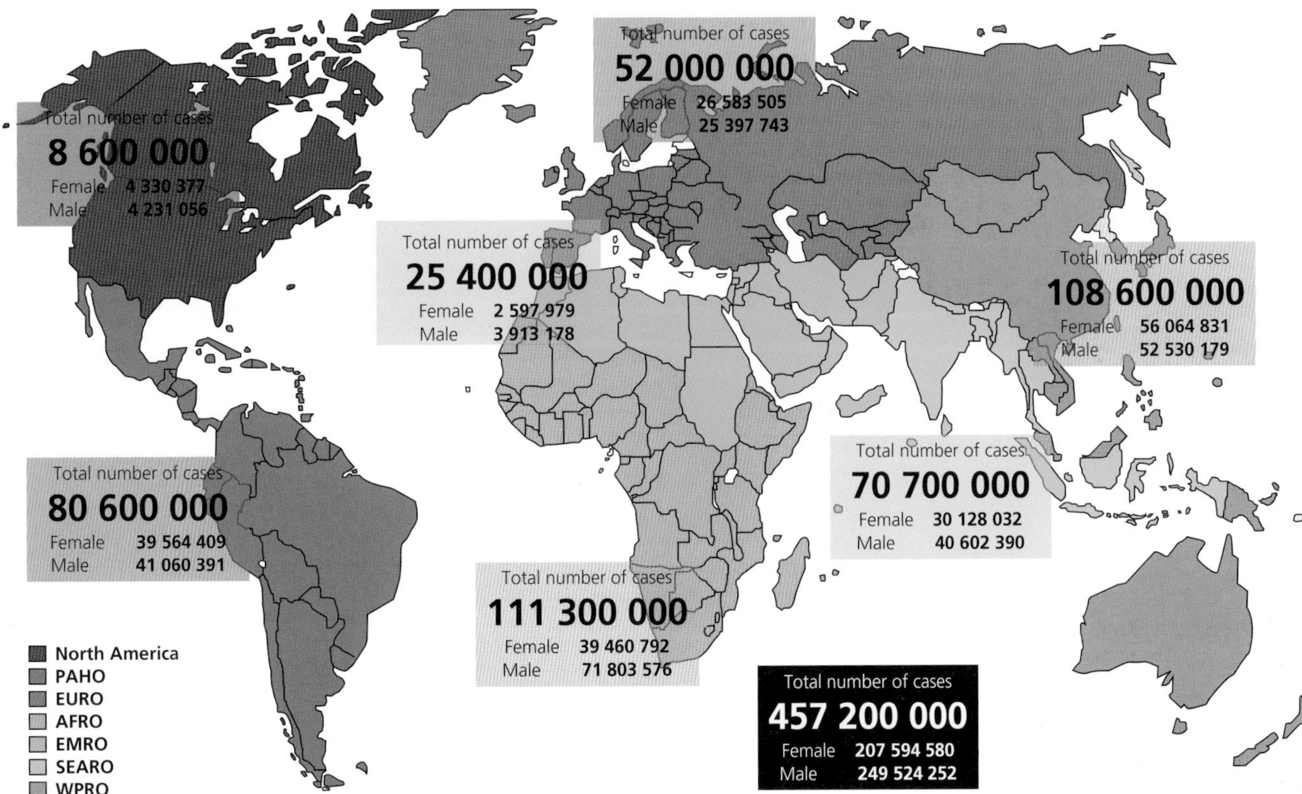

Figure 1.1 Global incidence of selected STIs, 2005. *Source*: World Health Organization, 2009.

of economic losses caused by ill-health and rank among the top 10 reasons for health care visits. In the United States, STIs cost $16 billion annually to the health care system (Tables 1.4 and 1.5). Care for the complications of STIs accounts for a large proportion of tertiary health care in terms of screening and treatment of cervical cancer, management of liver disease, investigation of infertility, care for perinatal morbidity, childhood blindness, and chronic pelvic pain. Preventing a single HIV transmission would save £0.5–1 million in health benefits and costs.

The economic impact in resource poor settings is even greater where the majority of curable STIs and HIV occur, particularly South and South-East Asia and sub-Saharan Africa (Box 1.1). Delays in the diagnosis and treatment increase complications and mortality with a substantial economic impact. In countries with high HIV prevalence, morbidity and mortality from HIV has led to important changes in average household composition and population structure.

Table 1.2 Estimated prevalence and annual incidence of curable STI by region.

Region	Adult population (millions)	Infected adults (millions)	Infected adults per 1000 population	New infections in 1999 (millions)
North America	156	3	19	14
Western Europe	203	4	20	17
North Africa & Middle East	165	3.5	21	10
Eastern Europe & Central Europe	205	6	29	22
Sub-Saharan Africa	269	32	119	69
South & Southeast Asia	955	48	50	151
East Asia & Pacific	815	6	7	18
Australia & New Zealand	11	0.3	27	1
Latin America & Caribbean	260	18.5	71	38
Total	3040	116.5	–	340

Source: World Health Organization, 2001.

Box 1.1 **Factors influencing costs and cost effectiveness of STI treatment and care**

- Health system characteristics, service delivery by public or private sector
- Economies of scale, economies of scope
- Prevalence and incidence, epidemic phase
- Transmission efficiency
- Population composition and concentration
- Resource combinations and input prices
- Incentives to providers for high quality and quantity of service delivery
- Willingness to pay for treatment as a function of price, income, and distance
- Stigmatization
- Disutility of condom use

Source: adapted from Bertozzi & Opuni (2008).

Table 1.3 Major sequelae of STIs.

	Women	Men	Infants
Cancers	Cervical cancer Vulval cancer Vaginal cancer Anal cancer Liver cancer T cell leukaemia Kaposi's sarcoma	Penile cancer Anal cancer Liver cancer T cell leukaemia Kaposi's sarcoma	
Reproductive health problems	Pelvic inflammatory disease	Epididymitis	
	Infertility	Prostatitis	
	Ectopic pregnancy	Infertility	
	Spontaneous abortion		
Pregnancy related problems	Preterm delivery		Stillbirth
	Premature rupture of membranes		Low birth weight
	Puerperal sepsis		Pneumonia
	Postpartum infection		Neonatal sepsis
			Acute hepatitis Congenital abnormalities
Neurological problems	Neurosyphilis	Neurosyphilis	Cytomegalovirus
			Herpes simplex virus Syphilis associated neurological problems
Other common health consequences	Chronic liver disease	Chronic liver disease	Chronic liver disease
	Cirrhosis	Cirrhosis	Cirrhosis

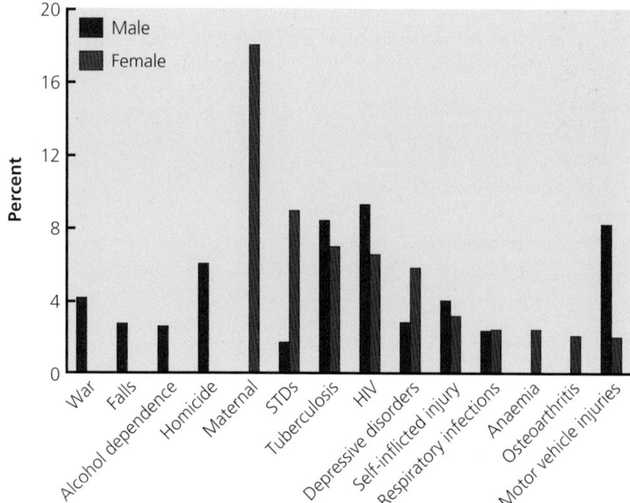

Figure 1.2 Top 10 causes of healthy life lost in young adults aged 15–44 years.

Table 1.4 Average (standard deviation) of estimated cost per unit output, by disease or syndrome and by type of output, 2001 US$.

Disease or syndrome	Treatment	Cure	Total
Syphilis	36.04 (5.91)	Not applicable	36.04 (5.91)
Urethral discharge	14.29 (20.68)	89.07 (0)	29.25 (37.94)
Genital ulcer	23.16 (21.73)	100.6 (83.74)	48.97 (59.56)
Venereal disease	25.47 (18.56)	82.65 (111.55)	31.83 (37.12)
Pelvic inflammatory disease	7.12 (3.09)	Not applicable	7.12 (3.09)
Vaginal discharge	48.23 (0)	102.92 (89.63)	81.04 (70.1)
Total	24.05 (19.04)	96.1 (73.44)	39.49 (47.23)

Source: Aral *et al*. (2005).

Table 1.5 Estimated annual burden and cost of STI in the United States.

STI	Estimated annual cases	Estimated annual direct cost (millions) US dollars
Chlamydia	2.8 million	$624
Gonorrhoea	718,000	$173
Syphilis	70,000	$22
Hepatitis B	82,000	$42
Genital herpes	1.6 million	$985
Trichomoniasis	7.4 million	$179
HPV	6.2 million	$5,200
HIV	56,300	$81,000
Total	18.9 million	$15.3 billion

Source: Centers for Disease Control and Prevention.

Size of the problem

In 2008 there were an estimated 33.4 million people living with HIV worldwide, 2.7 million new HIV infections, and 2 million HIV-related deaths (Figures 1.3 and 1.4; Table 1.6). Sub-Saharan Africa remains the region most heavily affected by HIV, accounting for 67% of all people living with HIV and for 70% of AIDS deaths in 2008. However, some of the most worrying increases in new infections are now occurring in populous countries in other regions, such as Indonesia, the Russian Federation, and various high-income countries. The rate of new HIV infections has fallen in several countries, including 14 of 17 African countries, where the percentage of young pregnant women (15–24 years) living with HIV has declined since 2000. As treatment access has increased over the last 10 years, the annual number of AIDS deaths has fallen. Globally, the percentage of women among people living with HIV has remained stable (at 50%) for several years, although women's share of infections is increasing in several countries.

Table 1.6 Prevalence of STIs among 14- to 19-year-old US females, NHANES, 2003–2004.

	All		Sexually experienced	
	Number	Prevalence (%)	Number	Prevalence (%)
HPV (HR6,11)	652	18.3	357	29.5
Chlamydia	793	3.9	396	7.1
Trichomonas	695	2.5	371	3.6
HSV-2	729	1.9	370	3.4
'Any STI'	612	25.7	347	39.5

Source: adapted from Forhan SE, Gottlieb SL, Sternberg MR, Xu F, Datta SD, McQuillan GM, *et al*. Prevalence of sexually transmitted infections among female adolescents aged 14 to 19 in the United States. *Pediatrics* 2009;**124**(6):1505–12.

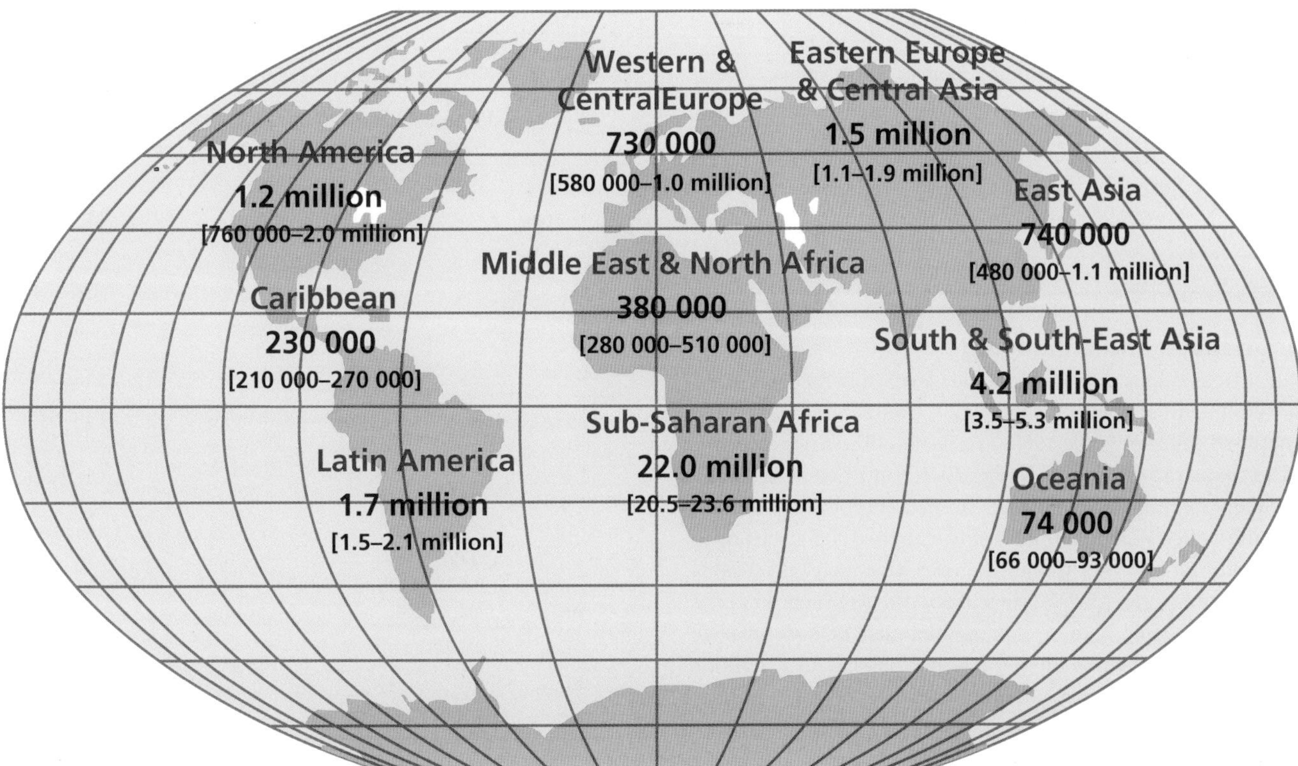

Figure 1.3 Adults and children estimated to be living with HIV, 2008. *Source*: UNAIDS, 2009.

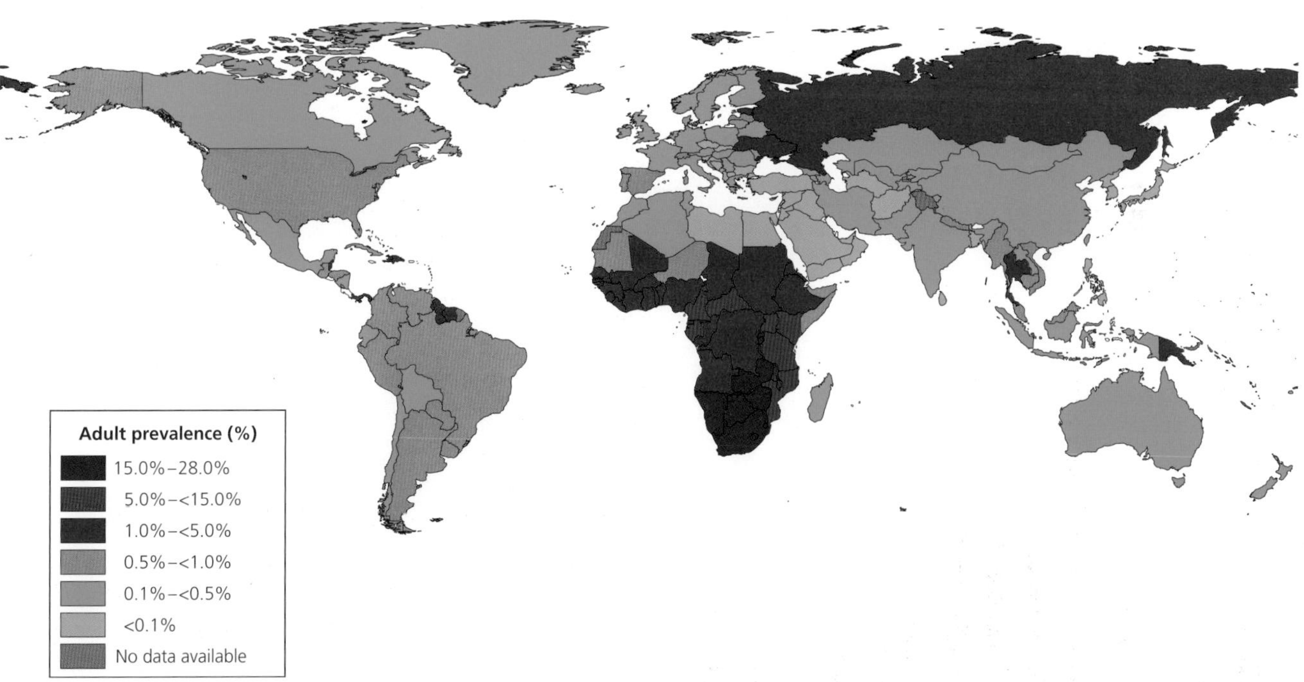

Figure 1.4 Global prevalence of Adult HIV prevalence, 2008. *Source*: UNAIDS, 2009.

Table 1.7 Number of new infections in 2005 (millions) in adult males and females between the ages of 15 and 49 (see also Figure 1.1).

WHO Region	Chlamydia	Gonorrhoea	Syphilis	*Trichomoniasis*	Total
AFRO	10.0	17.5	3.4	78.8	109.7
AMRO	22.4	9.5	2.4	54.9	89.2
EMRO	5.7	6.5	0.6	12.6	25.4
EURO	15.2	4.6	0.3	24.5	44.6
SEARO	6.6	22.7	2.9	38.6	70.8
WPRO	41.6	26.9	1.1	39.1	108.7
Total	101.5	87.7	10.6	248.5	448.3

Gonorrrhoea and Chlamydia

There is tremendous global geographic variation in the rates of the more common bacterial STI (Table 1.7). Gonorrhoea rates fell in westernised counties in the 1980s as a result of the AIDs epidemic leading to safer sexual practices (Figures 1.5 and 1.6). There was a subsequent increase in recent years in many European countries, but in the United Kingdom this has now stabilised and is starting to fall (Figures 1.7 and 1.8). Chlamydia rates have increased steadily in Europe and North America since 1996, with prevalence rates of 10% in young people. Because of the development of more sensitive tests, and screening programmes, it is not possible to determine whether this is a true increase in number of cases or not.

Genital herpes and genital warts

The total number of people aged 15–49 years who were living with herpes simplex virus 2 (HSV-2) infection worldwide in 2003 was

Table 1.8 Regional estimates of the prevalence of the herpes simplex virus type 2 infection among females, in 2003.

Region	Regional prevalence in millions, by age							
	15–19 years	20–24 years	25–29 years	30–34 years	35–39 years	40–44 years	45–49 years	Total
North America	0.9	1.5	2.0	2.6	3.2	3.8	3.9	17.9
Latin America and the Caribbean	2.6	4.5	5.8	6.4	6.7	6.6	6.0	38.6
North Africa and the Middle East	1.0	1.5	1.6	1.5	1.4	1.3	1.1	9.6
Sub-Saharan Africa	9.0	13.1	13.6	12.5	11.2	10.0	8.8	78.2
Western Europe	0.7	1.3	1.8	2.2	2.6	2.6	2.5	13.7
Eastern Europe and Central Asia	2.7	3.9	4.3	4.3	4.3	4.7	4.7	28.9
Eastern Asia	2.6	4.4	7.1	11.1	12.8	11.9	12.0	61.8
Japan	0.4	0.6	0.7	0.7	0.6	0.6	0.6	4.1
Pacific	0.03	0.04	0.05	0.06	0.06	0.06	0.05	0.3
South Asia	4.1	5.4	5.5	5.4	4.9	4.3	3.7	33.2
South-East Asia	1.7	3.1	4.0	4.6	4.9	4.8	4.4	27.6
Australia and New Zealand	0.03	0.06	0.09	0.1	0.2	0.2	0.2	0.9
Total	25.8	39.4	46.5	51.5	52.9	50.8	47.9	314.8

Source: Looker KJ, Garnett GP, Schmid GP. An estimate of the global prevalence and incidence of herpes simplex virus type 2 infection. Bull World Health Organ. 2008;**86**(10):805–12, A.

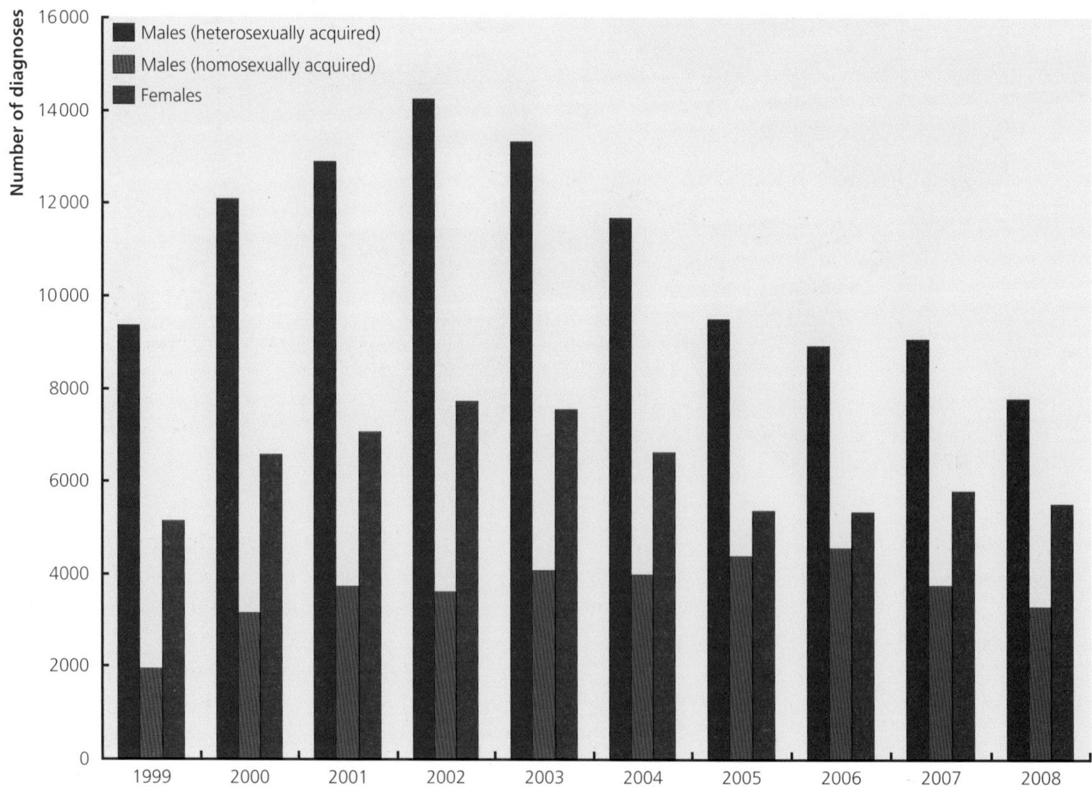

Figure 1.5 Cases of uncomplicated gonorrhoea seen in genitourinary medicine clinics by sex and male sexual orientation in England, Wales, and Northern Ireland, 1998–2008. *Source*: adapted from Health Protection Agency (www.hpa.org.uk), Communicable Disease Surveillance Centre. Data from KC60 statutory returns.

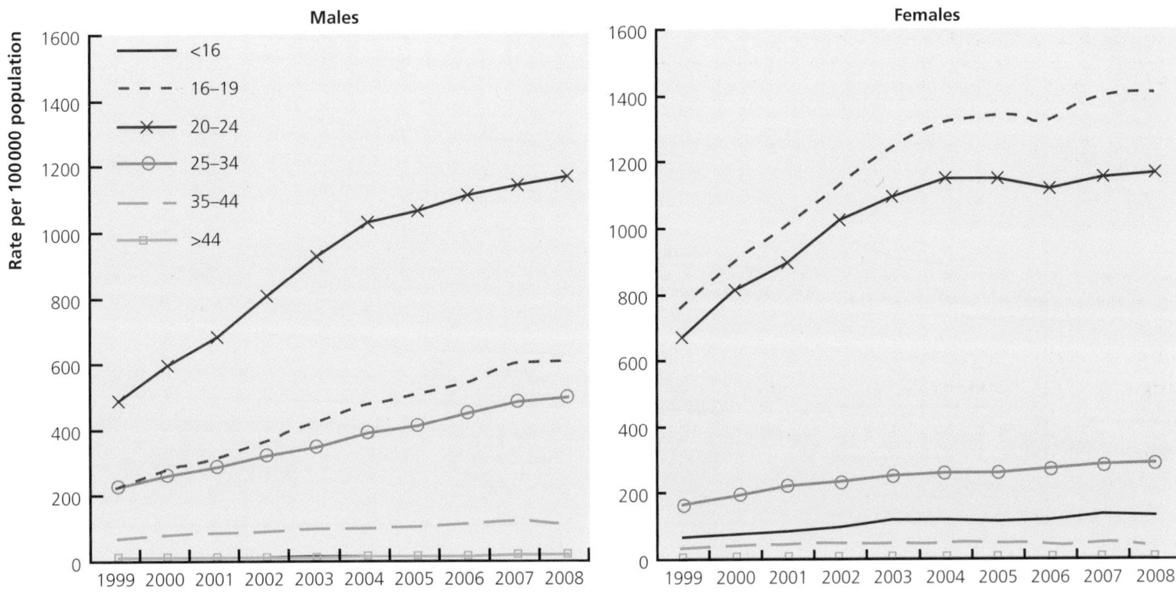

Figure 1.6 Diagnoses of uncomplicated genital chlamydial infection in genitourinary medicine clinics by sex and age group in the United Kingdom, 1999–2008. *Source*: adapted from Health Protection Agency (www.hpa.org.uk), Communicable Disease Surveillance Centre. Data from KC60 statutory returns and ISD(D)5 data.

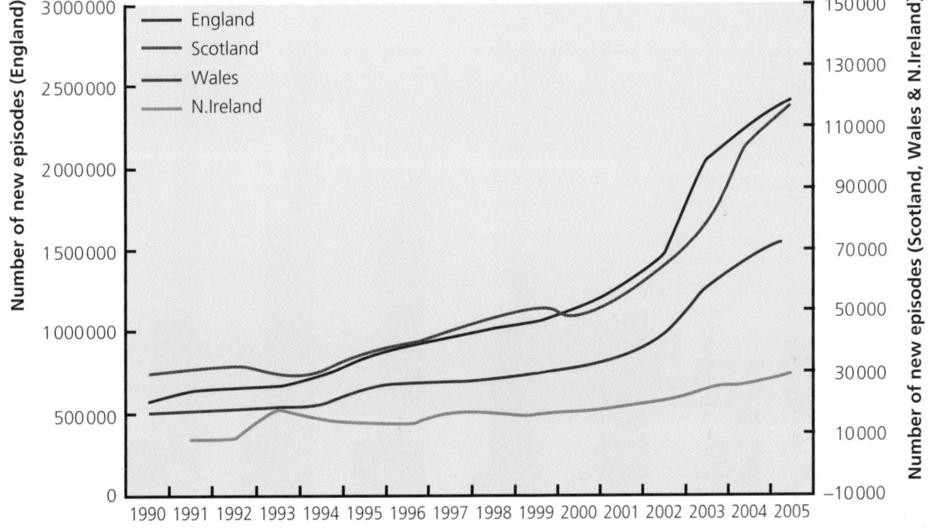

Figure 1.7 All diagnoses and workload at genitourinary medicine clinics by country, 1990–2005. *Source*: adapted from Health Protection Agency (www.hpa.org.uk), Communicable Disease Surveillance Centre. Data from KC60 statutory returns and ISD(D)5 data (http://www.hpa.org.uk/webc/HPAwebFile/HPAweb_C/1194947357259).

estimated to be 536 million, with the total number of people who were newly infected with HSV-2 in 2003 estimated to be 23.6 million. HSV-2 prevalence is highest in Africa and the Americas, and lowest in Asia. HSV-2 and -1 prevalence, overall and by age, varies markedly by country, regions within countries, and population subgroup (Table 1.8). Age-specific HSV-2 prevalence is usually higher in women than men and in populations with higher risk sexual behaviour. The number infected increases with age. Genital warts remain a major problem, but dramatic declines have been shown in parts of Australia following the introduction of the quadrivalent HPV vaccine in that country.

Syphilis and lymphogranuloma venereum

Despite the existence of simple tests, effective prevention measures, and cheap treatment options, syphilis remains a major global problem, with an estimated 10.6 million people becoming infected every year (Figure 1.9). Although syphilis remains relatively rare in developed countries, there has been a recent resurgence in rates of disease, particularly among men who have sex with men (MSM), and more recently among heterosexuals. Lymphogranuloma venereum (LGV), until recently considered a tropical STI, is now a significant problem in MSM in the United Kingdom and other westernised countries, and has a strong association with HIV.

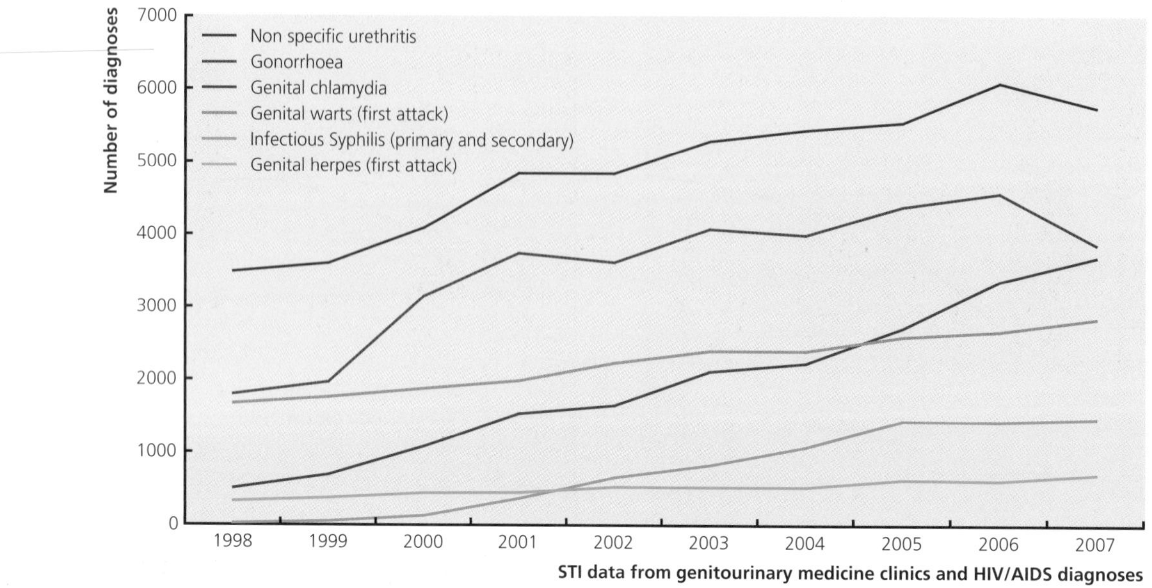

Figure 1.8 New diagnoses of selected STIs in men who have sex with men, England and Wales, 1998–2007. *Source*: adapted from Health Protection Agency (www.hpa.org.uk), Communicable Disease Surveillance Centre (http://www.hpa.org.uk/webc/HPAwebFile/HPAweb_C/1194947357259).

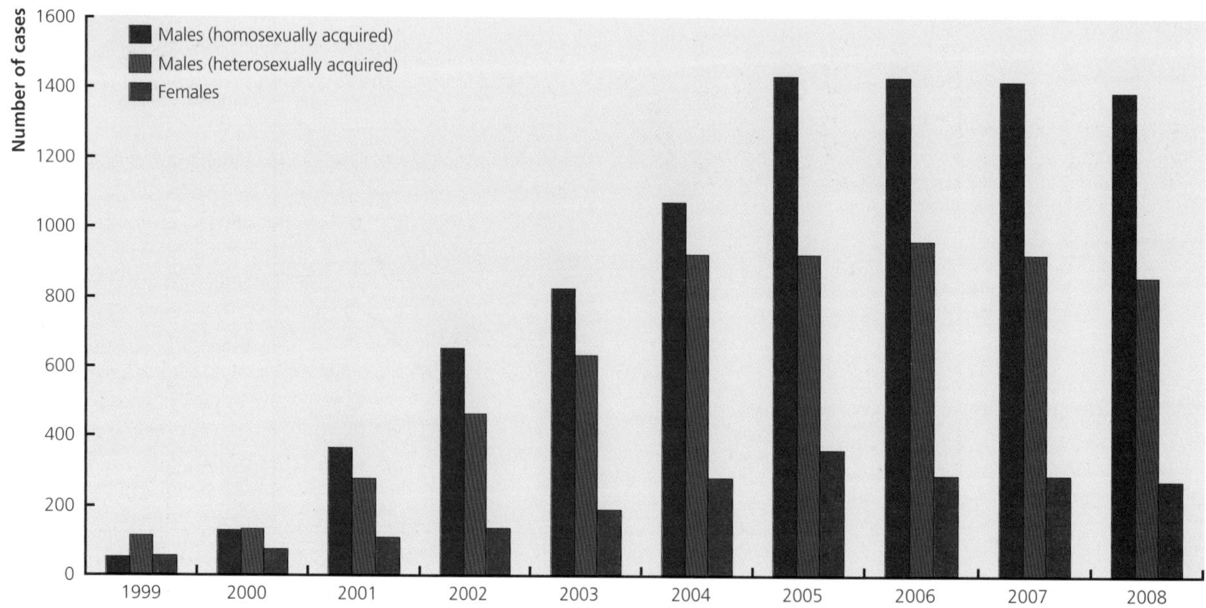

Figure 1.9 Cases of infectious syphilis (primary and secondary) seen in genitourinary medicine clinics by sex and male sexual orientation in England, Wales, and Northern Ireland, 1999–2008. *Source*: adapted from Health Protection Agency (www.hpa.org.uk), Communicable Disease Surveillance Centre.

Who gets STIs and why?

Globally, the highest rates of STIs occur among 20- to 24-year-olds, followed by 15- to 19-year-olds (Figure 1.10). One in 20 young people is believed to contract a bacterial STI in any given year. In the United States, up to 1 in 4 adolescent females have an STI. In the United Kingdom, 16- to 24-year-olds are the age group most at risk of being diagnosed with an STI, accounting for 65% of all chlamydial infections, 55% of genital warts, and 52% of gonorrhoea. MSM represent the majority of primary and secondary syphilis cases and racial and ethnic minorities bear a disproportionate burden of bacterial STIs including chlamydia and gonorrhoea.

At the individual level, biological and behavioural factors influence the risk of acquiring or transmitting an STI, including age, presence of other STIs, circumcision status, engaging in unprotected sex, riskier sex practices, and number of partners (Figure 1.11). Synergy between STIs and HIV affect risk. STIs are associated with increased risk of HIV transmission, at a population and individual level, and STIs increase the risk of both acquiring and transmitting HIV (Box 1.2). The British National Survey of Sexual Attitudes and Lifestyles shows an increase in many risk factors including number

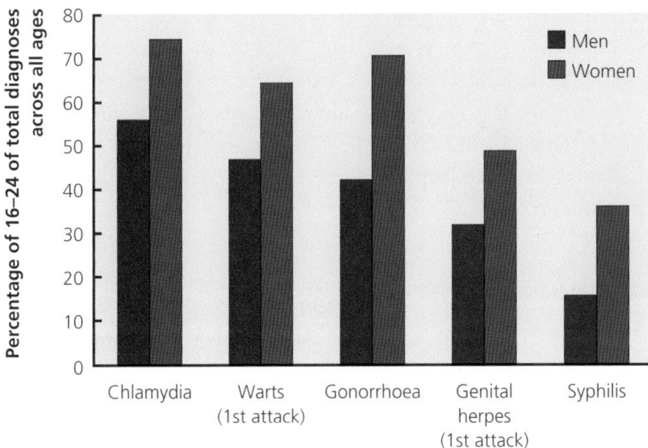

Figure 1.10 Percentage of STIs diagnosed among young people (16–24 years), United Kingdom, 2008.

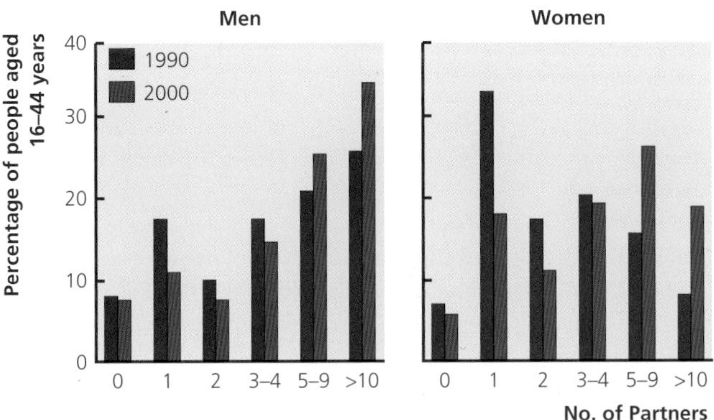

Figure 1.11 Percentage distribution of heterosexual partners in lifetime by sex, 1990 and 2000. *Source*: adapted from National Survey of Sexual Attitudes and Lifestyles, 2000.

of partners, concurrency rates, same sex partnerships, and anal sex (Figures 1.12 and 1.13). Additionally, the age of first sex has decreased in the UK, with 25% of teenagers sexually active by their sixteenth birthday. These behavioral changes may explain some of the increasing STIs seen in the UK over the past two decades.

> Box 1.2 **Role of STIs in the acquisition of HIV**
>
> - HIV acquisition increases by two- to fivefold in the presence of other STIs
> - Ulcers disrupt mucosal integrity and increase the presence or activation, or both, of HIV susceptible cells (e.g. CD4 lymphocytes)
> - Non-ulcerative STIs (such as gonorrhoea, chlamydia, *Trichomonas vaginalis*, and bacterial vaginosis) increase the presence or activation, or both, of HIV-susceptible cells

There is a strong association with number of lifetime and recent sexual partners, the rate of new sex partner acquisition, and partner concurrency (having overlapping sexual partnerships). Other factors include the type of partnership, the gender power dynamics within it, intimate partner violence, and cultural pressures.

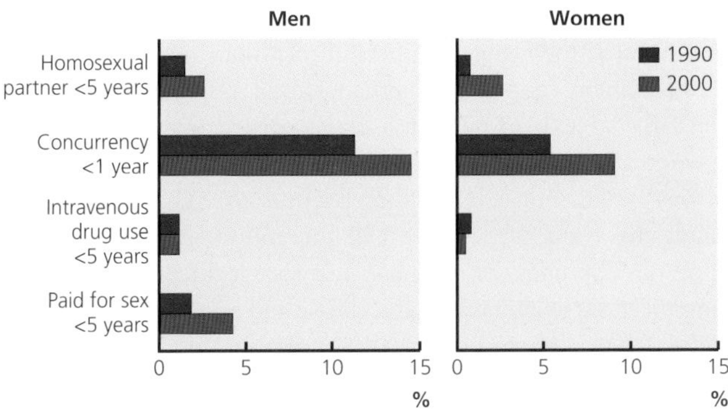

Figure 1.12 Changes in behaviour over time. *Source*: adapted from National Survey of Sexual Attitudes and Lifestyles, 2000.

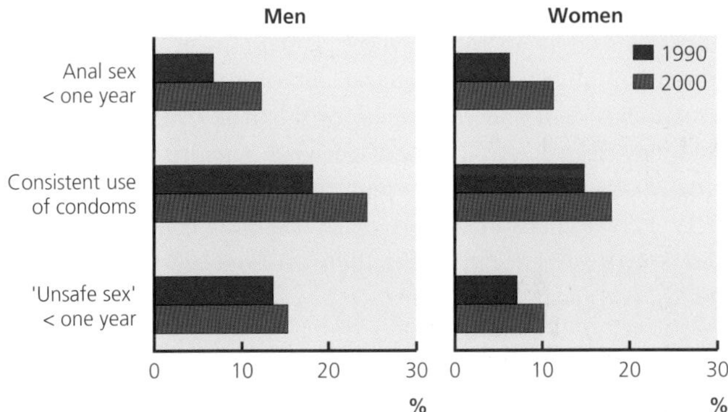

Figure 1.13 Changes in behaviour over time. *Source*: adapted from National Survey of Sexual Attitudes and Lifestyles, 2000.

Sexual networks

Sexual networks are groups of individuals who are directly or indirectly sexually connected to each other. The patterns of linkages between individuals in the network influence the paths through which STIs may be transmitted. Sexual networks can be affected by community norms about sexual behaviour, social upheaval, travel, and migratory patterns. The location of individuals within a network can be more important than their personal sexual behaviour, because it can increase the prevalence of infection in those to whom they are directly sexually connected. The existence of sexual bridges also influences the distribution of STIs in a population. The importance of networks is shown with the rapid spread of HIV in the early 1980s, outbreaks of LGV and syphilis among HIV-positive MSM in many western European countries, and the hyperendemic levels of bacterial STIs within racial and ethnic groups in developed country settings. In the latter, assortative sexual mixing by race/ethnicity combined with failure to break transmission chains within networks are key drivers for the persistent racial/ethnic health disparities in the United States and United Kingdom.

Societal burden and impact

Political conflict, economic and social disruption, and migration lead to the breakdown of existing social structures and the formation of new ones. In fast-growing cities, factors including high incarceration rates, the higher numbers of men than women, the lack of employment for women, and the social disruption resulting from large streams of migration are associated with increases in sex work.

Other population-level factors relevant to STI transmission include the availability and cost of prevention services (e.g. sex education, condoms, or treatment clinics), legislation regarding commercial sex workers, and educational and occupational opportunities for women. National HIV/STI prevention policies driven by religious or conservative social mores, can negatively impact on prevention programmes such as provision of free condoms.

Prevention

There are many actions individuals can take to protect themselves from STIs and their consequences: abstain from sex; be in a long-term, mutually monogamous relationship with an uninfected partner; consistent and correct use of the male condom; getting tested and treated for STIs; and receiving hepatitis B and HPV immunizations. For individuals with chronic viral conditions such as HIV, HSV, or hepatitis B and C, early diagnosis, counselling, and referral for treatment can reduce the risk of onward transmission to sexual partners.

Conclusions

Sexually transmitted infections are a major individual, societal, and public health concern. Their social, health, and economic costs are substantial and affect the lives and well-being of individuals, relationships, communities, and societies with disproportionate impacts among the young, socioeconomically deprived, or those with high levels of risk behaviours and their partners. Understanding the nature and determinants of this burden are the first steps in articulating their importance to the public and policy makers, and justifying scarce health resources for their management.

Further reading

Aral SO, Padian NS, Holmes KK. Advances in multilevel approaches to understanding the epidemiology and prevention of sexually transmitted infections and HIV: an overview. *J Infect Dis* 2005; **191**(Suppl 1): S1–6.

Bertozzi SM, Opuni M. An economic perspective on sexually transmitted infections including HIV in developing countries. In Holmes KI, Sparling PF, Stamm WE, Piot P, Wasserheit JN, Corey L, Cohen MS, Watts DH (eds). *Sexually Transmitted Diseases*, 4th edn. McGraw Hill, New York, 2008, pp. 13–26.

Fenton KA, Breban R, Vardavas R, Okano JT, Martin T, Aral S, Blower S. Infectious syphilis in high-income settings in the 21st century. *Lancet Infect Dis* 2008;**8**(4):244–53.

Joint United Nations Programme on HIV/AIDS (UNAIDS) and World Health Organization (WHO) 2009. AIDS epidemic update: November 2009. Available at http://data.unaids.org/pub/Report/2009/2009_epidemic_update_en.pdf.

Schmid G. Global incidence and prevalence of four curable sexually transmitted infections (STIs): New Estimates from WHO. Presentation at the 2nd Global HIV/AIDS Surveillance Meeting. March 2009. Bangkok, Thailand. Available at http://hivsurveillance2009.org/pages/presentations.html. Last accessed 19 January 2010.

World Health Organization. *Global Prevalence and Incidence of Curable STIs*. WHO, Geneva, 2001 (WHO/CDS/CDR/EDC/2001.10).

CHAPTER 2

STI Control and Prevention

Frances Cowan [1] *and Gill Bell* [2]

[1]University College London, London, UK
[2]Genitourinary Medicine, Royal Hallamshire Hospital, Sheffield, UK

OVERVIEW

- Primary prevention of STIs aims at keeping people uninfected
- Secondary preventions aims to prevent onward transmission of an STI from an infected person
- Partner notification is an essential part of STI management
- Novel methods of partner notification may increase its success

Pattern of spread

Several factors are known to be important in maintaining STI spread within communities. A simple arithmetic formula has been developed which makes it possible to anticipate the pattern of spread of STIs within communities under certain circumstances (Box 2.1). If the average number of infections resulting from one infection is more than one, then overall the rate of that STI will increase within the community (Figure 2.1). Conversely, if the average number is less than one then the rate of the STI will fall. In theory, reducing any of these parameters at a community level will decrease the average number of new infections resulting from one infection within that community. In reality, of course, it is not quite as simple as this, and factors such as who is having sex with whom (sexual networks) and the extent to which partnerships overlap (concurrency) are also critical.

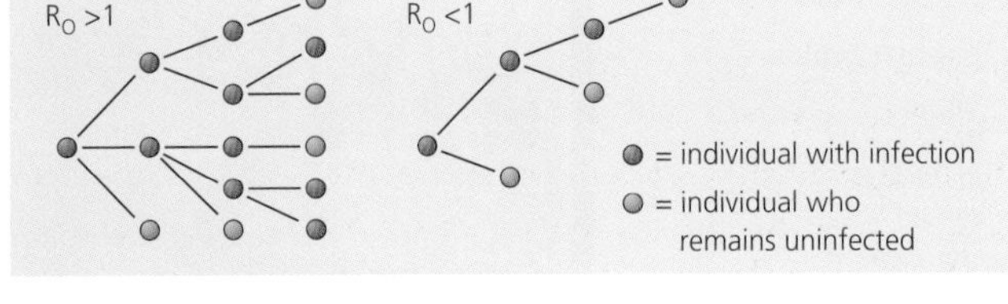

Figure 2.1 Pattern of spread.

Box 2.1 **Determinants of STI spread**

$R_o = \beta cd$
R_o = average number of new infections resulting from one infection
β = transmissability
c = average rate of acquiring partners
d = duration of infection

Principles of control

The approach to the control of STIs and the emphasis placed on different components will depend on the local pattern and distribution of STIs within the community and whether one is working in a resource rich or resource poor setting. However, the same general principles will apply (Box 2.2). Prevention can be aimed at uninfected people within the community, to prevent them acquiring infection (primary prevention; Figure 2.2, Boxes 2.3 and 2.4) or at people who are already infected, to prevent the onward transmission of their infection to their sexual partners (secondary prevention; Box 2.5). While effective primary prevention can theoretically reduce the prevalence of both viral and bacterial STIs, secondary prevention is much more effective at reducing the prevalence of bacterial STIs (which are all curable using antibiotics). In fact, the population prevalence of a bacterial STI can be dramatically reduced entirely through effective secondary prevention activities without any reduction in risky sexual behaviour occurring.

Box 2.2 **Principles of effective STI control**

Reduce infectiousness of STI

- Condoms

Reduce duration of infection

- Encourage early diagnosis and treatment of both symptomatic (encourage health seeking behaviour) and asymptomatic infection (screening, partner notification, mass or targeted treatment)

Reduce risky behaviour

- Reduce rate of partner change
- Reduce concurrency
- Delay onset of sexual intercourse

Countries that combine primary and secondary prevention approaches at both an individual and population level have managed to reduce substantially the burden of infection within their population. Effective implementation of prevention programmes

ABC of Sexually Transmitted Infections, Sixth Edition.
Edited by Karen E. Rogstad.

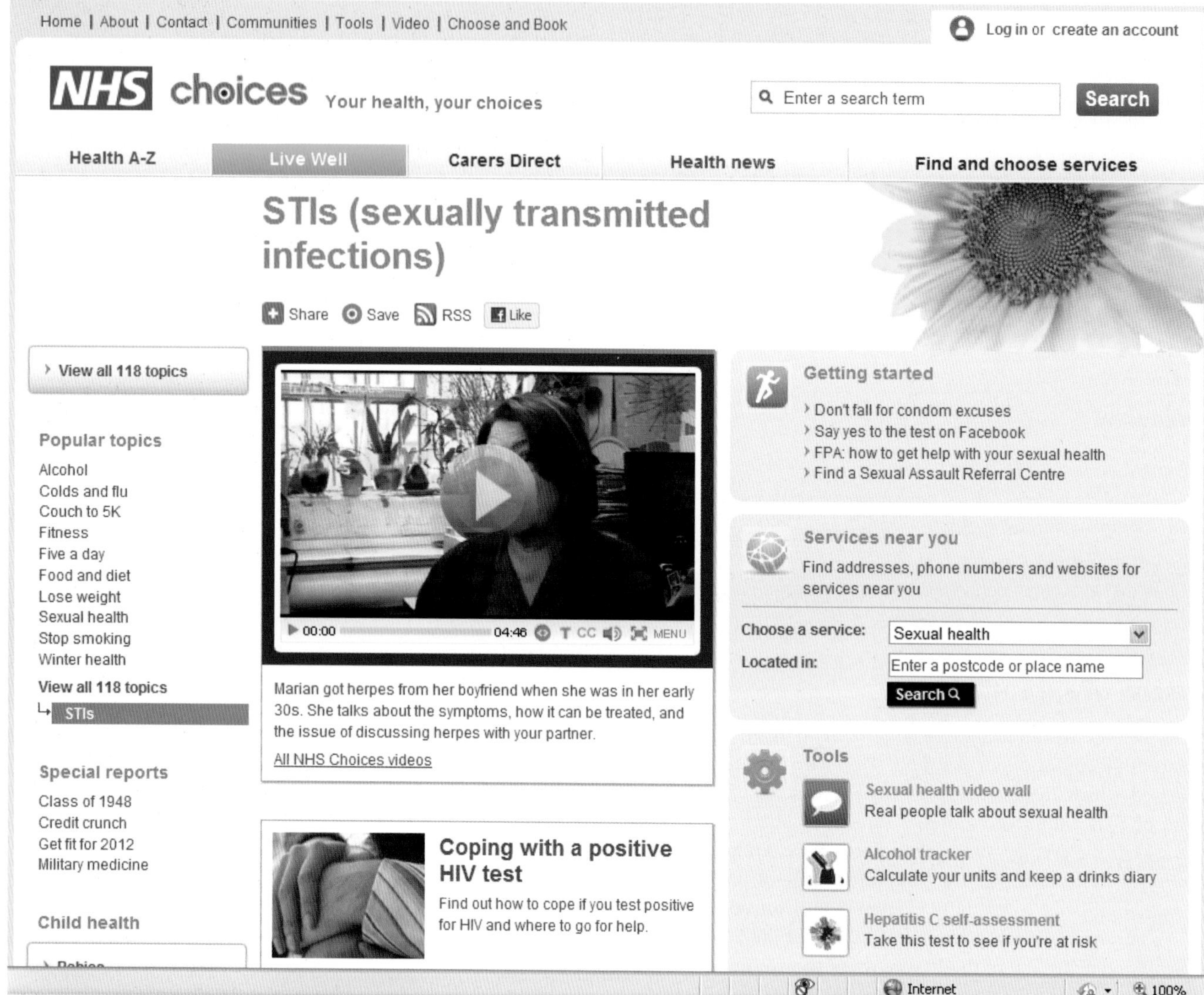

Figure 2.2 From http://www.nhs.uk/Livewell/STIs/Pages/STIs-hub.aspx entitled 'Condoms don't fit me and other excuses'. *Source:* Reproduced by permission of Department of Health (www.nhs.uk).

requires strong political leadership and genuine commitment, without which the most well-designed and appropriate programmes are likely to founder. Countries such as Thailand, Brazil, Uganda, Zimbabwe, and Senegal have made dramatic impacts on their rates of STIs and HIV, greatly facilitated by the political support at the highest level.

Box 2.3 **Primary prevention**

- **Behavioural interventions:** aimed at enhancing knowledge, skills, and attitudes to help individuals protect themselves against infection (e.g. health promotion to encourage decrease in rates of partner change and increase condom use)
- **Structural interventions:** aimed at broader the societal and economic issues that drive the spread of STIs
- **Biomedical interventions:** condoms, vaccines, vaginal microbicides, pre-exposure prophylaxis, post-exposure prophylaxis, or male circumcision to prevent acquisition of infection

Box 2.4 **Ways for an individual to reduce their risk of contracting an STI**

- Abstain
- Mutually monogamous relationship with someone who is uninfected
- Careful partner selection – select individuals whose behaviour past and current behaviour puts them at low risk of infection. Consider encouraging screening of both partners prior to unprotected sex
- Reduce the number of sexual partners
- Reduce number of overlapping sexual partnerships
- Avoid sex with people who have symptoms of an STI or oral 'cold sores'
- Use condoms consistently, on every occasion with all partners
- Negotiated safety – some couples in open relationships agree to have only non-penetrative or protected sex outside their main relationship

Box 2.5 **Secondary prevention**

- Enhancing health seeking behaviour
- Improving access to STI diagnosis and treatment
- Ensuring appropriate case management
- Early detection and treatment of symptomatic and asymptomatic infection
- Partner notification (contact tracing)

Interventions that seek to reduce the rate of STIs can be aimed at the entire community, or be targeted at specific groups who are at high risk of, or are particularly vulnerable to, infection. One-to-one prevention interventions can take place in clinic settings.

Primary prevention

Primary prevention interventions aim to keep those people who are uninfected uninfected. As outlined in Box 2.3, primary prevention interventions can be **educational** (Figure 2.3) and aim to modify knowledge, skills, attitudes, and behaviour, **structural** (Box 2.6) and aim to alter environmental and societal factors that increase STI risk, or **biomedical** and aim to physically reduce the infection risk of each sexual encounter. These approaches are obviously not mutually exclusive. It is likely that individual behaviour change will be best sustained within a community that is broadly supportive. In addition, the broader cultural perspective of the community will greatly influence the feasibility of delivering education within that community and will also affect how people respond to it.

Box 2.6 **Structural interventions**

These can take place at various levels, including:

- **Community level:** for example, legislating to change the age of consent to sex, legality of homosexual sex or inheritance laws
- **Organisational level:** for example, providing reproductive health clinics in schools or the workplace
- **Individual level:** for example, microfinance initiatives that seek to train women to become less economically dependent

Education and information

The aim of sexual health promotion is broader than minimising the risks associated with sexual intercourse and other sexual practices; it also aims to facilitate development of healthy sexual behaviour patterns and relationships. While supplying appropriate and timely factual information is very important and the first step in this process, there is evidence that providing information alone is not enough to bring about behaviour change. Interventions that are likely to be effective are those that draw on social psychological theories of behaviour change, derived from research that seeks to understand the origins and control of sexual behaviour. Of note, there is considerable evidence that providing information

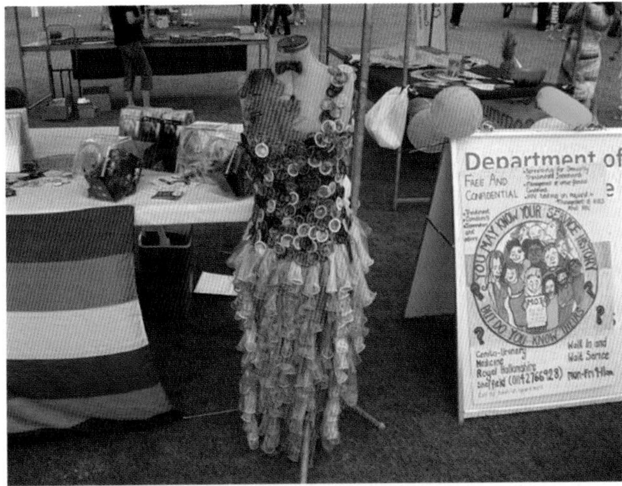

Figure 2.3 Condom dress: promoting awareness of sexual health.

about STIs (or about contraception) does no harm – it does not encourage immoral or promiscuous behaviour.

Health education needs to inform people of the advantages of discriminate and safer sex and the means to prevent or reduce the risk of infection (Boxes 2.4 and 2.5). While the best way to avoid sexually transmitted infections is to avoid sexual intercourse, this is not a realistic or acceptable message for many people. People need messages that are tailored to their lifestyles and their needs, which allow them to make informed choices about their behaviour. However, factors other than lack of knowledge contribute to an individual's ability to practice safer sexual behaviour including perception of health risk, low self-esteem, poor self-efficacy, peer pressure, and power and gender inequalities. Drug and alcohol use are also associated with poor sexual decision-making. Increasingly, health promotion interventions aim to address some or all of these factors.

It is also important that health promotion campaigns address the issues directly related to the infections themselves including what the various infections are, how to recognise their symptoms, what the short and long-term consequences may be, and where to access appropriate advice, diagnosis, and treatment. People also need to be aware that they cannot rely on symptoms alone to distinguish infected from uninfected individuals and that they can be infected even if asymptomatic.

Structural or societal interventions

Clearly, it may be unrealistic to expect individual behaviour change when the broader societal and cultural context is not supportive of this change. Structural factors that may hinder behaviour change include physical, social, cultural, organisational, economic, and legal or policy aspects of the environment. For example, interventions that promote condom use and partner reduction strategies for impoverished heterosexual women in developing countries may be impractical because women lack the power to negotiate condom use, particularly with their regular partners or husbands, and because they maybe economically dependent on sex work to provide income for basic necessities such as food or their children's school fees. In this scenario, interventions need to include men (e.g. through couples counselling and testing) and more broadly to tackle women's rights regarding inheritance, owning property, and earning income legitimately.

Structural interventions can take place at various levels including community level (e.g. legislating to change the age of consent for homosexual men or inheritance laws), organisational level (e.g. providing reproductive health clinics within the workplace or within schools), or at an individual level (e.g. microfinance initiatives which seek to train women to become less economically dependent) (Box 2.6). Recent research suggests that regular cash transfers can be used to promote behaviour change and even to reduce rates of STI and HIV acquisition.

Biomedical interventions

Male condoms, if used properly and consistently, have been shown to reduce the risk of transmission of many sexually transmitted infections. However, they are more effective for some STIs than for others, and their use does not guarantee that infection will not occur. Female condoms are also advocated to reduce STI and HIV transmission and can be attractive in some settings because women have more control over their usage, although evidence of their effectiveness is less than for the male condom.

The number of effective biomedical prevention interventions is slowly increasing. Hepatitis B vaccine is highly effective and vaccination against human papillomavirus (HPV) infection is now available. In a large trial of male circumcision conducted in Uganda, men who were circumcised were significantly less likely to acquire herpes simplex virus type 2 and/or HPV infection, although there was no effect on risk of acquiring syphilis. Vaginal microbicides continue to be evaluated for their effect on both HIV and STI acquisition. Recent data suggest that the topical antiretroviral product tenofovir gel is likely to be effective in preventing acquisition of both HIV and some STIs. Antiretrovial drugs reduce the risk of vertical transmission of HIV and likely sexual transmission although the evidence for this is not yet conclusive.

Secondary prevention

Secondary prevention interventions aim to reduce the risk of individuals infected with an STI transmitting this infection to their sexual partners. It involves increasing screening and appropriate treatment of symptomatic and asymptomatic individuals, encouraging health seeking behaviour and tracing, screening and treating sexual partners of infected individuals (contact tracing, also known as partner notification). Other more experimental approaches have included presumptive treatment of individuals at high risk of infection.

Screening and treatment

Early diagnosis and treatment are cheap but the late sequelae of untreated disease are expensive. For example, if gonorrhoea and chlamydial infection (a major cause of pelvic inflammatory disease) are well controlled, then pelvic inflammatory disease and all its serious long-term sequelae can be prevented.

In many parts of the world STI clinics have been established to provide screening and treatment for people with symptoms of, or who feel they are at risk of, an STI (Box 2.7).To be most effective, clinics should be open access and provide confidential, non-judgemental, and appropriate health care for which there is no charge. Waiting times should be minimal to avoid delay in access to care.

Box 2.7 **Specialist services for STIs in the United Kingdom**

- GUM (sexual health and HIV) – 269 clinics and 273 consultants
- Features of service
  - Open access and free
  - Confidential
  - Screening and treatment for STIs
  - Screening and treatment for HIV
  - Contraception and psychosexual problems
  - Miscellaneous care (e.g. for urinary tract infections and genital dermatological conditions)
  - Partner notification
  - Health promotion, counselling, and advice
  - Outreach and special services
  - Training and research

Widening the availability of STI testing and/or treatment to a range of health and non-health settings can improve timely access by providing patient choice of service and creating opportunities to offer screening to those at risk.

Postal kits for most STIs can be ordered via the internet or phone, collected from self-service bins, purchased through commercial outlets, or distributed by mailshot. However, making STI testing available from non-health care settings may undermine other aspects of control: individuals may be falsely reassured by negative results without appreciating the need for repeat testing if in a window period, screening for other STIs, or epidemiological treatment if a contact of chlamydia; health promotion opportunities for condom distribution and risk reduction discussion are also missed. Patients receiving treatment from non-specialist settings may not be offered adequate support with partner notification.

In countries without access to a laboratory, most people presenting to clinical services will be symptomatic and screening may be limited to clinical examination with or without microscopy. The sensitivity and specificity of clinical examination for distinguishing STI causes of genital symptoms from non-STI causes, particularly in women, has been shown to be poor but improved somewhat by use of a risk scoring system. For example, having had a new partner recently greatly increases woman's risk for an STI. Testing and treatment in resource poor settings is considered in Chapter 21.

Partner notification

Partner notification (also known as contact tracing) is an essential aspect of STI control because sexual partners may be asymptomatic and therefore unaware of their risk of developing complications or infecting others.

The need to inform partners should be discussed at the time the diagnosis or treatment is given. Ideally, the patient should have access to a specialist contact tracer with the expertise to prepare the patient for the sensitive task of informing a partner themselves (**patient referral**), or to inform the partner directly, without the patient's name being mentioned (**provider referral**). A hybrid alternative gives the patient an agreed period of time to refer partners before the contact tracer assumes responsibility (**contract or conditional referral**; Box 2.8). Patients electing to notify partners themselves should be followed up to check progress and repeat the offer of assistance if necessary. Partner notification interviews can take place by telephone if required, allowing a small team of contact tracers to manage partner notification for patients attending a variety of testing and treatment services, over a wide geographical area.

Box 2.8 **Partner notification**

- **Patient (index) referral:** whereby the patient informs their sexual partners
- **Provider referral:** whereby the index patient asks the health care worker to inform partners on their behalf
- **Contract (conditional) referral:** whereby the index patient undertakes to notify their partners in a given timeframe. If the partners are not notified in this period, the contact tracer or health adviser will attempt to notify them with the patient's consent. This uses a combination of patient and provider referral techniques

The effectiveness and acceptability of partner notification may depend on the degree of support and choice available to patients, which varies according to local resources, culture, and legislation. A provider referral option might be limited to patients in STI clinics, or chlamydia screening programmes, or to patients with more serious STIs such as syphilis or HIV. Conversely, in some areas, patients with serious STIs may be required to supply partner details for provider referral, which is a more effective, although more costly, method of securing partner attendance.

The cost and therefore availability of provider referral has prompted recent initiatives to improve the effectiveness of patient referral for chlamydia and gonorrhoea through expedited partner therapy. This may involve giving patients medication to pass on to partners, or prescriptions or referral cards for partners to collect treatment from a clinic or pharmacy. Treatment may be accompanied by optional testing kits, health promotion materials, and condoms. Trials have shown patient-delivered partner therapy increased the proportion of partners treated and reduced reinfection rates among index patients. However, it is not legal in some areas, including the UK, to prescribe medication without a consultation with the recipient. The negative impact on STI control of treating partners without testing, thereby missing opportunities to diagnose infection and trace their other partners, is under investigation.

Other initiatives found to improve the effectiveness of patient referral include giving written information, or home sampling kits, for partners.

Further reading

Corey L, Wald A. Genital herpes. In Holmes KI, Sparling PF, Stamm WE, Piot P, Wasserheit JN, Corey L, Cohen MS, Watts DH (eds). *Sexually Transmitted Diseases*, 4th edn. McGraw Hill, New York, 2008, pp. 399–438.

Des Jarlais DC, Semaan S. HIV Prevention research: cumulative knowledge or accumulating studies?: An introduction to the HIV/AIDS Prevention Research Synthesis Project Supplement. *J AIDS* 2002;**30**:S1–S7.

Guttmacher S. Strategies for partner notification for sexually transmitted diseases. *Cochrane Database Syst Rev* 2001;(4):CD002843.

Holmes KK. Human ecology and behaviour and sexually transmitted bacterial infections. *Proc Nat Acad Sci U S A* 1994;**91**:2448–55.

Mathews C, Coaetzee N, Zwarenstein M, Lombard C, Parker R, Easton D, Klein C. Structural barriers and facilitators in international research. *AIDS* 2000;**14**(Suppl 1):S22–32.

Sumartojo E, Doll L, Holtgrave D, Gayle H, Merson M. Enriching the mix: incorporating structural factors into HIV prevention. *AIDS* 2000; **14**(Suppl 1):S1–2.

Trelle S, Shang A, Nartey L, Cassell J, Low N. Improved effectiveness of partner notification for patients with sexually transmitted infections: systematic review. *Br Med J* 2007;**334**:354.

CHAPTER 3

Provision and Modernisation of Sexual Health Services

Christopher K Fairley

The Alfred Hospital and School of Population Health, Melbourne Sexual Health Centre, University of Melbourne, Australia

OVERVIEW

- Access to sexual health services for high risk or symptomatic individuals is a critical part of effective STI control
- Clinical services should include a thorough risk assessment which directs investigations, treatment, counselling, vaccination and partner notification; preferably all at a single visit
- Electronic health records with well-developed decision support programming will significantly improve the quality of sexual health services
- Computer-assisted sexual history-taking that is integrated into clinical care can improve both the quality and efficiency of services
- Many excellent web sites can significantly improve many aspects of sexual health services, particularly in relation to partner notification

Provision of sexual health services

Providing communities with effective and efficient sexual health services will put substantial downward pressure on the prevalence of sexually transmitted infections (STIs). Unfortunately, there are a number of examples where inadequate or poorly accessible services are or have been directly responsible for high rates of STI. The extraordinary high rate of STI among geographically isolated indigenous communities in Australia is a national disgrace. Other examples include the financial isolation among African-American populations in some parts of the United States or recently in the United Kingdom where inadequate funding to genitourinary medicine (GUM) clinics was temporally associated with rises in STIs. Unless individuals with symptoms of STI or those at high risk can access services, the prevalence of infection will rise.

Service delivery model

The structures of health care services in different countries will influence how STI services are delivered. For example, in the UK there are separate GUM clinics and the public is aware that these clinics should be consulted for STI, rather than their general practitioners (GPs). In contrast, in Australia GPs provide the bulk of services for STI and a smaller number of sexual health clinics deal only with those who do not wish to see their GPs. Other countries have private STI clinics. No matter which model is chosen, it is critical that sufficient clinical services are provided and are accessible to those at greatest risk.

Key elements of a clinical service

There are two elements to the design of sexual health services. The first is ensuring it serves the need of individual patients, and the second, and arguably more important, is ensuring that the service is designed to afford the community a low prevalence of STI (Boxes 3.1 and 3.2).

Box 3.1 **Key elements of sexual health service**

- Accessible to those at highest risk
- Free
- Confidential
- Comprehensive single consultation with no unnecessary follow-up

Box 3.2 **Accessibility of services**

- Geographically accessible to public and private transport
- Walk-in or same day appointment service
- Priority or triage system based on risk assessment and individual clinical need
- Opening hours that provide access for high risk individuals

There are a number of successful models that provide highly accessible services including walk-in triage systems or triage to a same day appointment system. All the evidence suggests that an appointment system that only allows bookings weeks into the future will fail because symptomatic individuals who cannot access treatment will continue to transmit their infections.

ABC of Sexually Transmitted Infections, Sixth Edition.
Edited by Karen E. Rogstad.

Clinical services should be comprehensive and targeted

Most services now aim to deal with all issues at one session and minimise the need for follow-up or review appointments unless they are absolutely necessary (Box 3.3). Individuals need a sexual history that provides a risk assessment and allows risk-based testing, treatment, immunisation, and counselling. For example, a low risk heterosexual man may only need a first pass urine test for chlamydia in most developed countries, while a man who has sex with men (MSM) may need throat, anal, urine tests, serology and vaccination for hepatitis A and B, with follow-up risk reduction counselling. Services need to be strictly confidential and not dependent on national insurance cards which exclude individuals such as young travellers who are often at significant risk.

Box 3.3 **Comprehensive consultation**

- Risk assessment that directs investigations (including HIV) and treatment
- Immediate microscopy
- Pharmacy for immediate and free medications including HIV post-exposure prophylaxis
- Contraceptive services
- Vaccinations
- Counselling services
- Partner notification services
- Phone follow-up for results

Efficient and cost effective services

The reality is that services for STIs are often under-funded in comparison with more prestigious and politically acceptable specialities (Box 3.4). It is therefore even more critical that STI services are run very efficiently. An essential element of this is the need for an ongoing critical evaluation of their practices. One of the best examples of this is the commendable way in which UK clinics have dramatically increased access for new clients by reducing the need to review patients; the follow-up to new client ratio has fallen from from 2.2 in 1990 to 0.75 in 2005.

Box 3.4 **Improving the cost effectiveness of clinical services**

- Match clinical expertise with services provided
- Minimise examinations unless required
- Maximise the use of self-collected samples
- Use brochures or videos for provision of information
- Use of electronic history-taking and risk assessment and self-collected samples in lower risk patients
- Minimise review appointments
- Ongoing process of evaluation

Recently, a number of studies have looked at better utilising the time patients spend in the waiting room. In one US study, educational videos and other materials were associated with a 10% reduction in STI notifications. Another study utilised videos for post-test counselling for HIV. These studies suggest clinics need a good reason not to show the videos in waiting rooms given the benefit they bestow at little or no cost (Figure 3.1).

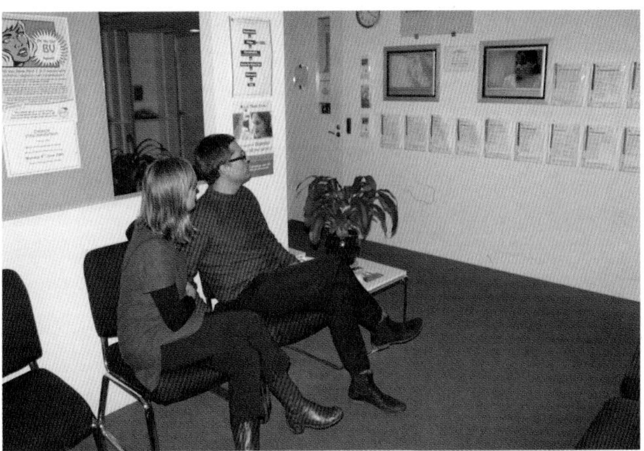

Figure 3.1 Viewing of health promotion videos in the waiting area.

Partner notification

Partner notification is a critical element of any STI management, but it is often not well carried out. Partner notification is particularly important for asymptomatic infections, because it prevents infected partners continuing to unknowingly transmit their infection. In many countries it relies on the practitioner remembering to ask patients to tell their sexual partners to get tested and treated while others countries have varying degrees of government funded personnel (e.g. termed health advisers or partner notification officers) whose specific role is to notify partners. More recently, innovative methods have been delivered such as partner delivered therapy which has shown to reduce reinfection rates in the index case. Disappointingly, in some areas partner delivered therapy remains illegal but is nevertheless often used as practitioners seek to do the best for their patients and their communities regardless of administrative obstructions. In the United Kingdom, azithromycin has recently become available through pharmacies without a prescription for the treatment of chlamydia and for epidemiological treatment of sexual partners (without a test for chlamydia) of someone with chlamydia. This is an important development that will increase the ease of partners accessing treatment. Other significant developments have occurred using information technology to assist in partner notification.

Quality of health care

Clinics should provide a high quality of care that is safe and effective. To date, the health industry has lagged significantly behind other industries such as the airline industry that have pioneered processes for improved safety. To do this clinics need to adopt an accepted quality framework that involves all the appropriate elements such as customer participation, comprehensive health records, infection control procedures, health care incident and feedback systems, risk management policies and systems, and detailed protocols. Some practical examples include a process for auditing the quality of care that individual practitioners provide, and a responsive confidential reporting system that identifies potentially near misses and corrects any systems faults that are allowing serious errors to occur.

Practitioners need to appreciate that when errors occur, they are almost always not the fault of an individual practitioner but occur because systems have not been designed to prevent them. Take for example a practitioner who prescribes a drug that interacts with another drug the patient is taking, in a clinic using paper prescriptions. This error could easily have been prevented by electronic prescribing software that alerted the practitioner of this interaction at the time it was being prescribed.

Modernisation of sexual health services

A health service that does not modernise necessarily moves backwards. The implications of this extend beyond the individual patient and may be reflected in an otherwise higher prevalence of STI in the community. It is important that all services retain some budget for this modernisation process despite the enormous clinical pressures many of them are under.

Advances in information technology over recent years have been enormous and provide perhaps the greatest opportunity to improve the quality of sexual health services. This can involve simply providing accessible resources through the intranet or internet on all clinic computers or more advanced processes such as specifically designing decision support software.

Provision of information for practitioners at the consultation

This is a central element of a high quality health service (Box 3.5). Up-to-date and comprehensive information should be available at the clinician's desk including treatment guidelines, policy and procedures, client brochures, diagnostic pictures, and extensive links to other resources (discussed below).

Box 3.5 **Intranet resources**

- Treatment guidelines
- Policy and procedures
- Clinical photographs to aid clinician
- Patient brochures, contact letters, and educational aids
- Links to internet sites for patients (e.g. partner notification services)
- Links to national resources (e.g. HIV treatment guidelines, HIV resistance testing)
- Pharmaceutical resources

Electronic medical record

The electronic medical record (EMR) has the potential to make a very significant contribution to the quality of sexual health care. There is clear evidence that the recording of consultations in EMR is superior to their paper counterparts with more words, more diagnosis, and more management plans which are more legible. Importantly, if designed well, the EMR provides the opportunity to support clinical decisions through decision support software. These can be simple such as reminders for vaccination in certain risk groups (e.g. hepatitis A and B vaccine in MSM), or investigations that are triggered by diagnoses (e.g. *Mycoplasma genitalium* with pelvic inflammatory disease).

However, the EMR will only work well in sexual health medicine if it includes the right data to allow these alerts to work. For example, to be reminded to vaccinate MSM, there must be a field in the software for the sex of the client and the sex of their partners. Individual users can request alerts in commercially available software but because these have been priced for pharmaceutical companies their cost is prohibitive for public good alerts. In contrast, clinics with their own specifically developed software can create simple alerts in less than 5 minutes.

Computer-assisted sexual interviewing

Sexual health medicine lends itself particularly well to a computer-assisted interviewing (CASI). This is because a risk assessment is such an important step in management of patients and there are relatively few questions that are required for a thorough risk assessment. There are now a number of clinics where CASI forms part of the initial assessment of clients and the results of CASI determine the outcome of triage. In the UK for example, CASI is used in some clinics so low risk asymptomatic patients who need only chlamydia screening leave a self-collected sample without seeing a clinician (Figures 3.2 and 3.3).

CASI provides an almost endless opportunity to improve the provision of health care. For example, clients can be asked if they would like a text message reminder for frequent screening if, for example, they are at high risk of syphilis, such as MSM with many partners. At a public health level it also provides the opportunity for detailed risk assessment.

These CASI systems can also be adapted for routine HIV care before patients see the practitioner. Patients can be asked about adherence to HIV medication, screened for depression, and assessed for the need for STI screening or cardiovascular risks such as smoking. A summary of this information could alert practitioners to issues before patients are seen. A web-based system is already in existence directed specifically to patients with HIV (healthmap.org.au).

Using the internet to improve sexual health services

At the very least, one web site in each country should have detailed authoritative information for partitioners and the public.

The San Francisco Public Health Department has led web-based interventions for partner notifications (www.inspot.org) and others have followed (www.letthemknow.org.au), (www.whytest.org), and (thedramadownunder.info). At the inspot web site over one-quarter of recipients of messages accessed sexual health information.

Other web pages have been designed specifically for practitioners at the time they are giving a positive result to patients (e.g. www.gpassist.org.au). This site appears with positive chlamydia results from laboratories and contains brochures for practitioners

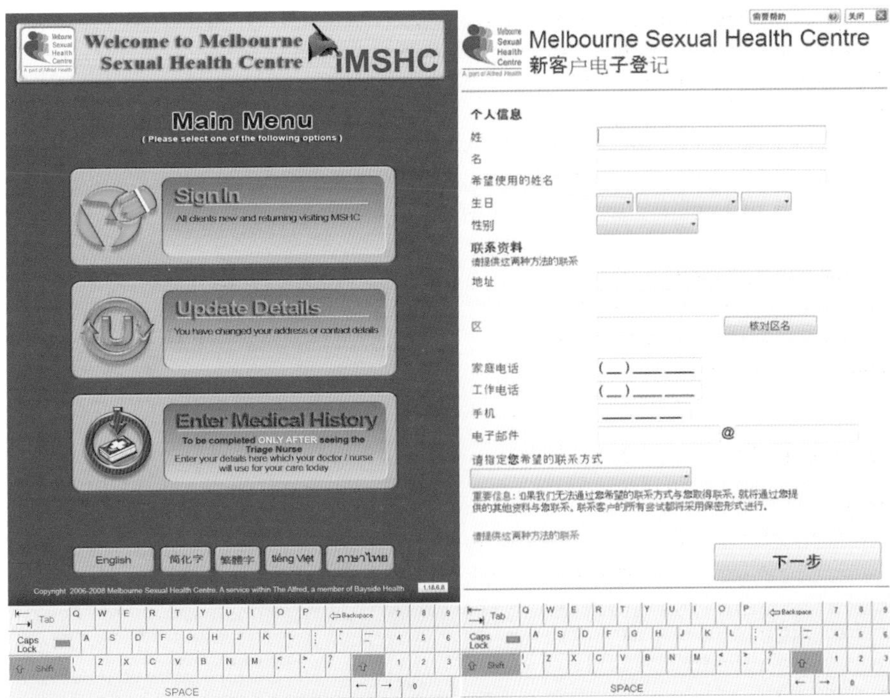

Figure 3.2 Computer-assisted sexual interviewing (CASI).

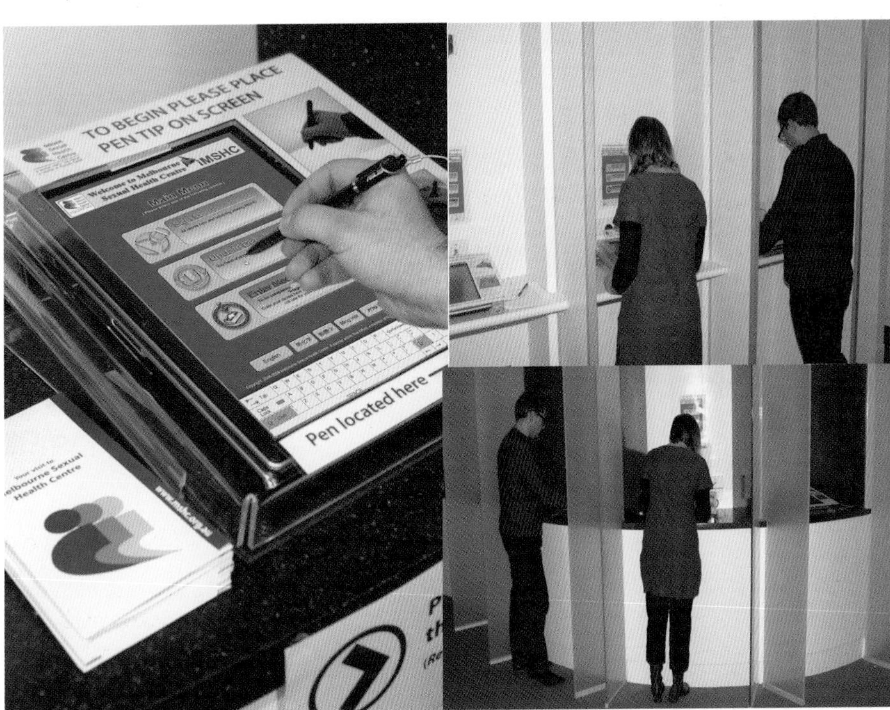

Figure 3.3 Computer-assisted sexual history taking.

that include the 'let them know' web site above, treatment guidelines, and letters for patients to give their partners and may be particularly useful for GPs.

Another novel idea to improve the appropriate testing for STIs is a web site that uses a web-based questionnaire to preform a risk assessment on asymptomatic individuals and prints out a list of recommended tests for an STI screen (www.checkyourrisk.org.au) that they then take to their GP. Other web sites have been designed to assist patients with symptoms to make their own diagnosis (www.gumnewcastle.nhs.uk/checklist.asp?id = 51), and others allow patients to obtain STI test kits (www.iwantthekit.org or www.boots.com).

Provision of results electronically

Automated text messages or web-based results are particularly cost effective if no other interventions (e.g. counselling) are required with the results. A number of centres around the world have now effectively implemented this.

In the United States, at www.cdc.gov/std/program/default.htm, there are many guidelines, STD treatment guidelines and clinic guidelines, videos for waiting rooms, and other useful resources and information.

In the United Kingdom, the British Association for Sexual Health and HIV (BASHH) have formed a **Clinical Effectiveness Group** whose role is to produce and update evidence-based National Guidelines and standards for UK specialists in genitourinary medicine (www.bashh.org). This site also has a number of other excellent resources.

Further reading

French P. BASHH 2006 National Guidelines – consultations requiring sexual history-taking. *Int J STD AIDS* 2007;**18**:17–22.

Robinson AJ, Rogstad K. Modernization in GUM/HIV services:what does it mean? *Int J STD AIDS* 2003;**14**:89–98.

Rogstad KE, Ahmed-Jushuf IH, Robinson AJ. Standards for comprehensive sexual health services for young people under 25 years. *Int J STD AIDS* 2002;**13**:420–4.

CHAPTER 4

The Sexual Health Consultation in Primary and Secondary Care

Cecilia Priestley

Dorset County Hospital NHS Foundation Trust, Dorchester, UK

OVERVIEW

- The clinical process for diagnosis and treatment of STIs has changed in the last few years, as a result of increased demand and the availability of non-invasive testing
- Patients are increasingly tested for STIs in settings outside genitourinary medicine (GUM) clinics
- For symptomatic patients seen in settings outside GUM, the decision to test a patient for STIs should be based on their clinical presentation rather than their perceived risk
- Sexual history-taking will identify patients at increased risk of infection, and patients who might need to be retested
- Clinicians should be aware of the limitations of STI testing, particularly non-invasive tests
- The principles of open access, confidentiality, and free treatment, along with effective partner notification, remain important for STI control

The principles of STI control in the UK were established by the Venereal Diseases Regulations (1916), one of the most progressive pieces of legislation in the last century. The principles of open access, confidentiality, on-site diagnostic facilities, and free treatment have remained unchanged since then, and the only thing that has significantly altered (apart from attitudes to women; Figures 4.1 and 4.2) is the responsibility for provision of services, from County Councils to NHS Trusts. However, the clinical process has altered significantly, as a result of modernisation and advances in diagnostic methods (Table 4.1).

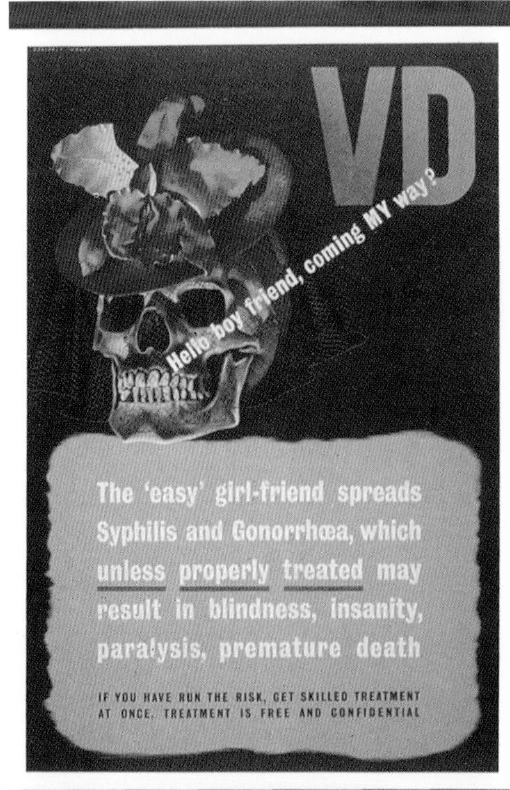

Figure 4.1 The responsibility for spreading STIs then.

Who to test

The number of patients presenting to GUM clinics with STIs represents the tip of the iceberg, and there are opportunities to diagnose STIs in many clinical settings (Table 4.2). The majority of STIs are asymptomatic, and many cases will remain undiagnosed in the community (acting as a reservoir for spread). When symptomatic, STIs have many manifestations, and patients can present to almost any medical specialty (Table 4.3).

For symptomatic patients, the decision to test for STIs, including HIV, in settings outside GUM, should be based on their clinical presentation rather than their perceived risk. Inclusion of STI testing as part of routine diagnostic testing ('We test everyone with pelvic pain/abnormal vaginal bleeding for chlamydia' or 'We test everyone with tuberculosis/oral thrush for HIV') will reduce stigma and adverse outcomes from late diagnosis.

However, sexual history-taking will identify patients at increased risk of infection, those who require additional tests and STI prophylaxis, and patients who might need to be retested if they are within the window period before the infection can be diagnosed.

ABC of Sexually Transmitted Infections, Sixth Edition.
Edited by Karen E. Rogstad.

Chlamydia.
Now available in easy
to open packets.
For your inconvenience, this sexually transmitted infection is now available everywhere. Unwittingly supplied by 1 in 14 young people, it's easily treated with antibiotics. But if left, it can cause problems with pregnancy or infertility. (This offer not open to those who always use condoms.) For more information, call the confidential fpa helpline on 0171 8374044 or visit www.lovelife.hea.org.uk
Protect yourself from Chlamydia. Always use a condom.
fpa

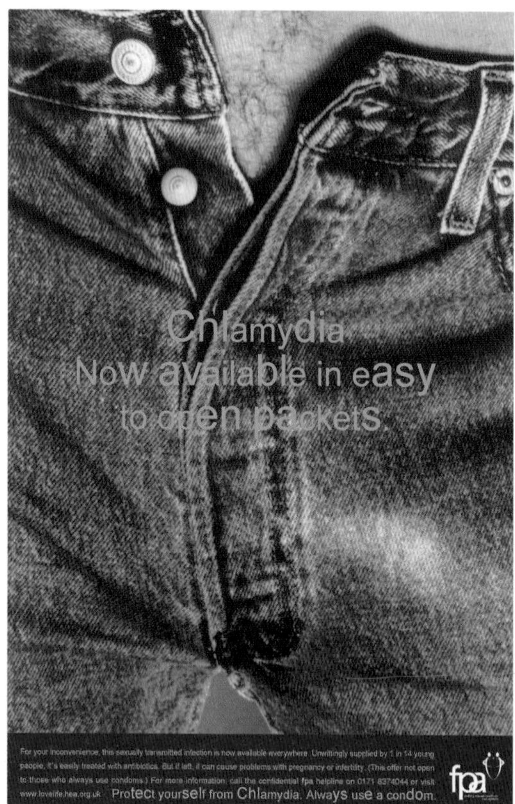

Figure 4.2 The responsibility for spreading STIs now – men as well as women. *Source:* Reproduced by permission of FPA © 2009.

Table 4.1 The clinical process and key principles of STI care.

Access to care	Easy, rapid, and free; direct access or referral; walk-in or appointment clinics
Triage or streaming	By patient or staff; asymptomatic screening or assessment and investigation of symptoms
Consultation	Non-judgmental sexual history-taking and risk assessment; the confidential nature of the service (including for under 16 s) should be made clear
Examination	Genital ± general. In the UK, a chaperone is mandatory for a male clinician seeing a female patients, and desirable for all intimate examinations
Investigations	Invasive or non-invasive; should support but not delay care
Diagnosis	Immediate (microscopy, near patient testing) or delayed (laboratory); diagnosis before treatment is preferable
Treatment	Preferably easy to adhere to (single dose if possible), and provided directly to the patient free of charge
Health promotion	Sexual health education, risk reduction (e.g. one-to-one intervention), condom provision
Partner management	Partner notification by patient or provider
Follow-up	Confirm whether this will be by texting results, telephone consultation, or in person. At follow-up, symptom resolution, treatment adherence, further sexual exposure, and treatment of partners should be explored. A microbiological test of cure may be performed

Table 4.2 Diagnosis of STIs.

Diagnostic setting	Example
Patient request for screening	Concern about risky behaviour such a 'one night stand' or partner's infidelity
	New relationship
Opportunistic screening	Consultation for contraceptive provision, pregnancy counselling or antenatal clinic, travel advice
National screening programme	Chlamydia screening programmes
With symptoms of an STI	For most STIs, only 30–50% have symptoms
As a contact of an STI	Patient or provider notification
With complications of an STI	See Table 4.3

The sexual health consultation

It is easy to take a sexual history – if you have been trained to do so, and are seeing a patient in a sexual health clinic, where consultations are facilitated by:

- Patient expectation
- Staff training
- Time
- Confidentiality
- Privacy

The patient will probably have attended because they have a concern about their sexual health, and such questioning will not be unexpected. Within a minute of meeting a nervous patient, a trained, sensitive, and empathetic clinician will have established a rapport with the patient, and will be asking intimate questions about their sex life, which will generally be responded to openly and honestly. Most patients will leave the clinic feeling better than when they arrived.

In the UK, confidentiality extends beyond that of other medical specialties. Patients may attend anonymously if they wish; clinic numbers are used as patient identifiers for clinical specimens; notes and IT systems are separate from other hospital departments; and general practitioners will usually only receive communication with the patient's consent.

To attempt to take a sexual history from a patient in the middle of a busy ward, accident and emergency department, or general practice surgery offers a challenge to any clinician, not least one without training and experience, and can result in embarrassment or even offence to the patient. However, even a short amount of practice and experience will increase confidence.

In taking a sexual history, you should aim to get to the direct question, 'When did you last have sex?' as sensitively and efficiently as possible, without making assumptions about the patient's sexual behaviour or their partner's gender or relationship (Table 4.4).

If you have asked directly when they last had sex, the next question should be 'Was that with a regular partner?' This allows them to say 'yes' or 'no', without causing offence to someone in a long-standing relationship. You should identify the type of sex,

Table 4.3 Presentation of sexually transmitted infections (excluding HIV) to other medical specialties.*

Cardiology	Cardiovascular syphilis, pericarditis
Dermatology	Warts, secondary syphilis, scabies, skin lesions of gonorrhoea, and SARA
ENT	Oropharyngeal ulceration
Gastroenterology	LGV, HPV-related AIN, hepatitis
General medicine	Secondary or tertiary syphilis, systemic gonococcal infection
General surgery	PID presenting as appendicitis, Fitz-Hugh–Curtis syndrome (peri-hepatitis associated with PID, often chlamydia)
Gynaecology	PID, infertility, pelvic pain, dyspareunia, ectopic pregnancy, HPV-related CIN, or VIN
Haematology	Unexplained lymphadenopathy due to syphilis or LGV
Neurology	Herpes simplex meningitis; neurosyphilis
Oncology	Genital intra-epithelial neoplasia, HPV-related cancer
Ophthalmology	Conjunctivitis (chlamydial, gonococcal, or associated with Reiter's syndrome), iritis (Reiter's syndrome)
Paediatrics	Neonatal conjunctivitis (chlamydial, gonococcal) or pneumonitis (chlamydial), laryngeal papillomatosis, genital gonorrhoea or chlamydia, TV, herpes; congenital syphilis
Psychiatry	Neurosyphilis, dementia
Rheumatology	Sexually acquired reactive arthritis (Reiter's syndrome), gonococcal arthritis
Urology	Epididymitis, prostatitis, HPV-related PIN, retention of urine (herpes simplex)

AIN, anal intra-epithelial neoplasia; CIN, cervical intra-epithelial neoplasia; ENT, ear, nose, and throat; HPV, human papillomavirus; LGV, lymphogranuloma venereum; PID, pelvic inflammatory disease; PIN, penile intra-epithelial neoplasia; SARA, sexually acquired reactive arthritis; TV, trichomoniasis; VIN, vulval intra-epithelial neoplasia.
*This table does not include the presentation of patients with HIV, who may also present to any medical specialty – see BASHH guidelines and BHIVA audit.

Table 4.4 Sexual history-taking.

Good questions	Questions to avoid
What can I do for you?	I'm sorry to ask you this ...
I need to ask you some routine questions	Don't be embarrassed but ...
Do you have a regular partner?	Are you married?
When did you last have sex?	When did you last make love?
Was that with a regular partner?	Was that with your boyfriend/girlfriend or a one night stand?
(If regular) How long have you been with them?	How long have you been with him/her?
What is their name?	
Do (did) you use condoms at all?	Do you always use condoms/protection?
Have you had any accidents?	
Is your partner OK?	Have they been unfaithful?
When did you last have sex with anyone other than them?	Have you been unfaithful? Have you had a one night stand?

whether condoms were used, their partner's gender, and whether their partners have any symptoms. The partner's gender can usually be established without asking directly (e.g. 'How long have you been with them? What is their name? Are they OK?') but you may need to ask directly if their partner is a man or a woman. If they are not in a regular relationship, you should identify in addition whether the partner is known to them ('Was it someone you know?') and, if so, any details that will facilitate contact tracing.

Once you have the details of their last sexual contact, the question 'When did you last have sex with anyone other than them?' should be asked. This will allow someone in a long-term relationship to respond 'Ten years ago' or 'Two weeks ago', without causing offence – which the question 'Have you been unfaithful to them?' would invariably do. If their previous sexual contact was recent, obtain details as above.

Other components of the sexual history are listed in Table 4.5 and examples of proformas for taking a male and female history are provided (Appendix 1 and 2).

Table 4.5 Components of a sexual history.

Component	Rationale
Reason for attendance	Identify patient's concerns; establish a rapport before asking more intrusive questions
Symptom review	Guide examination and testing
Last sexual intercourse, partner relationship and gender, sites of exposure, condom use	Identify sites that need to be tested and risky behaviours
Previous sexual partner, details if recent	Identify the risks of an STI
Past medical and surgical history	Identify conditions that may be associated with or influence the management of an STI
Past history STIs	Identify the risk of complications from previous STIs
	Allow the interpretation of positive syphilis serology in patients who have previously been treated
Drug history and history of allergies	Identify drugs that cannot be given safely
Risk assessment for HIV, hepatitis B and C	Assess the risk of infection, need for retesting if exposure was within the window period, and facilitate health promotion
Women: menstrual history, LMP, contraceptive and cytology history	Identify pregnancy or pregnancy risk Determine whether to offer cervical cytology
Under 16 or vulnerable: assess competency, child protection concerns	Consider whether liaison with local child protection team is indicated
Explanation of the need for and nature of a clinical examination and tests	Enable patient to give informed consent to testing
Establish the mode of communicating the results to the patients	Ensure that patients with a positive result can be contacted to enable treatment to be given

LMP, last menstrual period.

Investigations

Examination and investigations are covered in detail in Chapters 5 and 18.

Traditionally, STI testing has involved examination of the patient and taking swabs in men from the urethra (and throat and rectum if indicated), and in women from the urethra, vagina, and cervix. The introduction of nucleic acid amplification tests (NAATs) has permitted non-invasive testing for chlamydia and gonorrhoea, using urine specimens in men and self-taken vulvo-vaginal or urine specimens in women. Many GUM clinics operate a triage system, so that patients presenting for routine 'asymptomatic screening' can be seen by a nurse for rapid non-invasive STI testing (see Appendix).

There is some debate about whether on-site microscopy is cost effective in asymptomatic patients. If a clinic has the capacity to provide a 'gold standard' service, immediate diagnosis and treatment of urethritis or cervicitis may reduce the risk of:

- Delayed treatment of an STI (e.g. a patient with asymptomatic gonorrhoea, who could infect another partner before receiving the result and attending for treatment)
- Untreated STI (e.g. a patient with chlamydia who does not return for treatment)
- Undiagnosed STI (e.g. *Mycoplasma genitalium*, which may cause urethritis or pelvic inflammatory disease (PID), but cannot be diagnosed using routine laboratory methods)

However, if the demand for STI testing outstrips the capacity of a service, there is a valid argument that wider provision of a less than 'gold standard' service will provide a greater public health benefit. For example, chlamydia screening programmes (CSPs) have been shown to reduce the prevalence not only of chlamydia, but of its consequences such as ectopic pregnancy.

In future, near patient testing (other than microscopy) will have an increasing role in the management of patients, facilitating immediate diagnosis and treatment. Several point of care tests for STIs are already available, although their use needs to be carefully considered because of concerns about low sensitivity or specificity, reproducibility, and quality control.

Potentially, STI testing and treatment could take place without patients attending a sexual health clinic. Patients may obtain a postal chlamydia testing kit from the CSP or internet, and those with proof of a positive result may purchase azithromycin from pharmacies without a prescription. Giving treatment to the patient for their partner is also under consideration, although this is not currently legal in the UK.

Limitations of STI testing

It is important to remember that the majority of STIs can remain latent for many years, without symptoms, but still potentially transmissible. STIs may present in long-standing monogamous relationships:

- One or the other partner may have brought the infection into the relationship
- Tests for STIs are neither 100% sensitive nor specific
- There are some infections that may not be diagnosed by a routine STI screen (Table 4.6)

The clinician should never cause unnecessary stress in a relationship by wrongly implying that the diagnosis of an STI, or discordant results in a couple, implies infidelity.

Treatment

Treatment of individual STIs is covered in the relevant chapters. National and international STI treatment guidelines are also readily available on the internet (Box 4.1); these are evidence-based and regularly updated.

Adherence to therapy is extremely important in the control of STIs; hence the principles of free treatment and, wherever possible, single dose therapy. Single dose therapy is available for most uncomplicated bacterial STIs, but treatment of viral STIs, for which there is no cure, may be more complicated.

Table 4.6 Sexually transmitted conditions that may not be diagnosed during a routine sexual health check.

Infection	Diagnosis
Chlamydia	NAAT; good, but not 100%, sensitivity and specificity
Gonorrhoea	Culture or NAAT. Culture is 100% specific but not 100% sensitive; NAATs have good sensitivity but high false positive rates in a low prevalence population
Mycoplasma genitalium	By PCR in research settings; routine testing not available. May cause some cases of NSU and pelvic inflammatory disease; these will be missed by non-invasive testing
NSU	Microscopy of a urethral swab in men; cannot be diagnosed by urine NAAT testing for chlamydia and gonorrhoea. NSU cannot be tested for in female partners, who should be given epidemiological treatment
PID	Clinical or by laparoscopy in women; in up to 70%, no specific infective cause can be identified. It cannot be tested for in male partners, who should be given epidemiological treatment
Epididymitis	Clinically in men; some, but not all, will also have urethritis. It cannot be tested for in female partners, who should be given epidemiological treatment
HPV	Diagnosis of genital warts is clinical; subclinical or latent HPV infection cannot be diagnosed by routine screening
HSV	Clinical or by viral culture or PCR if symptomatic; culture is difficult and not very sensitive. Routine screening does not exclude latent infection. Serology may be of value in some cases
TV	Microscopy or culture of a vaginal swab in women; if available, PCR is more sensitive. Rarely diagnosed in male partners, who should be given epidemiological treatment
HIV	Blood test, usually HIV antibody/antigen; 100% sensitive as long as patient is not within the 'window period' before antibody development (3 months; less if a 4th generation test is used)
Syphilis	Blood test, usually syphilis antibody; this may be negative in early or primary infection or if HIV infected

HPV, human papillomavirus; HSV, herpes simplex virus; NAAT, nucleic acid amplification test; NSU, non-specific urethritis; PCR, polymerase chain reaction; PID, pelvic inflammatory disease; TV, trichomoniasis.

Instructions to contact:

You have had sex with somebody who has an infection which can be passed on through sexual contact. As most of these infections do not cause symptoms, it is important that you are tested and receive treatment, even if you feel well.
We recommend that you do not have sex again until you have been tested and treated.

Please attend either:

- Your local GUM clinic (telephone NHS Direct 0845 46 47 for your nearest clinic) ***or***
- Your GP

Please give slip(s) to your patient, asking that they pass it on to any person they have had sex with in the previous 6 months (or the most recent partner if over 6 months).

Patient code / initials: ______

Date: ______

Instructions to practice / clinic who see and treat contact:

- Please screen the contact as appropriate; however as current tests are unreliable, empirical treatment should be given even if the results are negative.
- Telephone your local Dept of GUM for advice if needed
- If local arrangements are in place, inform the Community Sexual Health Adviser that the contact has been treated.

Infection(s) (please tick)		Recommended treatment for contact:
Chlamydia	☐	Azithromycin 1g stat
Non-specific urethritis (NSU)	☐	Azithromycin 1g stat
Pelvic inflammatory disease (PID)	☐	Azithromycin 1g stat
Epididymitis	☐	Azithromycin 1g stat
Trichomoniasis	☐	Metronidazole 2g stat
Gonorrhoea	☐	Seek advice

Figure 4.3 An example of a partner notification slip.

Box 4.1 **STI treatment guidelines**

- British Association for Sexual Health and HIV (BASHH): Clinical Effectiveness Group guidelines http://www.bashh.org/guidelines
- International Union against STIs (IUSTI): European guidelines http://www.iusti.org/regions/europe/euroguidelines.htm
- Centers for Disease Control and Prevention (CDC): Sexually transmitted infections treatment guidelines http://www.cdc.gov/std/treatment/2006/toc.htm
- World Health Organization (WHO): Guidelines for the management of sexually transmitted infections http://www.who.int/hiv/pub/sti/pub6/en/

It is important that patients treated for a bacterial STI understand that they must not have unprotected sex with any untreated sexual partners, to avoid being reinfected. Generally, patients are advised to abstain completely, but as this seems to be very difficult for some, a pragmatic compromise would be 'Don't have sex, but if you cannot avoid it, make sure you use a condom.' For most infections, abstinence is recommended for a week after both the patient and partner have completed their therapy, or after confirmation of cure. Women taking the combined oral contraceptive pill should be advised that it will not be effective while taking the antibiotics and for 7 days afterwards.

Patients taking antibiotics for a non-specific infection such as PID or epididymitis should be advised that if their tests are negative, this does not exclude an infection (for the reasons given in Table 4.6), and they should complete the treatment and return for follow-up.

Discussion of the nature and rationale of treatment should be accompanied by provision of verbal and written information about the condition, partner notification if appropriate (by patient or provider; Figure 4.3), and confirmation of follow-up arrangements. The diagnosis of an STI, or recognition by the patient that they have been at risk of one, can provide quite a jolt, and this is often an ideal opportunity for providing health promotion and education on a one-to-one basis. This may be undertaken by the clinician who has seen the patient, or in some GUM clinics by a health adviser who has had specific training in counselling and motivational interviewing techniques.

The future of sexual health services

In the UK, the drive for the future is for the provision of integrated sexual health services, employing staff qualified to provide effective contraception and STI testing and treatment, and for the development of sexual health networks, linking these and other sexual services such as abortion, sexual dysfunction, health promotion, and HIV, to ensure that patients receive truly holistic sexual health care.

Further reading

British Association for Sexual Health and HIV (BASHH): Clinical Effectiveness Group Guidelines. http://www.bashh.org/guidelines.

Clutterbuck D. Sexually transmitted infections: the sexual health consultation. In Clutterbuck D (ed.) *Sexually Transmitted Infections and HIV*. Elsevier Mosby, 2004.

UK National Guidelines for HIV Testing, 2008.

UK National Guidelines on Undertaking Consultations Requiring Sexual History Taking 2006. http://www.bashh.org/documents/84/84.

UK National STI Screening and Testing Guideline. 2006. http://www.bashh.org/documents/59/59.

CHAPTER 5

Examination Techniques and Clinical Sampling

Katrina Perez and Vincent Lee

Manchester Centre for Sexual Health, Central Manchester University Hospitals NHS Foundation Trust, Manchester, UK

OVERVIEW

- Examination must be carried out in a sensitive manner, ensuring privacy and a chaperone as necessary
- General examination is often required to look for systemic manifestations
- All patients require tests for *Neisseria gonorrhoeae* and *Chlamydia trachomatis*
- Further tests will be dictated by the history and examination findings
- Blood test for HIV and syphilis should be routinely offered as part of the sexual health screen

Patients should be given clear instructions about the examination procedure, ensuring verbal agreement is given. In certain situations such as biopsy, local anaesthetic, or photography, written consent is required. A warm and private environment must be created for the patient to undress below the waist and a gown or drape provided. The United Kingdom General Medical Council recommends a chaperone should be offered irrespective of the gender of the patient and the examiner; preferably not a relative and acceptance or refusal should be documented in the patient's notes. The chaperone can also aid specimen collection and offer reassurance to the patient. A pre-arranged trolley should be set up for the examination with a speculum warmed with water for the female patient. Lubricant gels should be avoided as there is evidence to suggest they can interfere with the growth of *Neisseria gonorrhoeae*.

Examination is usually confined to the genitals; however, a fuller examination may be required in cases of HIV, syphilis, and other suspected systemic manifestations of sexually transmitted infections (STIs) (Box 5.1). Frequently, this will involve examining the mouth, skin, and lymph nodes. Genital lesions may also be a feature of dermatological diseases.

Box 5.1 **General examination**

- **Skin**
  - Scabies – rash which favours wrists, interdigital web, buttocks, and areolae
  - Secondary syphilis and HIV seroconversion illness – generalised rash with characteristic lesions on palms and soles
- **Lymph nodes**
  - Secondary syphilis, HIV, and primary herpes simplex – generalised lymphadenopathy
- **Mouth**
  - Secondary syphilis – snail track ulceration and mucous patches
  - HIV – ulceration in primary HIV disease, oral hairy leukoplakia, oral candidiasis, Kaposi's sarcoma
  - Herpes simplex – ulceration
  - Warts

Examining the female patient

Inspect the pubic hair and entire perineal area for evidence of pediculosis pubis, ulcers, warts, molluscum contagiosum, and inflammation (Figures 5.1 and 5.2). Palpate for enlarged and/or tender inguinal lymphadenopathy. Part the labia minora and examine for any ulcers, discharge, Bartholin's cysts, and warts. Urethral specimens for *N. gonorrhoeae* can be obtained using a small cotton tip or plastic loop. This can then be gram stained and cultured.

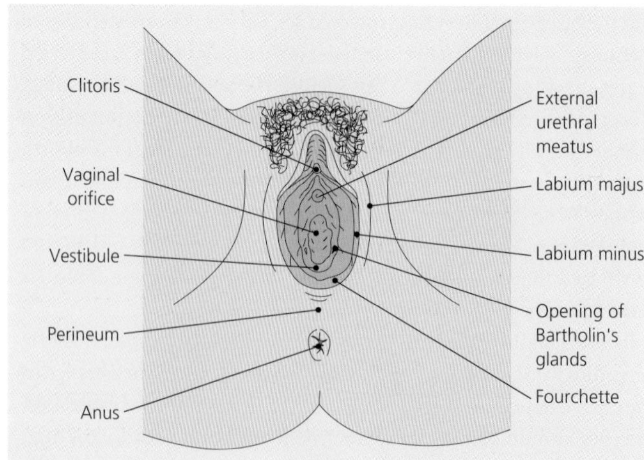

Figure 5.1 Female external genitalia. Source: adapted from *Sexually transmitted infections: history taking and examination*, CD, The Wellcome Trust, 2003.

ABC of Sexually Transmitted Infections, Sixth Edition.
Edited by Karen E. Rogstad.

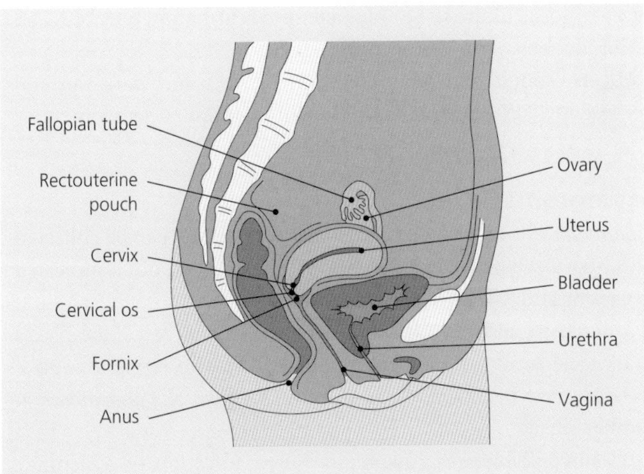

Figure 5.2 Female internal genitalia. Source: adapted from *Sexually transmitted infections: history taking and examination*, CD, The Wellcome Trust, 2003.

There is only a small additional benefit in doing this sample and it may be uncomfortable.

Gently introduce the speculum lubricated with warm water to examine the vagina and cervix. Look for abnormal discharge, inflammation, and mucosal lesions. Using a cotton tip or loop take a sample of discharge from the lateral vaginal walls and test the pH using narrow range pH paper. Elevated pH ($\geq$5.0) indicates either bacterial vaginosis or *Trichomonas vaginalis* infection. Then prepare a dry slide from this specimen which is gram stained and examined for bacterial vaginosis and candida. Collect the pool of vaginal secretions in the posterior fornix with a loop and prepare a wet slide using a drop of saline and cover slip. This is examined further for clue cells, candida, and *T. vaginalis*. A high vaginal swab can be sent for culture in women with abnormal discharge. For candida this has a better sensitivity and typing, and sensitivity for non-responders to treatment can be requested.

Cervical cytology should be performed at this stage if required. Use a large cotton mop to clean the cervix then take an endocervical specimen for gram stain smear and culture for *N. gonorrhoeae*. This is done by rotating a cotton tip or loop in the cervical os. A second specimen is then collected from the endocervical canal for *C. trachomatis* and *N. gonorrhoeae* using a nucleic acid amplification test (NAAT) kit. A vulvo-vaginal swab (preferably high vaginal) is also suitable and forms the basis of asymptomatic screening both in the hospital and community settings. A pelvic and abdominal examination should be performed for all women who have abdominal symptoms or signs to exclude pelvic inflammatory disease or pelvic masses.

Urine collection may be required if a pregnancy test is indicated, or mid-stream urine for any symptoms of urinary tract infection. *C. trachomatis* and *N. gonorrhoeae* testing can be done on the first 20 mL urine if necessary; however, the sensitivity is much lower and most women will perform a self-taken vulvo-vaginal swab as an alternative.

Ulcers should be examined and prompt wider examination for signs of syphilis. A swab should be taken for herpes simplex virus (HSV) polymerase chain reaction (PCR) test. Treponemal PCR tests can be requested on the same sample and this is useful for atypical lesions. Dark ground microscopy should be peformed on any lesions (excluding the mouth due to commensal treponemes) suspicious of early syphilis including possible chancre and condylomata lata.

Pharyngeal specimens for *N. gonorrhoeae* culture are obtained in symptomatic individuals, victims of sexual assault, or those whose partners have *N. gonorrhoeae*. Specimens are obtained by wiping a swab over the posterior pharynx, tonsils, and tonsillar crypts and plated directly on to a culture medium. Tests for *C. trachomatis* should be carried out for patients presenting with symptoms suggestive of STI and victims of sexual assault who have reported oral penetration or attempted penetration. NAAT is generally used although this still does not have Food and Drug Administration (FDA) approval for pharangeal or rectal sites in women or men.

If there are anal symptoms or a history of receptive anal sex, the perianal region is examined for warts, inflammation, or ulcers. Rectal swabs are collected for *N. gonorrhoeae* using cotton tips for gram stain and culture and for *C. trachomatis* and *N. gonorrhoeae* using NAAT. Rectal swabs for *N. gonorrhoeae* should be taken when patients are named contacts of an infected patient.

Asymptomatic women

Chlamydia trachomatis and *N. gonorrhoeae* NAAT can be collected either with endocervical swab with the addition of *N. gonorrhoeae* culture **or** self-taken vulvo-vaginal swab. Further tests are only carried out if indicated by examination.

Trichomoniasis is relatively uncommon and usually symptomatic but testing is required to fully exclude it. It is not possible to exclude genital herpes infection by 'screening'. Lesions should be present to warrant taking a test for herpes.

In asymptomatic patients, at the present time, there is no value in taking samples for bacterial vaginosis and candida, neither of which are strictly sexually transmitted.

Examining the male patient

Inspect the areas covered with hair for pediculosis pubis and the entire genital area for ulcers, inflammation, masses, warts, and molluscum contagiosum (Figure 5.3). Palpate the inguinal region for lymphadenopathy. Palpate the testes and epididymis to look for tenderness or swelling. The shaft of the penis is examined for lesions such as herpes, warts, or papules from scabies. The prepuce, if present, is retracted. The glans, frenum, coronal sulcus, and prepuce are examined. Examine the urethral meatus for discharge, meatitis, intrameatal warts, and ulcers.

Visible exudate, a history of dysuria, discharge or gonorrhoea contact requires a urethral specimen for gram stain smear. A swab or plastic loop is gently placed in the meatus. Sample material from the urethra by applying gentle lateral pressure on withdrawing the swab. Massaging the meatus for discharge by the patient or examiner (explain what you are about to do and why) may be required. Ideally, the patient should have held urine for over 4 hours (2 hours is often adequate). This specimen is then plated on to selective *N. gonorrhoeae* culture media. If urine has not been held, still test but explain a retest will be needed if testing is negative.

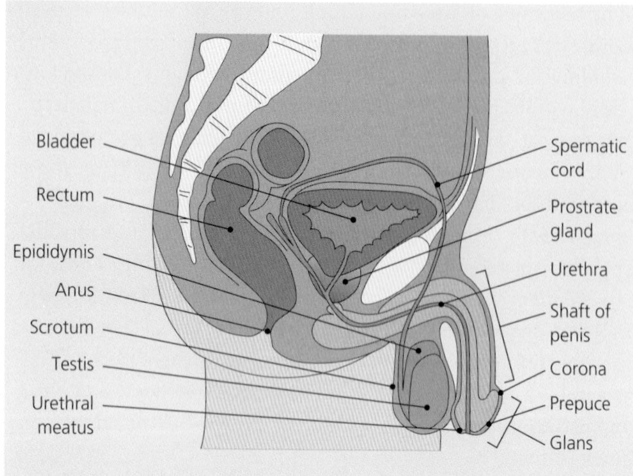

Figure 5.3 Male genitalia including scrotal contents. Source: adapted from *Sexually transmitted infections: history taking and examination*, CD, The Wellcome Trust, 2003.

Direct observation by wet mount of urethral smear, spun urine microscopy, urethral culture or culture of first-void urine can be taken when patients are named contacts of someone infected with *Trichomona vaginalis.* If there are anal symptoms or history of receptive anal sex or receptive oro-anal sex, the perianal region is examined for warts, inflammation, or ulcers.

Proctoscopy is performed to examine anal and rectal mucosa for inflammation, pus, and warts and to improve specimen collection. Blind anal swabs are acceptable in patients without anal symptoms.The use of lubricant gels should be avoided as there is some evidence to suggest an inhibitory effect on gonorrhoea growth. Rectal swabs are collected for *N. gonorrhoeae* using cotton tips for gram stain and culture and *C. trachomatis* and *N. gonorrhoeae* using NAAT. Prostatic digital examination may be required to examine for inflammation and prostatic enlargement. Prostatic massage examinations are not widely used in clinical practice as reliability of this test is not known.

Urine is collected for *C. trachomatis* and *N. gonorrhoeae* NAAT. The first 20 mL is collected after the urine has been held for a minimum of 1 hour. A second mid-stream specimen can be collected for analysis (for leucocytes, nitrites, blood, and protein) and culture if there are symptoms suggestive of a urinary tract infection. The two glass test, looking for threads in the first as an indicator of urethritis, is now less useful in the management of urethritis.

Pharyngeal specimens for *C. trachomatis* and *N. gonorrhoeae* NAAT and culture are obtained in men who have sex with men, symptomatic individuals, victims of sexual assault, or those found to have *N. gonorrhoeae* at another site. Specimens are obtained as for women.

A positive NAAT for gonorrhoea should prompt referral to a specialised STI service (level 3 in the United Kingdom) for a gonorrhoea culture to be obtained for confirmation purposes and antibiotic sensitivities prior to treatment.

Ulcers should be examined and tested for dark ground microscopy, HSV PCR and treponemal PCR test as per women.

Asymptomatic men

Chlamydia trachomatis and *N. gonorrhoeae* NAAT can be collected with first-catch urine. Further tests are only carried out if indicated by examination. Tests for *N. gonorrhoeae* and *C. trachomatis* should be offered to all men who report receptive anal sex. Likewise, a pharyngeal swab can be carried out on men who report receptive oral sex, have been assaulted, or found to have *N. gonorrhoeae* at another site.

It is not possible to exclude genital herpes infection by 'screening'. Lesions should be present to warrant taking a test for herpes.

It is important to liaise with your local microbiology laboratory to ensure the correct collection and transport of specimens.

Blood tests

All patients should be offered HIV and syphilis testing routinely. Hepatitis B and C tests should be offered where indicated. Risk assessment should be performed routinely; however, lengthy pre-test HIV counselling is not required unless a patient needs or requests this. HIV pre-test discussion is primarily to establish informed consent, explain the individual benefits of testing if they decline testing, and how results will be given. This opt-out approach with verbal consent documented is now routine practice in STI and antenatal clinics in the United Kingdom. There is no longer any need for HIV testing to be restricted to specialist services. Testing is discussed further in Chapter 17.

Patients with high risk of hepatitis B infection should be screened and offered vaccination at their first visit.

Further reading

BASHH. Sexually Transmitted Infections: UK National Screening and Testing Guidelines, August 2006.

BASHH. Microscopy for sexually transmitted infections. An educational DVD for health care professionals available via www.bashh.org.

McMillan A, Young H, Ogilvie MM, Scott GR. *Clinical Practice in Sexually Transmissible Infections*. Saunders, 2002.

Pattmen R, Snow M, Handy P, Sankar KN, Elawad B. *Oxford Handbook of Genitourinary Medicine, HIV, and AIDS*. Oxford University Press, 2007.

UK National Guidelines for HIV testing 2008. http://www.bhiva.org/documents/Guidelines/Testing/GlinesHIVTest08.pdf

CHAPTER 6

Main Presentations of Sexually Transmitted Infections in Male Patients

John Richens

Centre for Sexual Health and HIV Research, University College London, London, UK

OVERVIEW

- Frank urethral discharge in a sexually active male most commonly results from gonorrhoea or chlamydia infection
- Involvement of the upper genital tract in males by sexually transmitted infections may manifest as epididymitis
- Infections of the prostate present with pain and voiding symptoms; sexually transmitted pathogens are rarely identified in such patients
- Men who have sex with men (MSM) are at risk of anorectal infection with syphilis, herpes, gonorrhoea, chlamydia, and lymphogranuloma venereum
- Asymptomatic pharyngeal colonization by *Neisseria gonorrhoeae* is common among MSM

Some sexually transmitted infections (STIs), such as gonorrhoea and chlamydial infection, have very different presentations in the two sexes because of differences in genital anatomy. This chapter focuses on infections of the male urethra, epididymis, testis, and prostate. Anal and oral symptoms are also covered because these are encountered more often among men, especially men who have sex with men (MSM).

Urethral discharge and dysuria

Spontaneous discharge of fluid from the urethral meatus is usually most noticeable after holding the urine overnight (Figures 6.1 and 6.2). It is often accompanied by burning discomfort during urination (dysuria), and strongly indicates a sexually acquired urethral infection (Box 6.1).

Symptomatic gonorrhoea usually develops within 2–5 days of exposure; chlamydia infections take 1–2 weeks. Mild infections may cause urethral discomfort and dysuria without discharge and may be confused with cystitis.

In clinics with laboratory facilities, the usual approach is to test for gonorrhoea and chlamydial infection (Boxes 6.2 and 6.3). The first step is microscopy of a urethral smear. Optimal results for gram stain and culture are obtained from patients who have held their urine for 4 hours or more (Figure 6.3).

Urethritis is confirmed if the urethral smear shows five or more polymorphs per high power field. If the smear shows gram-negative intracellular diplococci (Figure 6.4), the patient is treated for gonorrhoea and chlamydia to cover the possibility of a mixed infection. Meanwhile, confirmatory tests for gonorrhoea and chlamydia are carried out (see Chapter 18). These include nucleic acid

Box 6.1 **Causes of urethritis in men**

Common diagnoses among men with urethritis

- Gonorrhoea
- Chlamydial infection
- Non-specific urethritis

Less common diagnoses among men with urethritis

- *Mycoplasma genitalium* infection
- Trichomoniasis
- Herpes simplex virus infection
- Adenovirus infection
- *Escherichia coli* infection
- Urinary tract infection
- Trauma
- Foreign body
- Urethritis associated with reactive arthritis and allied conditions

Box 6.2 **Management of urethritis in male patients**

1. Take history, including sexual history
2. Examine, looking especially for evidence of discharge
3. Take samples from urethra or test urine
4. Treat for gonorrhoea and chlamydia if urethral gram stain is positive for gram-negative intracellular diplococci
5. Give treatment for chlamydia if the urethral smear shows five or more polymorphs per high power field and the gram stain does not suggest gonorrhoea
6. Explain diagnosis, treatment, and methods of prevention
7. Advise to avoid sex until treatment and follow-up are completed
8. Advise partner treatment
9. Review patient after treatment for symptoms, adherence, and treatment of partners

ABC of Sexually Transmitted Infections, Sixth Edition.
Edited by Karen E. Rogstad.

Box 6.3 **Overview of chlamydial and gonorrhoea infection**

Chlamydia

Cause

- *Chlamydia trachomatis*, types D–K (see also lymphogranuloma venereum). *C. trachomatis* is an obligate intracellular bacterium

Initial sites of infection

- Epithelial cells of urethra, cervix, rectum, pharynx, and conjunctiva, depending on mode of exposure

Incubation period

- Less than 4 weeks for men; unknown in women
- Asymptomatic infections are common in both sexes and can persist for many months

Main symptoms in men

- Urethral discharge and dysuria

Less common symptoms in men

- Proctitis, conjunctivitis, epididymo-orchitis, and reactive arthritis

Main symptoms in women

- Dysuria, vaginal discharge, and intermenstrual bleeding

Less common symptoms in women

- Pelvic inflammatory disease (with sequelae of infertility and ectopic pregnancy), peri-hepatitis (Fitz-Hugh–Curtis syndrome), conjunctivitis, reactive arthritis

Symptoms affecting neonates

- Conjunctivitis and pneumonia

Main methods of diagnosis

- Nucleic acid amplification tests (NAAT) or enzyme immunoassay (see Chapter 17)

Recommended treatments for uncomplicated chlamydia

- See Chapter 22

Gonorrhoea

Cause

- *Neisseria gonorrhoeae*, a gram-negative coccus
- Initial sites of infection: columnar epithelium of urethra, endocervix, rectum, pharynx, or conjunctiva depending on mode of exposure

Incubation period

- Two to five days in 80% of men who develop urethral symptoms
- Asymptomatic infections common in both sexes, especially infections of pharynx, cervix, and rectum

Main symptoms in men

- Urethral discharge, dysuria, and tender inguinal lymph nodes

Less common genital symptoms in men

- Epididymo-orchitis, abscesses of paraurethral glands, and urethral stricture

Main symptoms in women

- Vaginal discharge, dysuria, abnormal bleeding
- Examination may show mucopurulent discharge from the cervical os, urethra, Skene's glands, or Bartholin's glands

Less common genital symptoms in women

- Lower abdominal pain, bartholinitis and vulvo-vaginitis (pre-pubertal girls)

Extragenital symptoms and complications that affect both sexes

- Pharyngitis, rectal pain and discharge, and conjunctivitis
- Disseminated infection involving skin, joints, and heart valves, secondary infertility after damage to fallopian tubes, or epididymis

Main methods of diagnosis

- Detection of gram-negative intracellular diplococci in smears and culture for *N gonorrhoeae*. PCR testing of urine samples is a useful screening tool

Treatments recommended for uncomplicated gonorrhoea in the following guidelines

- Choice of treatment should take into account local susceptibility data (Figures 6.5–6.7)
- Treatment schedules: see Chapter 22

Follow-up

- A test of cure culture is no longer recommended

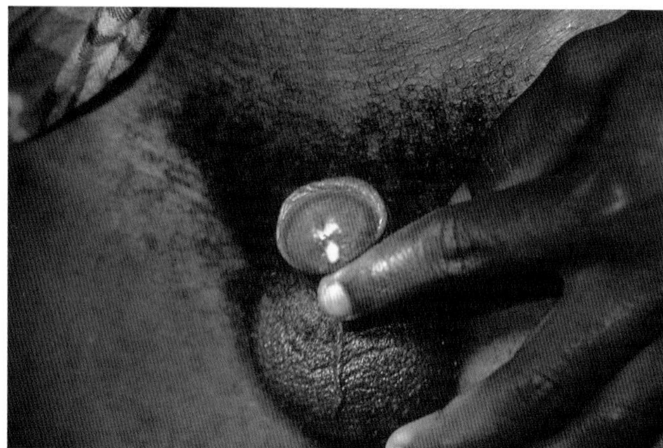

Figure 6.1 Gonococcal urethral discharge.

amplification tests (NAATs) on first pass urine and gonorrhoea from the urethra in symptomatic men.

Patients without evidence of gonorrhoea receive azithromycin (1 g single dose), doxycycline (100 mg twice daily for 1 week), or erythromycin (500 mg twice daily for 2 weeks), which are active against chlamydial infection and other pathogens associated with non-gonococcal urethritis. Doxycycline can cause photosensitivity. Absorption is impaired by antacids, iron, calcium, and magnesium salts. Gastrointestinal upset is common with erythromycin and azithromycin.

This approach will relieve symptoms in most patients, but some will report persistent symptoms or show a persistently abnormal smear without symptoms. The options are then to investigate for treatment failure or reinfection or for infection by less common pathogens (e.g. *Trichomonas vaginalis and Mycoplasma*

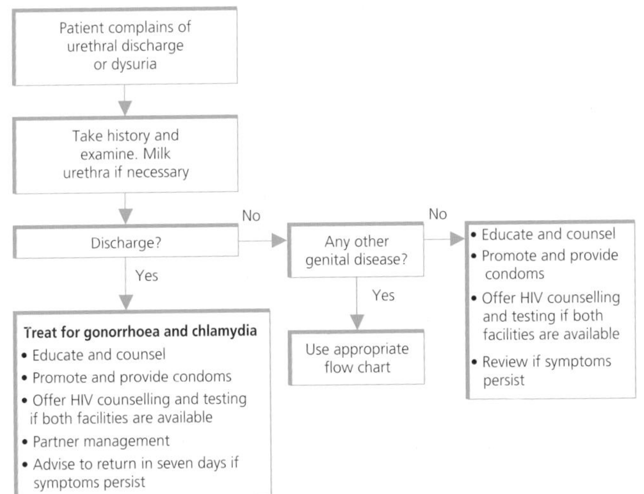

Figure 6.2 Urethral discharge flow chart. Source: World Health Organization.

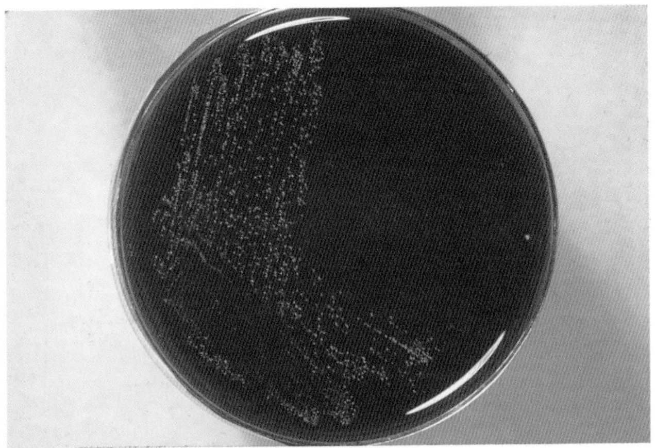

Figure 6.3 *Neisseria gonorrhoeae* culture.

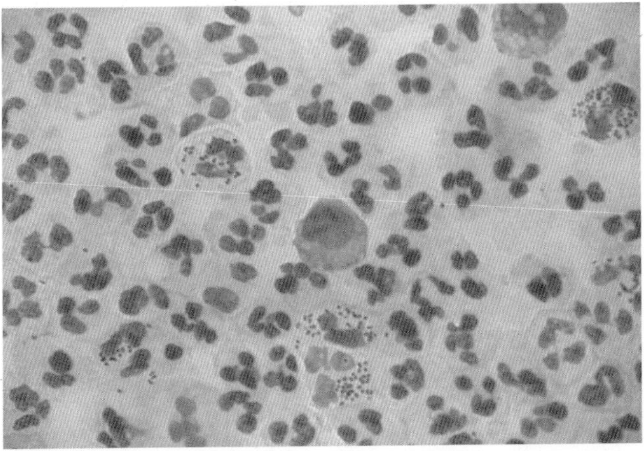

Figure 6.4 Gram-negative intracellular diplococci. Courtesy of CDC/Joe Miller.

genitalium) and to repeat, continue, or change the antibiotic therapy or await spontaneous resolution of symptoms.

When access to laboratory testing is not available, for example in resource poor settings (see Chapter 21), the simplest approach to managing urethritis is to administer blind treatment for gonorrhoea and chlamydia (syndromic management) (Figure 6.2).

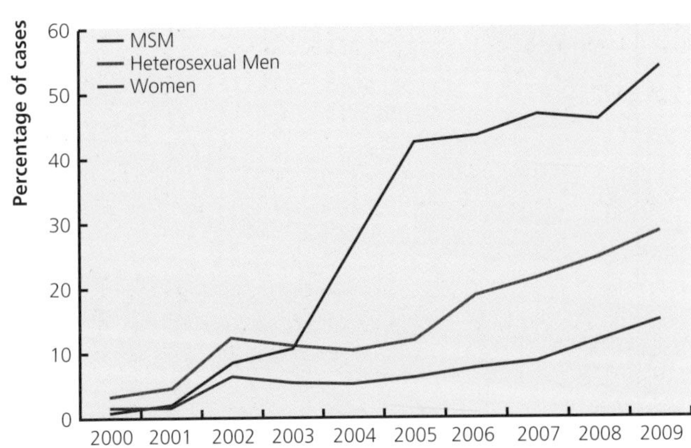

Figure 6.5 Antimicrobial resistance of *N. gonorrhoeae* resistance to ciprofloxacin. Source: Gonococcal Resistance to Antimicrobials Surveillance Programme (GRASP) in England and Wales: report of 2009 data by courtesy of the Health Protection Agency.

Scrotal swelling and pain

Mild testicular discomfort in the absence of abnormal physical signs is encountered commonly in young male attenders in STI clinics. Many such patients can be reassured if testicular examination and a screen for STIs are carried out and found to be normal. In some cases, anxiety about infection, sexual function, or cancer is present. More marked scrotal pain has a variety of causes (Box 6.4).

Box 6.4 **Causes of scrotal swelling and pain in adults and adolescents**

- Infections of testis and epididymis: gonorrhoea, chlamydia, tuberculosis, mumps virus, and gram-negative bacteria
- Torsion of testis (mainly adolescents) or appendix testis (mainly 3- to 7-year-olds)
- Hydrocoele, spermatocoele, varicocoele
- Vasculitis: Henoch–Schönlein purpura, Kawasaki's disease, and Buerger's disease
- Amiodarone therapy
- Tumour
- Hernia
- Trauma

Acute epididymo-orchitis (usually unilateral) in young men is usually caused by gonorrhoea or chlamydia (Figure 6.8). In men over 35 years, *Escherichia coli*, *Klebsiella*, *Pseudomonas*, and *Proteus* subsequent to a urinary tract infection are found more often. The first consideration in diagnosis is to exclude acute torsion, which requires emergency surgery. Torsion predominates in the teenage years, usually has an acute onset, and is often accompanied by vomiting. An immediate surgical opinion should be sought for any possible case. Doppler scanning is useful for demonstrating impaired blood flow. The distinguishing features of a mumps orchitis are usually onset several days after parotid swelling,

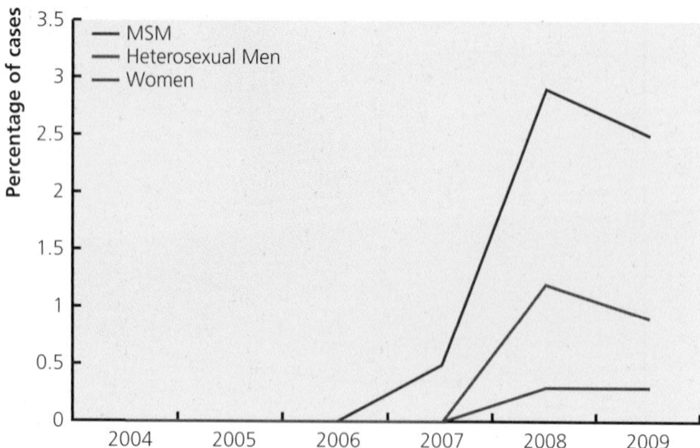

Figure 6.6 Antimicrobial resistance of *N. gonorrhoeae* resistance to cefixime. Source: Gonococcal Resistance to Antimicrobials Surveillance Programme (GRASP) in England and Wales: report of 2009 data by courtesy of the Health Protection Agency.

severe testicular pain (which may be unilateral or bilateral), and marked systemic symptoms, although the parotitis may be absent. Useful tests for cases of suspected epididymo-orchitis are a urethral smear, mid-stream urine culture, and investigations for gonorrhoea and chlamydia. Paired sera for mumps antibodies may be helpful. Presumptive treatment for gonorrhoea and chlamydia is appropriate in younger males while waiting for results. Severe cases require treatment in hospital with parenteral antibiotics. Analgesia, scrotal support, and elevation may reduce discomfort and promote recovery.

Painless swellings in the scrotum are common. Most of these are small, round, epididymal cysts or spermatocoeles that require no investigation or treatment. Lesions in the testis can be caused by tuberculosis, syphilis, or malignancy and require urgent ultrasound examination. Varicocoeles feel like a bag of worms in the scrotum and can be associated with infertility. Referral to a urologist is advised if pain, testicular atrophy, infertility, or the threat of infertility are concerns. Larger swellings of the scrotum include hydrocoele and hernias.

Pelvic pain in the male

The prostate can be affected by a variety of infectious and poorly defined non-infectious conditions that present with acute or chronic pelvic pain with a range of accompanying urinary and systemic symptoms (Box 6.5). Gonorrhoea, chlamydial infections, and trichomoniasis can affect the prostate, but most acute infections are caused by other bacteria such as *E. coli, Proteus, Streptococcus faecalis, Klebsiella*, and *Pseudomonas*. STIs and non-sexually transmitted bacterial infections of the prostate account for only a few painful prostatic syndromes. Most patients with prostatic pain fall into a category recently designated 'chronic pelvic pain syndrome' (CPPS) by the National Institutes of Health (NIH) classification of prostatitis syndromes.

Box 6.5 **Differential diagnosis of prostatic disease**

NIH classification of prostatitis syndromes

I Acute bacterial prostatitis
II Chronic bacterial prostatitis
III Chronic prostatitis (CP)/chronic pelvic pain syndrome (CPPS)
IIIA CPPS, inflammatory (leucocytes in prostatic secretion, semen, or urine after prostatic massage)
IIIB CPPS, non-inflammatory (as above without leucocytes)
IV Asymptomatic inflammatory prostatitis

Other causes of pelvic pain or prostatic symptoms

- Specific and non-specific granulomatous prostatitis
- Pudendal neuralgia (sometimes caused by tumour)
- Bladder outlet obstruction
- Bladder tumours
- Urinary stone disease
- Ejaculatory duct obstruction
- Seminal vesicle calculi
- Irritable bowel syndrome

In patients who present with pelvic pain, the prostate should be examined for enlargement and tenderness. Patients with prostatitis

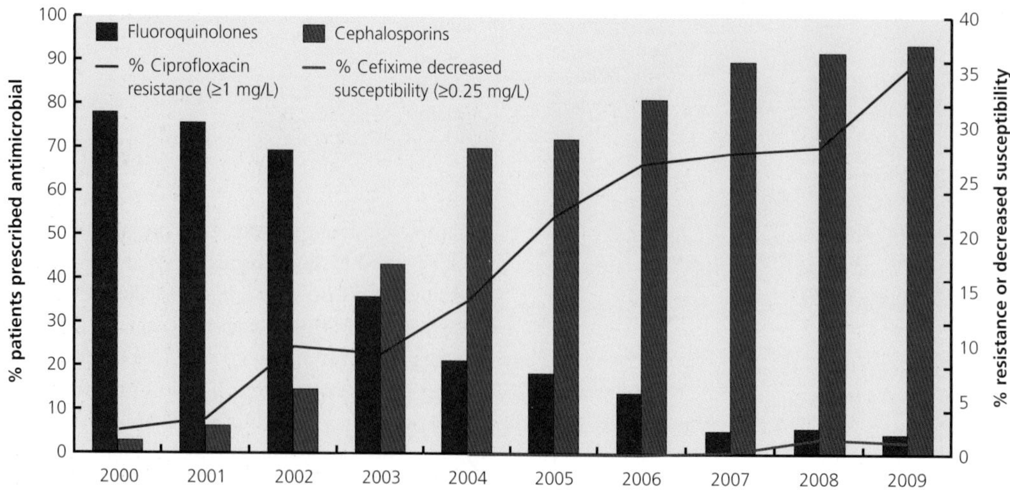

Figure 6.7 Antimicrobial resistance of *Neisseria gonorrhoea* and antibiotic use. Source: Gonococcal Resistance to Antimicrobials Surveillance Programme (GRASP) in England and Wales: report of 2009 data by courtesy of the Health Protection Agency.

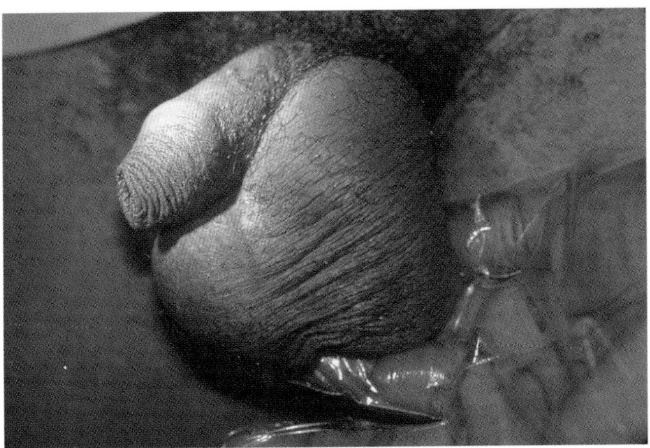

Figure 6.8 Acute epididymo-orchitis due to STI.

should undergo a normal screen for STIs. The value of subjecting patients to the unpleasant procedure of prostatic massage to examine prostatic secretions for bacteria and inflammatory cells is now questioned by many experts.

Transrectal ultrasonography, urodynamic studies and biopsy are helpful in some patients. Confirmed infections respond well to antibiotics, the first choice often being a 28-day course of a quinolone or tetracycline, which have better prostatic penetration than other antibiotics.

Treating the more common CPPS is difficult. None of the treatments are well validated, and response rates are often poor. A recently published NIH symptoms index for chronic prostatitis is a useful way to record and monitor symptoms.

Anal symptoms

Anorectal STIs

Sexually transmitted infections can be transmitted by penile–anal contact, oroanal contact, or with fingers, resulting in asymptomatic infection, ulceration (e.g. herpes and syphilis), warts, or proctitis, the main manifestations of which are pain, tenesmus (a uncomfortable sensation of needing to pass stool even when the bowel is empty), bleeding, discharge and, rarely, diarrhoea. Anorectal infections are a potent cofactor for HIV transmission. Ulceration is investigated in the same way as genital ulceration (see Chapter 12). Discharges require investigation by proctoscopy, during which samples can be taken from the rectum to test for gonorrhoea and chlamydia (including lymphogranuloma venereum (LGV)) and herpes. Herpes proctitis is usually readily distinguished by the presence of perianal vesicles or erosions. Within the anal canal, erosions have a white or yellow appearance, but with primary herpes the proctitis may be too severe to permit the insertion of a proctoscope. When rectal gonorrhoea is identified, co-treatment for chlamydia should be offered (Figure 6.9). Evidence has recently emerged that all types of rectal chlamydia infections may respond better to doxycyline than azithromycin. Males with symptomatic non-gonococcal proctitis should receive the 3-week courses of antibiotics recommended to eliminate LGV.

Anal intercourse can lead to the transmission of a wide variety of other organisms normally transmitted by the faeco-oral route:

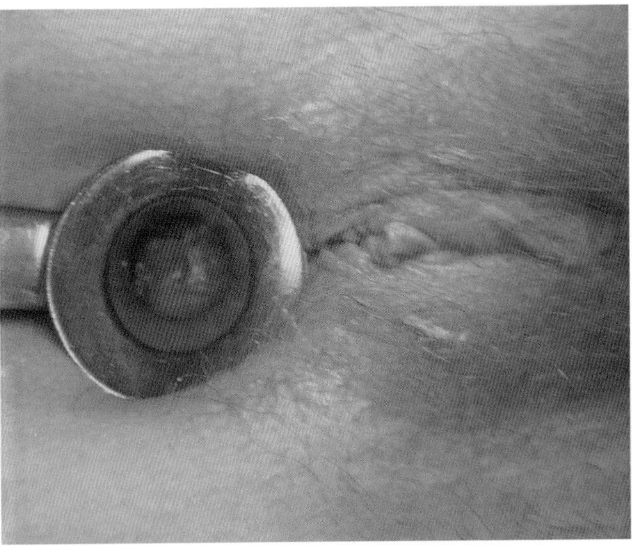

Figure 6.9 Rectal gonorrhoea.

hepatitis A, *Shigella*, *Salmonella*, and *Giardia*. In the absence of specific infection, and where symptoms persist despite antibiotics, then investigation and treatment should focus on inflammatory bowel disease.

Anal intra-epithelial neoplasia and invasive carcinoma may follow infection with oncogenic subtypes of human papillomavirus.

Infections in MSM are covered further in Chapter 20

Non-infectious anal conditions

Patients who practise receptive anal sex often present to STI services with anal fissure, haemorrhoids, perianal haematomas, and pruritus ani. It is important to provide training and guidelines for the management and referral of these common conditions in clinics that see clients who practise anal sex.

Oral and perioral symptoms

Oral STIs are usually asymptomatic. Gonorrhoea and chlamydia infect the pharyngeal mucosa readily but rarely cause acute

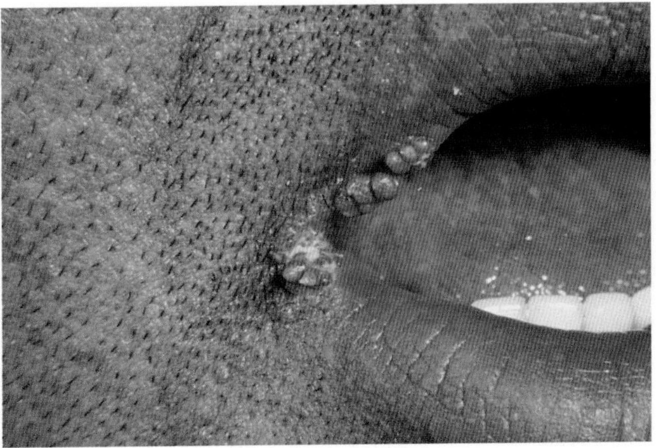

Figure 6.10 Perioral warts. With permission from the Wellcome Trust.

inflammation. Primary syphilis may present on the tongue or lips, and secondary syphilis can produce an oral mucositis. HIV has an important array of oral manifestations that include oral candidiasis (both erythematous and pseudomembranous), angular cheilitis, gingivitis, oral hairy leucoplakia, and Kaposi's sarcoma. Warts may develop in and around the mouth as a result of orogenital sexual activity (Figure 6.10).

Further reading

Alexander RB, Propert KL, Schaeffer AJ, *et al.* Ciprofloxacin or tamsulosin in men with chronic prostatitis/chronic pelvic pain syndrome: a randomized, double-blind trial. *Ann Intern Med* 2004;**141**:581–9.

Bradshaw CS, Tabrizi SN, Read TR, Garland SM, Hopkins CA, Moss LM, Fairley CK. Etiologies of nongonococcal urethritis: bacteria, viruses, and the association with orogenital exposure. *J Infect Dis* 2006;**193**:336–45.

Bruce AJ, Rogers RS. Oral manifestations of sexually transmitted diseases. *Clin Dermatol* 2004;**22**:50–7.

Geisler WM, Krieger JN. Epididymitis. In Holmes KI, Sparling PF, Stamm WE, Piot P, Wasserheit JN, Corey L, Cohen MS, Watts DH (eds). *Sexually Transmitted Diseases*, 4th edn. McGraw Hill, New York, 2008, pp. 1127–45.

Rompalo AM, Quinn TC. Sexually transmitted intestinal syndromes. In Holmes KI, Sparling PF, Stamm WE, Piot P, Wasserheit JN, Corey L, Cohen MS, Watts DH (eds). *Sexually Transmitted Diseases*, 4th edn. McGraw Hill, New York, 2008, pp. 1277–308.

www.bashh.org.uk Management of prostatitis *and* Management of epidymo-orchitis.

CHAPTER 7

Other Conditions Affecting the Male Genitalia

Sarah Edwards [1] and Chris Bunker [2]

[1]Department of Genitourinary Medicine, West Suffolk Hospital, Bury St Edmunds, UK
[2]Department of Dermatology, University College and Chelsea & Westminster Hospital, London, UK

OVERVIEW

- Patients with genital skin diseases commonly present to sexually transmitted infection clinics. They more common and more florid in the uncircumcised
- All men presenting with balanoposthitis should be screened for sexually transmitted infections and diabetes
- Candida is a common opportunist on the uncircumcised penis and its presence may not be the cause of the dermatosis
- It is crucial to maintain a high threshold of suspicion for precancerous and cancerous situations
- There are an increasing number of pharmacological treatments for erectile dysfunction and premature ejaculation

Conditions affecting the glans and prepuce

Inflammation of the glans is known as balanitis and inflammation of the prepuce as posthitis. Appearances can vary from minimal to florid erythema, which may be generalised or appear as red patches or plaques. These conditions are commonly seen in sexually transmitted infection clinic attendees, and their aetiology is multifactorial (Table 7.1). Problems are less frequent in circumcised men and a non-retractile foreskin (phimosis) may be a contributing factor, or symptoms may be secondary to an inflammatory dermatosis such as lichen sclerosus. A paraphimosis results from prolonged retraction of the prepuce, which leads to constriction of the distal shaft and oedema of the glans.

Normal variants

There are three commonly seen normal variants: pearly penile papules, angiokeratomas, and Fordyce spots. Pearly penile papules are angiofibromas that are found around the coronal margin of the glans and are smooth, papular, and flesh coloured, and may be seen in nearly 50% of men (Figure 7.1). Angiokeratomas are small blue papules common on the scrotum, less often found on the penis around the meatus (Figure 7.2). Fordyce spots are prominent sebaceous glands commonly seen on the penile shaft and scrotum (Figure 7.3).

Table 7.1 Conditions affecting the glans and prepuce.

Normal variants	Inflammatory dermatoses	Premalignant/ malignant change	Infection
Pearly penile papules (hirsutes papillaris penis)	Eczema (including irritant, allergic and seborrheic)	Erythroplasia of Queyrat	Anaerobes
Fox–Fordyce spots	Psoriasis	Bowen's disease	Streptococci
Angiokeratomas	Lichen planus	Bowenoid papulosis	Staphylococci
	Lichen sclerosus	Squamous cell carcinoma	Candida
	Zoon's balanitis		

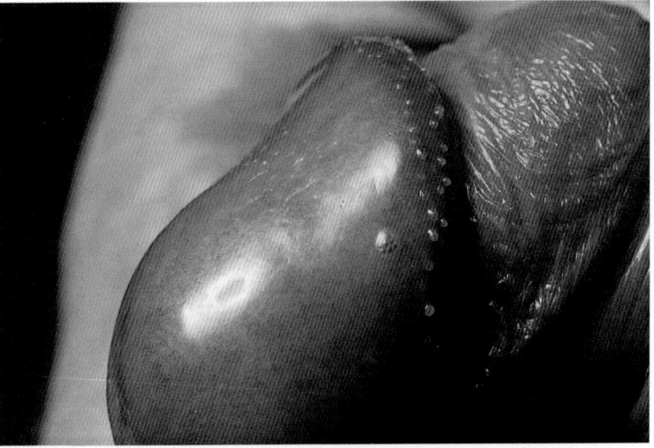

Figure 7.1 Pearly penile papules. *Source*: From Bunker C.B. and Neill S.M. In *Rook's Textbook of Dermatology*, 2010. With permission from Wiley-Blackwell. Courtesy of Dr D.A. Burns, Leicester, UK.

Inflammatory dermatoses

Irritant dermatitis is possibly the most common cause of balanoposthitis seen in sexually transmitted infection clinics and

ABC of Sexually Transmitted Infections, Sixth Edition.
Edited by Karen E. Rogstad.

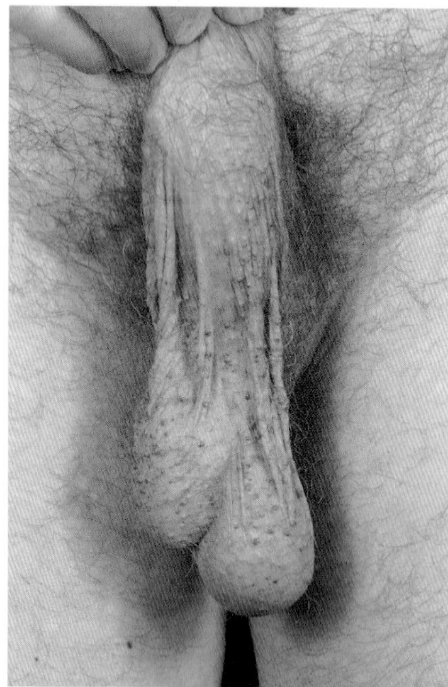

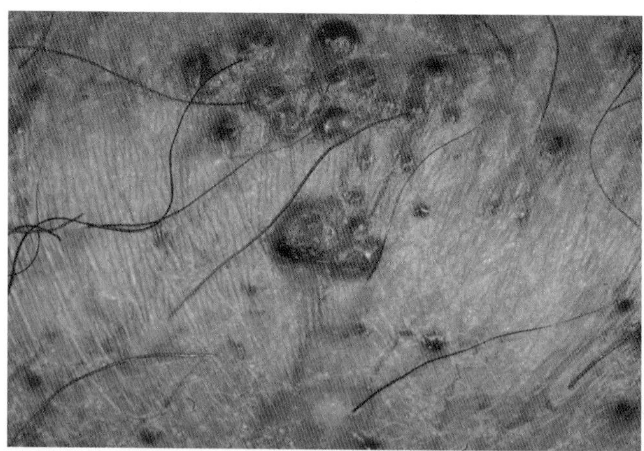

Figure 7.2 Angiokeratoma affecting the scrotum. With thanks to Professor C.B. Bunker and permission from Medical Illustration UK Limited.

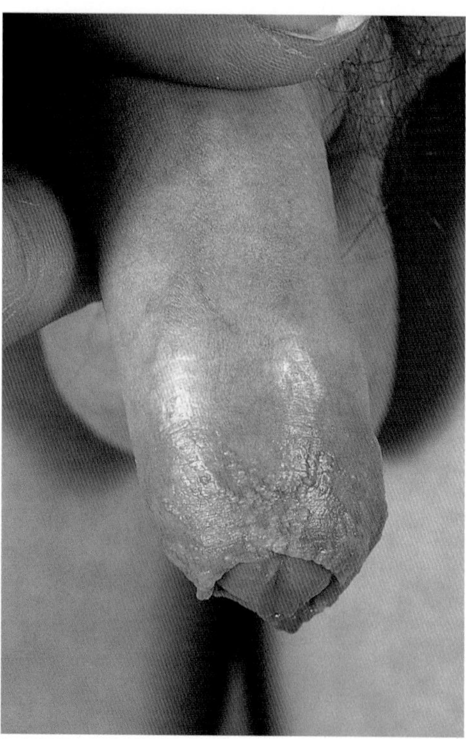

Figure 7.3 Prominent sebaceous glands on the prepuce. Courtesy of Dr F.A. Ive, Durham, UK.

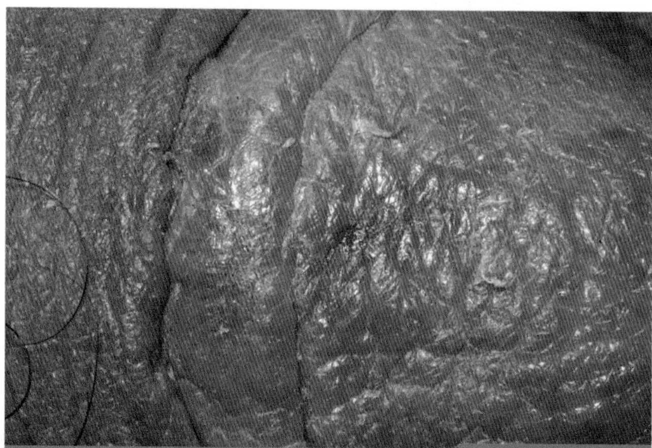

Figure 7.4 Light eczematisation of the glans penis and distal shaft from exogenous irritant contact dermatitis (over-washing with soap). With thanks to Professor C.B. Bunker and permission from Medical Illustration UK Limited.

often causes mild generalised inflammation (Figure 7.4). A specific irritant may not be identified, but advice about toiletries and avoidance of overwashing or poor hygiene can help. In severe cases, superinfection should be excluded and patch testing may be indicated if allergic contact dermatitis (e.g. to rubber latex) is suspected. Seborrheic dermatitis can also cause a mild non-specific balanoposthitis, and the diagnosis may be supported by clinical evidence at extragenital sites. A mild to moderate topical steroid combined with an antifungal may be required.

Psoriasis also has a predilection for the male genitalia, causing well-demarcated erythematous patches or plaques, without the characteristic scale in uncircumcised men (Figure 7.5). There are often clinical clues elsewhere: scalp, elbows, nails. The circinate balanitis of Reiter's syndrome is more micropapular but still psoriasiform in nature (Figure 7.6). Treatment is with mild to moderately potent topical steroids. The plaques of lichen planus are also clearly demarcated but more red–purple in colour: there may be Wickham's striae or erosions (Figure 7.7). Full dermatological examination may assist in diagnosis if the appearances are not

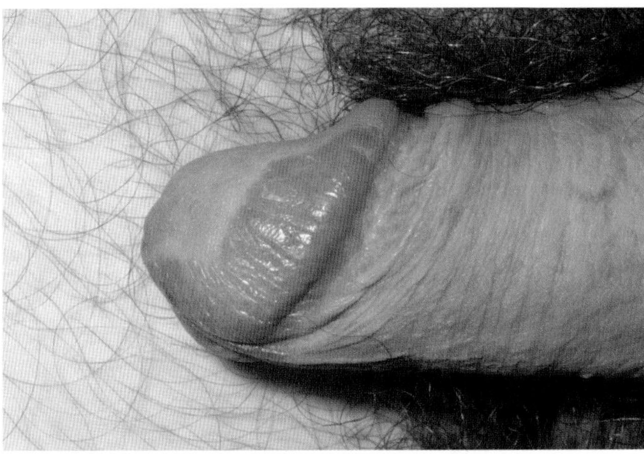

Figure 7.5 Well-demarcated salmon-pink patches of psoriasis on the coronal rim. With thanks to Professor C.B. Bunker and permission from Medical Illustration UK Limited.

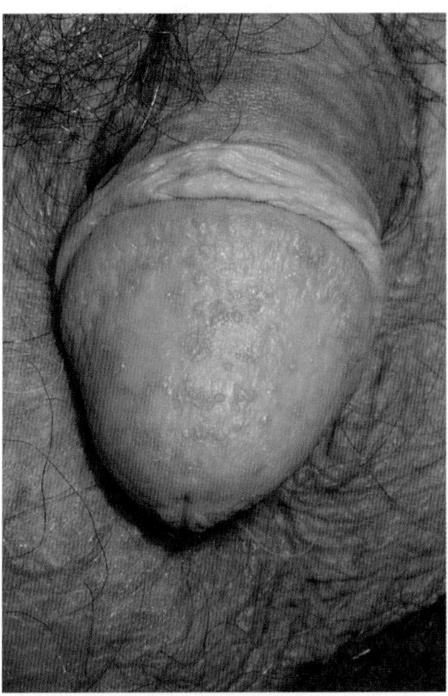

Figure 7.6 Circinate psoriasiform balanitis (HLA B27 positive). With thanks to Professor C.B. Bunker and permission from Medical Illustration UK Limited.

typical of the condition as seen elsewhere on the body. Topical treatment is with potent topical steroids.

Lichen sclerosus is a chronic inflammatory condition, in men only affecting the uncircumcised genitalia. It has variable symptomatology amounting to dyspareunia and dysuria and is a cause of phimosis (Figure 7.8). Symptoms include itch, soreness, and splitting. There is a symmetrical lichenoid balanoposthitis with white atrophic plaques and purpuric change (Figure 7.9). Very potent topical steroids are required to control the inflammation and reverse the sclerotic changes. Circumcision may be required if maximal medical treatment fails. The objectives of treatment are to normalise sexual and urinary function and mitigate the risk of penile cancer.

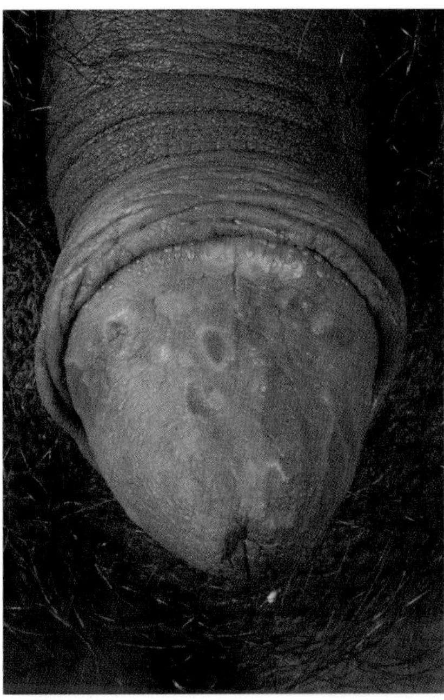

Figure 7.7 Lichen planus with coalescing papules and plaques and Wickham's striae. With thanks to Professor C.B. Bunker and permission from Medical Illustration UK Limited.

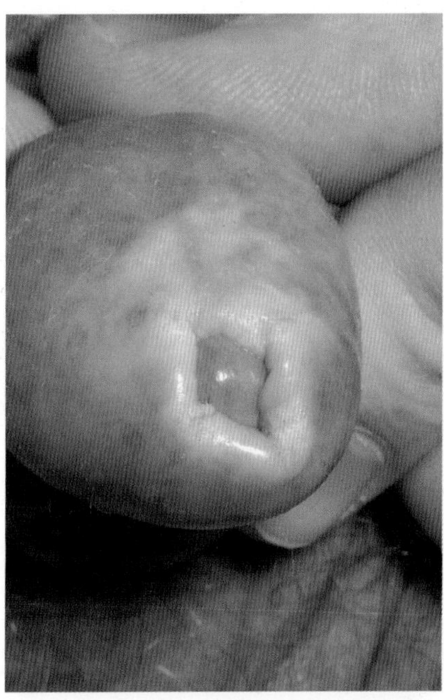

Figure 7.8 Lichen sclerosus with phimosis ('muzzling'). With thanks to Professor C.B. Bunker and permission from Medical Illustration UK Limited.

Zoon's balanitis occurs in uncircumcised men and is characterised by well-demarcated, moist, orangy-red patches in a symmetrical distribution on the glans and internal aspect of the foreskin (Figure 7.10). Despite its florid appearance it is minimally symptomatic, although a blood-stained discharge can occur. Topical treatments may help, but it tends to be a chronic condition unless treated with circumcision. Zoonoid inflammation may attend other dermatoses, especially lichen sclerosus and carcinoma

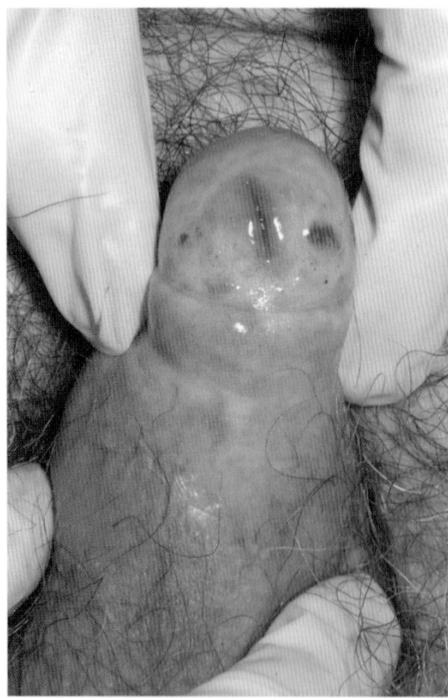

Figure 7.9 Severe lichen sclerosus with etiolation of the glans, a low grade lichenoid balanoposthitis, constrictive posthitis with sclerotic 'waisting', with Zoonoid telangiectasia. With thanks to Professor C.B. Bunker and permission from Medical Illustration UK Limited.

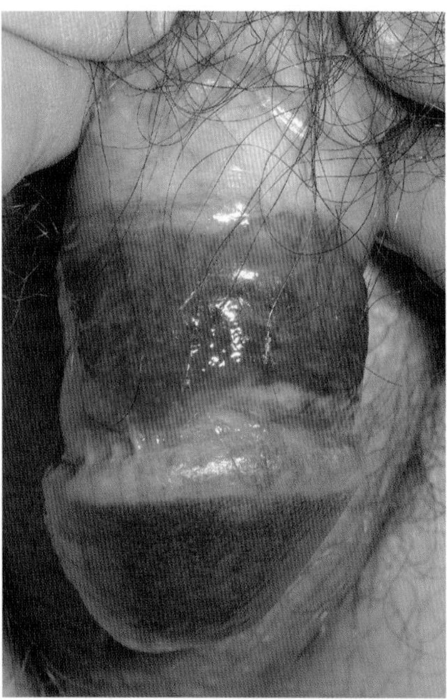

Figure 7.10 Zoon's balanitis, symmetrical inflammation with purpura. With thanks to Professor C.B. Bunker and permission from Medical Illustration UK Limited.

in situ, so Zoon's balanitis should only be diagnosed in the presence of classic features.

Infection

Primary infective balanoposthitis is relatively uncommon, and if clinically severe should prompt investigation for an underlying condition. Phimosis is a predisposing cause and subpreputial infection is an indication for circumcision. Diabetes mellitus should be excluded in all men presenting with balanoposthitis or clinically significant candida, but other causes of immunosuppression and iron deficiency may also predispose to candidosis. Other infective agents include anaerobes, staphylococci, and group A streptococci (group B streptococci are common commensals). Topical and/or oral treatment may be required.

Premalignant conditions

The important differential diagnosis of patches, plaques, and papules on the penis is carcinoma *in situ* (PCIS). It is seen in three forms: erythroplasia of Queyrat, Bowen's disease of the penis, and Bowenoid papulosis. An asymmetrical distribution of lesions is unusual in lichen sclerosus and Zoon's balanitis and any persistent asymmetric balanoposthitis of undetermined aetiology should be biopsied as should unexplained erosion and ulceration or hyperkeratosis or papulonodular change. Several or sequential biopsies may be required if a large area is affected or initial histology is inconclusive.

Erythroplasia of Queyrat is characteristically red and velvety and occurs on the glans or foreskin of uncircumcised men (Figure 7.11). Bowen's disease is more scaly, raised, and may be pigmented, occurring anywhere on the penis of circumcised men (but only possible by definition on the proximal penile shaft of uncircumcised men; Figure 7.12). Bowenoid papulosis is warty in appearance but with atypical features such as pigmentation, smoother surface change, and more coalescent lesions. A high proportion of PCIS is associated with human papillomavirus infection. All clinical variants have similar histology, with full thickness dysplasia. Treatments include topical 5-fluorouracil, imiquimod, cryotherapy, and surgery; circumcision is usually an obligatory part of management.

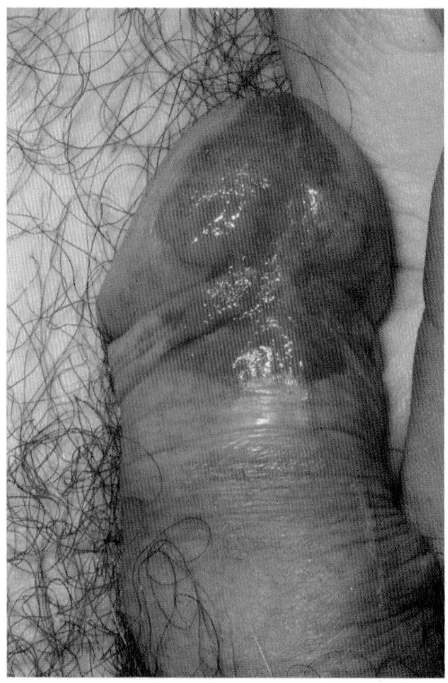

Figure 7.11 Erythroplasia of Queyrat. With thanks to Professor C.B. Bunker and permission from Medical Illustration UK Limited.

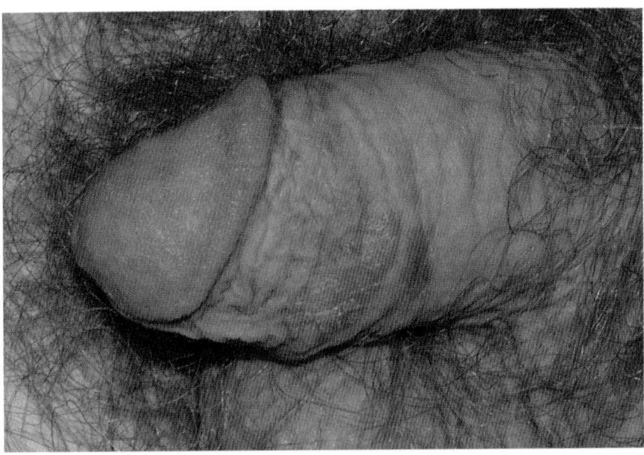

Figure 7.12 Bowen's disease of the mid-penile shaft presenting as a psoriasiform patch. With thanks to Professor C.B. Bunker and permission from Medical Illustration UK Limited.

Squamous cell carcinoma of the penis is rare but very serious and may be a cause of litigation because of missed or delayed diagnosis. There are about 400 cases per year in the United Kingdom and approximately 100 deaths. A long history of genital symptoms (dysuria, dyspareunia, balanoposthitis, or phimosis) is often presented. Risk factors are shown in Box 7.1. About 50% are due to human papillomavirus and 5% are associated with lichen sclerosus (Figure 7.13).

Box 7.1 **Risk factors for penis cancer**

- Uncircumcised state
- Phimosis
- Poor hygiene
- Chronic irritation, inflammation, scarring
- Smoking
- Multiple sexual partners
- Lichen sclerosus, lichen planus, squamous hyperplasia
- HPV
- HIV
- Photochemotherapy
- Iatrogenic immunosuppression

Asymmetrical, irregular nodular, and ulcerative morphology is found on examination. Background Bowen's disease/erythroplasia of Queyrat/Bowenoid papulosis, lichen sclerosus, or lichen planus may be present. Inguinal lymphadenopathy due to carcinoma confers a poor prognosis. Treatment by circumcision and glansectomy may be curative but penile amputation is sometimes necessary.

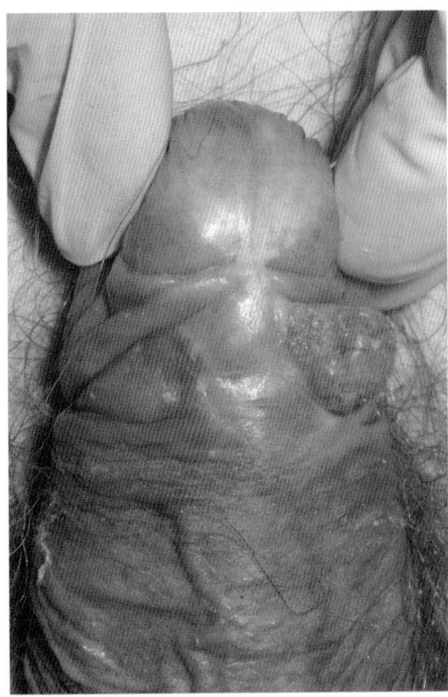

Figure 7.13 Nodular squamous carcinoma of the left ventral penile shaft. Note severe background lichen sclerosus. With thanks to Professor C.B. Bunker and permission from Medical Illustration UK Limited.

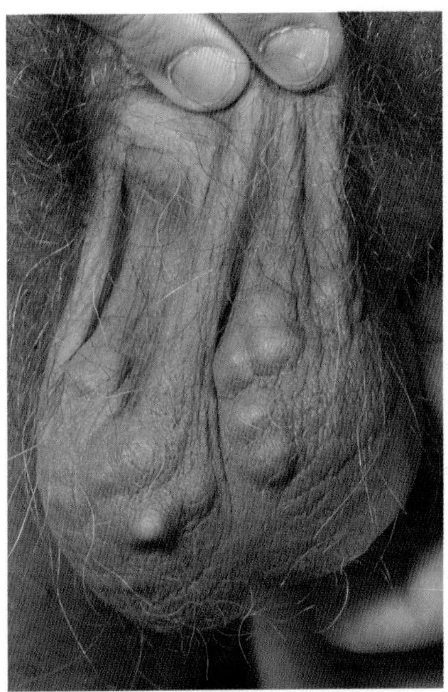

Figure 7.14 Idiopathic scrotal calcinosis. With thanks to Professor C.B. Bunker and permission from Medical Illustration UK Limited.

Conditions affecting the scrotum and groins

Prominent sebaceous glands on the scrotum and angiokeratomas have already been mentioned. Reassurance is usually all that is required.

The scrotum can be affected by other skin conditions, but the most common is probably lichen simplex. The skin becomes thickened because of an uncontrolled vicious circle of itching and scratching and can appear nodular, but in a more confluent pattern than scabetic nodules. Treatment aims to alleviate itching and includes soap substitution, a moisturiser, and a short course of potent topical steroids. Idiopathic scrotal calcinosis (Figure 7.14) can be the cause of considerable upset and embarrassment. Patients have one to dozens of firm, white to flesh coloured papules and nodules on the scrotum. They require surgical removal but frequently recur.

Inflammation in the flexures of the groins is defined as an intertrigo. The main causes are tinea cruris, candidosis, and erythrasma. All can present as erythematous areas extending from the groins. Erythrasma is classically velvety red and scaly but extends symmetrically from the groins, whereas tinea may have satellite lesions, central clearing, and more active inflammation at the edge. Atypical appearances of tinea are common as appearances can be altered by the use of topical steroids. Erythrasma can be differentiated by its coral pink fluorescence under Wood's light. The definitive treatment of erythrasma is with oral erythromycin. Tinea may require treatment with oral antifungals if topical agents fail. Both conditions may recur. Candidosis tends to cause raw, erythematous areas and is usually associated with a predisposing condition, such as obesity or diabetes. Extramammary Paget's disease (EMPD) is a rare disease presenting as burning or sore intertriginous psoriasiform patches or plaques in the groins, on the scrotum, perianally, and, less commonly, on the penile shaft. It is often mistaken for psoriasis. The differential diagnosis includes PCIS. EMPD is intra-epithelial adenocarcinoma *in situ*. Invasion of the dermis carries a poor prognosis. There may be a contiguous underlying carcinoma or carcinoma elsewhere, usually of the lower gastrointestinal or genitourinary tracts.

Other conditions affecting sexual function

Patients may present with other conditions that are causing difficulties with sexual intercourse, including physical problems, such as the penile curvature found in Peyronie's disease, problems with erectile function, and problems with the duration of intercourse.

Peyronie's disease

This is a deformity of the penis that is caused by fibrosis in the tunica alba. The affected side becomes shortened and the penis deviates toward that side when erect, and this may be painful. In severe cases the condition may cause difficulty with sexual intercourse which is an indication for surgical treatment. The diagnosis is made by palpation of the fibrotic plaque.

Erectile dysfunction

Erectile dysfunction (ED) is the inability to achieve or maintain an erection that is satisfactory for sexual intercourse. The condition is common and is estimated to have a prevalence of 19–26%. Risk factors include age, obesity, smoking, and hypercholesterolaemia, and ED itself is a risk factor for cardiovascular events. In addition, psychological and relationship issues can predispose to erectile problems (Table 7.2).

A careful history should elicit predisposing, precipitating, and risk factors, and whether early morning erections and successful masturbation are still occurring. Physical examination should include a genital examination, blood pressure, heart rate, and weight. Further investigation is warranted given the association with cardiovascular disease, and should include serum lipids, fasting blood glucose, and urinalysis. Measurement of morning testosterone levels is advised as hypogonadism is a treatable cause of ED and may reduce the effectiveness of phosphodiesterase inhibitors. Further investigations are not usually required unless abnormalities are found on screening tests, there is a history of trauma, or no response to medical therapies.

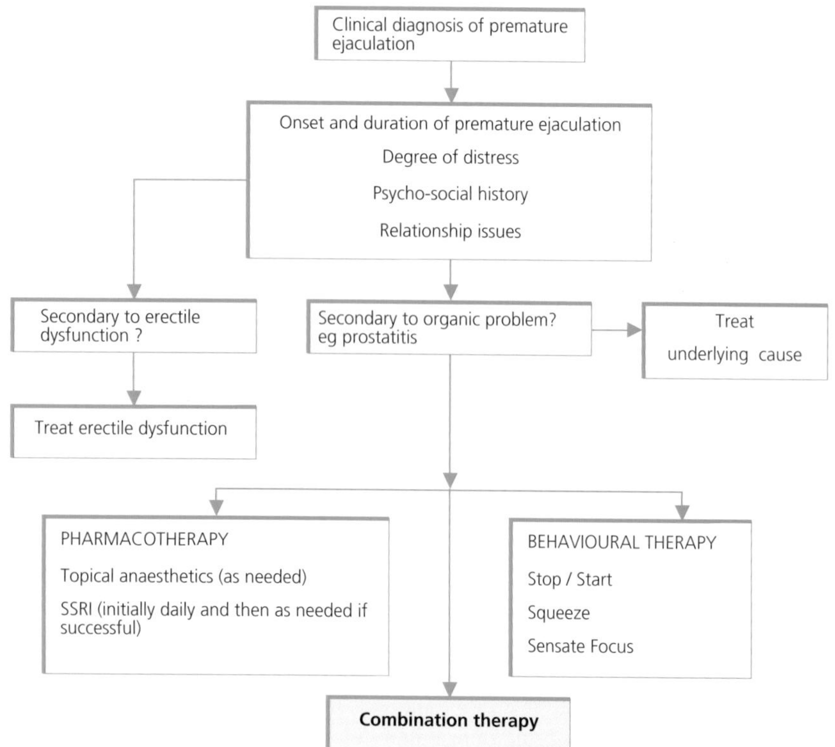

Figure 7.15 Flow diagram of clinical management of premature ejaculation. Source: BASHH Special Interest Group for Sexual Dysfunction. Recommendations for the management of premature ejaculation: BASHH Special Interest Group for Sexual Dysfunction. *Int J STD AIDS* 2006;**17**(1):1–6.

Table 7.2 Predisposing and trigger factors for erectile dysfunction.

Predisposing problems	Precipitating problems
Lack of sexual knowledge	New relationship
Poor past sexual experience	Acute relationship problems
Relationship problems	Family or social pressures
Religious or cultural beliefs	Pregnancy and childbirth
Restrictive upbringing	Major life events
Unclear sexual or gender preference	Partner's menopause
Previous sexual abuse	Acute physical or mental health problems
Physical or mental health problems	Lack of knowledge about normal changes of ageing
Other sexual problems in either partner	Other sexual problems in either partner
Drugs	Drugs

Source: Adapted from British Society for Sexual Medicine Guidelines on the Management of Erectile Dysfunction 2007.

Any underlying causes should be treated and psychosexual counselling may be required. Most patients who have low risk for cardiovascular disease can be treated with oral phosphodiesterase inhibitors such as sildenafil, tadalafil, or vardenafil, and these are effective in 75% of cases. In the remaining 25%, alternative treatments include intracavernosal or intra-urethral alprostadil, and mechanical or surgical devices.

Ejaculatory disorders

Both premature and retarded ejaculation can occur, although the latter is less likely to be a presenting complaint in sexually transmitted infection clinics. Premature ejaculation is also known as rapid ejaculation and is when ejaculation takes place shortly after or even prior to penetration (Figure 7.15). Psychosexual approaches include the 'pause and squeeze' technique, and sensate focus. Local anaesthetic gels may reduce sensitivity and delay ejaculation, and specific serotonin reuptake inhibitors (SSRIs) such as paroxetine, fluoxetine, and sertraline are effective in delaying ejaculation.

Further reading

Bunker CB. *Male Genital Skin Disease*. Elsevier Saunders, London, 2004.

Edwards SK, Handfield-Jones S. *2008 UK National Guideline on the Management of Balanoposthitis*. Clinical Effectiveness Group of the British Association for Sexual Health and HIV. http://www.bashh.org/guidelines

Hackett G, Dean J, Kell P, Price D, Ralph D, Speakman M, Wylie K. *British Society for Sexual Medicine Guidelines on the Management of Erectile Dysfunction*. http://www.bssm.org.uk/downloads/BSSMEDManagementGuidelines2007.pdf

Richardson D, Goldmeier D, Green J, Lamba H, Harris JR; BASHH Special Interest Group for Sexual Dysfunction. Recommendations for the management of premature ejaculation: BASHH Special Interest Group for Sexual Dysfunction. *Int J STD AIDS* 2006;**17**(1):1–6.

Tomlinson J. *ABC of Sexual Health*. BMJ Publishing Group, London, 2004.

CHAPTER 8

Vaginal Discharge: Causes, Diagnosis, and Treatment

Phillip Hay

Centre for Infection, St George's, University of London, London, UK

OVERVIEW

- Vaginal discharge may be normal or caused by a range of conditions
- Bacterial vaginosis is the most common cause of abnormal vaginal discharge in women
- Cervicitis can be caused by gonorrhoea, chlamydia, and *Mycoplasma genitalium*
- Although taking a history is helpful, investigations are necessary to determine the cause of discharge
- Candida apparently non-responsive to treatment should prompt consideration of an alternative diagnosis

Vaginal discharge is a common presentation and most women will develop an abnormal discharge at some point. Correct diagnosis is essential for appropriate treatment and advice. It may be concealed because of embarrassment, so sensitive history-taking is needed. For a few, recurrences are frequent and the condition can come to dominate their lives. The differential diagnosis is wide so that where syndromic management is used multiple treatments are prescribed to cover the most likely causes. Important questions for the history are shown in Box 8.1. Examination should be performed to aid diagnosis, which can readily be confirmed by microscopy, culture, or nucleic acid amplification test (NAAT) using appropriate swabs. It is important for practitioners to have an understanding of normal physiology when educating patients.

Physiology

In pre-menarchal girls the vagina is lined with a simple cuboidal epithelium. The pH is neutral and the vagina colonised with skin commensals. Under the influence of oestrogen at puberty, stratified squamous epithelium develops and Lactobacilli become the predominant organism (Figure 8.1). The pH falls to 3.5–4.5. Following the menopause, atrophic changes occur with a return to skin flora. The pH again rises to 7.0.

ABC of Sexually Transmitted Infections, Sixth Edition.
Edited by Karen E. Rogstad.

Box 8.1 **History-taking**

- Standard sexual history as described in Chapter 4
- Characteristics of discharge
  - Colour, consistency, amount (use of pads or tampons)
  - Smell
  - Bloodstained
- Associated symptoms
  - Dyspareunia: superficial or deep
  - Itching or soreness
- Has she had anything similar before, trigger factors, related to menstrual cycle
- Self-treatment, previous treatments, recent antibiotic use
- Washing practices, douching, antiseptics

Physiological discharge

Normal vaginal discharge is white or yellowish. It consists of epithelial cells, mucus, bacteria, and fluid transudate. Lactic acid comes from glycogen being metabolised by vaginal epithelium and lactobacilli. Physiological discharge increases mid-cycle. It

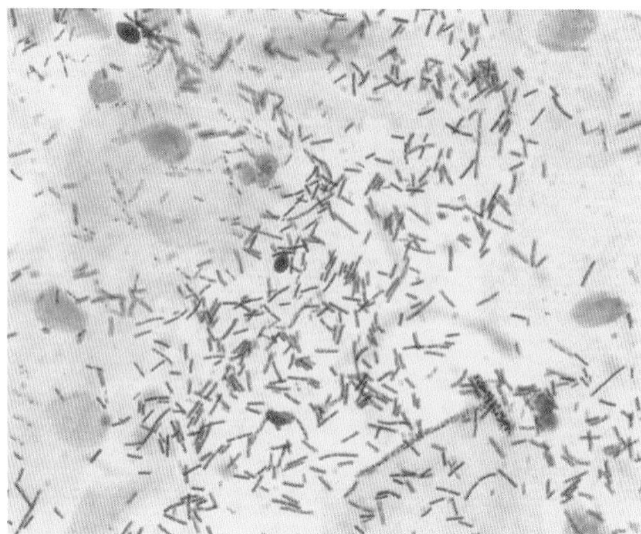

Figure 8.1 Gram-stained vaginal smear showing large gram-positive rods (Lactobacilli) and candida spores and pseudohyphae.

also increases in pregnancy, and sometimes when women start a combined oral contraceptive pill (Box 8.2). A cervical ectropion may be associated with excess mucus production causing persistent discharge. A gynaecologist can treat this with cautery.

Box 8.2 **What may influence physiological discharge?**

Age
- Pre-pubertal
- Reproductive
- Post-menopausal

Hormones
- Hormonal contraception
- Cyclical hormonal changes
- Pregnancy

Local factors
- Menstruation
- Postpartum
- Malignancy
- Semen
- Personal habits and hygiene

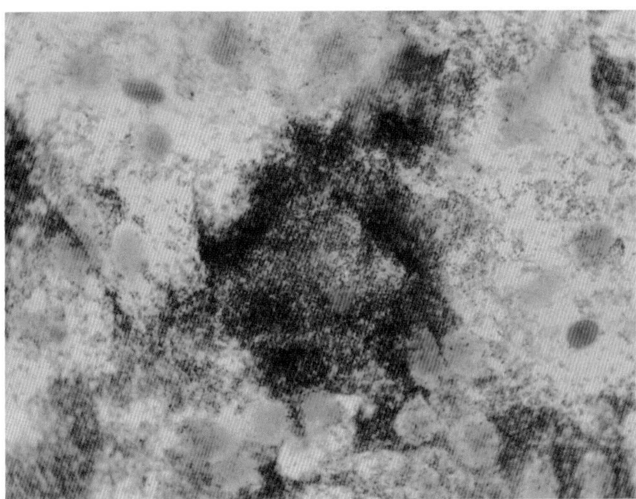

Figure 8.2 Gram-stained vaginal smear showing bacterial vaginosis. There is a 'clue cell' in the centre (a squamous epithelial cell coated with a thick layer of small bacteria). There are numerous small gram negative and positive cocci and rods.

Abnormal discharge

Vaginal discharge can originate from anywhere in the upper or lower genital tract. Discharge arising from the vagina itself can be physiological or pathological. The typical characteristics of the common infectious causes are summarised in Table 8.1. Less common causes are summarised in Box 8.3.

Box 8.3 **Less common causes of abnormal vaginal discharge**

Infective conditions
- Upper genital tract infection (e.g. pelvic inflammatory disease, post-partum endometritis)
- Primary syphilitic chancre
- Primary herpes

Non-infective conditions
- Retained tampon or condom
- Cervical ectropion or endocervical polyp
- Chemical irritation
- Intrauterine contraceptive device
- Allergic vaginitis
- Desquamative exudative vaginitis
- Atrophic vaginitis
- Physical trauma
- Fistula: recto-vaginal or vesico-vaginal
- Vault granulation tissue
- Neoplasia

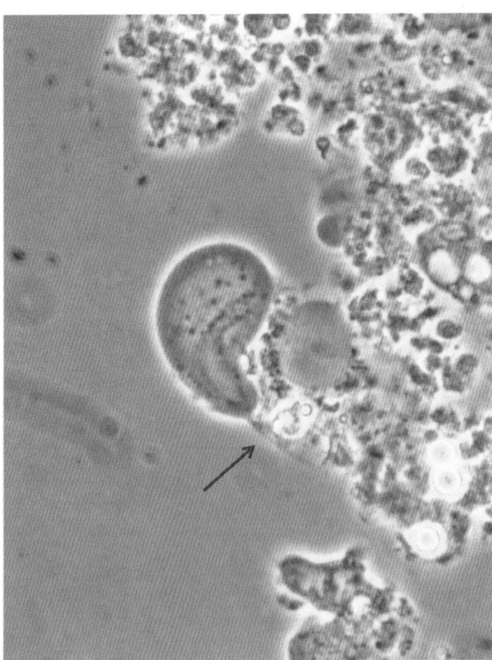

Figure 8.3 Vaginal wet mount (800) showing a *Trichomonas* in the centre with flagellae anteriorly (arrow). There is cellular debris and polymorphs in the right top corner.

Diagnostic tests

In specialised STI clinics (genitourinary medicine; GUM) in the United Kingdom, candida, bacterial vaginosis, and trichomoniasis are diagnosed by microscopy of a saline wet mount and gram-stained vaginal smear (Figures 8.2 and 8.3). This allows immediate diagnosis, subsequently supported by laboratory culture and NAAT as needed. In the absence of microscopy, vaginal pH can be measured simply with narrow range pH paper. Bacterial vaginosis and trichomoniasis are excluded by a pH <4.5, but a pH >4.5 is not very specific for a positive diagnosis. Testing must also be performed for gonorrhoea and chlamydia (by cervical gram stain and culture for gonorrhoea, NAAT for *Chlamydia trachomatis*, and gonorrhoea of cervix, vulvo-vaginal – which may be self-taken – or urine sample) as these cannot be distinguished clinically.

Vaginal candidiasis

Over three-quarters of women have at least one episode of vaginal candidiasis in their lifetime (Figure 8.4). At any one time,

Table 8.1 The differential diagnoses of the principal causes of abnormal vaginal discharge.

Symptoms and signs	Candidiasis	Bacterial vaginosis	Trichomoniasis	Cervicitis*
Itching or soreness	++	–	+++	–
Smell	May be 'yeasty'	Offensive, fishy	May be offensive	–
Colour	White	White or yellow	Yellow or green	White or green
Consistency	Curdy	Thin, homogeneous	Thin, homogenous	Mucoid
pH	<4.5	4.5–7.0	4.5–7.0	Any
Confirmed by	Microscopy and culture	Microscopy	Microscopy and culture	Microscopy, tests for chlamydia and gonorrhoea

*Cervicitis may be caused by infections such as chlamydia, gonorrhoea, *Mycoplasma genitalium*. A mucopurulent discharge is seen and the cervix is friable with contact bleeding.

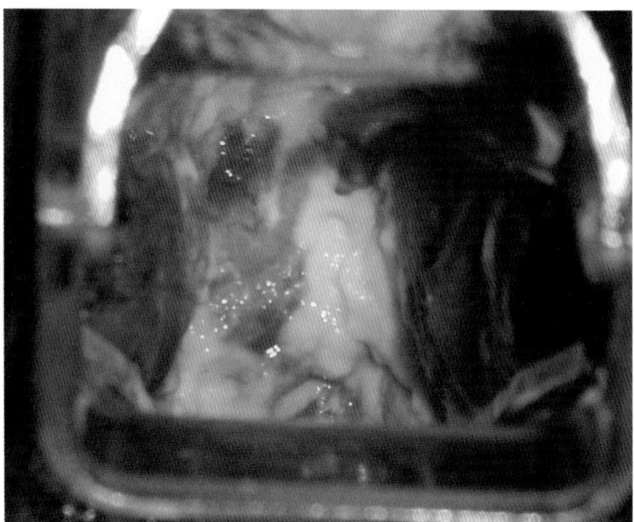

Figure 8.4 Speculum examination of a woman with vaginal candidiasis. There is a thick curdy discharge.

25% women have vaginal colonisation, but only a minority are symptomatic. *Candida albicans* is found in more than 80% of cases. Sexual acquisition is rarely important, although the physical trauma of intercourse may be sufficient to trigger an episode in a predisposed individual. It is oestrogen dependent so rarely seen in prepubertal girls or post-menopausal women. Predisposing factors are shown in Box 8.4.

Box 8.4 **Factors predisposing to vaginal candidiasis**

- Broad-spectrum antibiotic therapy
- Increased oestrogen
  - Pregnancy
  - High dose combined oral contraceptive pill
- Diabetes mellitus
- Underlying dermatosis (e.g. eczema)
- Immunosuppression
  - HIV
  - Immunosuppressive therapy (e.g. steroids)
- Vaginal douching, bubble bath, shower gel, tight clothing, tights (role uncertain)

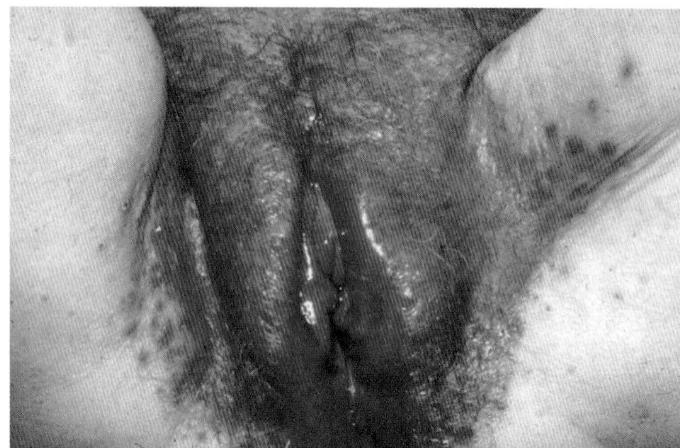

Figure 8.5 Vulval candidiasis.

Clinical features

- Itching, soreness, and redness of the vagina and vulva (Figure 8.5)
- Curdy white discharge which may smell yeasty but not unpleasant
- There may be fissuring and excoriations

Not all candida presents in the same way: in some cases there may be itching and redness with a thin watery discharge. The diagnosis can be confirmed by microscopy and culture of the vaginal fluid. Asymptomatic women from whom candida is grown on culture do not require treatment.

Treatment

Licensed treatments produce cure rates of 80–95% in non-pregnant women. Some women have a preference for oral therapy, particularly if required at the time of menstruation. Vaginal creams and pessaries can be prescribed at a variety of doses and durations of treatment. Commonly prescribed treatments are summarised in Box 8.5.

Complications and pregnancy

Oral azoles are not recommended in pregnancy.

Complications are uncommon. Occasionally, women become allergic to topical agents after regular application. In some women a severe episode of candida can trigger long-term vulvodynia.

Box 8.5 **Commonly prescribed treatments for vaginal candidiasis**

- A single dose topical azole (e.g. clotrimazole pessary 500 mg single dose)
- Oral fluconazole 150 mg tablet single dose

Longer courses of treatment (e.g. clotrimazole 100 mg/day for 6–7 days) are indicated

- In pregnancy
- When there are predisposing factors that cannot be eliminated, such as steroid therapy

Symptomatic candidal infection of male partners is uncommon, but men sometimes react to candida antigens, developing soreness and balanitis after intercourse.

Persistent or recurrent candida

Recurrent candida or candida not responding to treatment is relatively uncommon. Usually, those presenting with 'treatment-resistant candida' have an alternative diagnosis such as herpes simplex, vulvodynia, or dermatological conditions such as eczema or lichen sclerosus.

Genuine recurrent candida can be suppressed by various regimens such as weekly fluconazole 150 mg for 6 months. Unfortunately, this does not prevent further recurrences and treatment may need to be continued for longer.

If resistance to treatment is shown clinically and *in vitro*, referral to a specialist clinic is advised where new antifungal agents such as voriconazole may be used, or boric acid applied intravaginally.

Bacterial vaginosis

Bacterial vaginosis (BV) is the most common cause of abnormal vaginal discharge in women of childbearing age (Figure 8.2). Its reported prevalence has varied widely from as low as 5% in a selected group of asymptomatic college students to 50% of women in a large study in rural Uganda. Studies in antenatal and gynaecology clinics show a prevalence of approximately 12% in the UK. It is more common in women of black race and those who have an intrauterine contraceptive device (IUCD). It is probably more common in women with sexually transmitted infections but has been reported in virgins, and may be particularly common in lesbian women. The condition often arises spontaneously around the time of menstruation and may resolve mid-cycle.

When BV develops, predominantly anaerobic organisms increase in concentration up to a thousand-fold, and overwhelm the lactobacilli (Figure 8.2). Vaginal pH rises to 4.5–7.0. The microbiology is summarised in Table 8.2. Recently, novel organisms such as *Atopobium vaginae* have been identified using molecular techniques. Additionally, a biofilm, consisting predominantly of *Gardnerella* and *A. vaginae*, was described that places these organisms at the centre of pathogenesis.

Table 8.2 The organisms classically associated with bacterial vaginosis are shown in the left-hand column. These are present in levels >100-fold greater than in normal flora. Some of the newly described organisms, identified through molecular techniques, are in the right-hand column:

Gardnerella vaginalis	*Atopobium vaginae*
Bacteroides spp. (*Prevotella*)	BVAB*1–3 (Clostridiales)
	Megasphaera
Mycoplasma hominis	Sneathia
Mobiluncus spp.	Leptotrichia

BVAB, bacterial vaginosis associated bacteria.

Clinical features

- Offensive fishy-smelling discharge
- Discharge characteristically thin, homogenous, and adherent to the walls of the vagina
- It may be white or yellow
- The smell is particularly noticeable around the time of menstruation or following intercourse. Semen itself can give off a weak fishy smell

The diagnosis was traditionally made in clinical practice identifying at least three of the composite (Amsel) criteria:

- Vaginal pH >4.5
- Release of a fishy smell on addition of alkali (10% potassium hydroxide)
- A characteristic discharge on examination
- Presence of 'clue cells' on microscopy

Clue cells are vaginal epithelial cells so heavily coated with bacteria that the border is obscured (Figure 8.2). In GUM clinics, BV is now diagnosed from a gram-stained vaginal smear. Large numbers of gram-positive and gram-negative cocci are seen, with reduced or absent large gram-positive bacilli (lactobacilli). Culture is not useful for diagnosis as for instance *Gardnerella* can be grown from 50% of those who do not have BV.

Treatment

Bacterial vaginosis will resolve on treatment with antibiotics with good anti-anaerobic activity (Box 8.6). A comprehensive review was used to guide the 2006 Centers for Disease Control guidelines.

- Metronidazole 400 mg twice a day for 5 days is the preferred treatment

  Alternative treatments:
- Metronidazole 2 g as a single dose
- Metronidazole vaginal gel 0.75% applied daily for 5 days
- Clindamycin cream 2% applied nightly for 5–7 nights

Initial cure rates are greater than 80%, but up to 30% of women relapse within 1 month of treatment.

Complications

During pregnancy, women with BV are at greater risk of second trimester miscarriage and preterm delivery. This may result in perinatal mortality or cerebral palsy. The results of studies treating BV with metronidazole or clindamycin have been conflicting so current guidelines do not recommend routine screening and treatment.

Box 8.6 **Side effects and contraindications**

Antifungal agents

Fluconazole

- Monitor liver function with high doses or extended courses
- Avoid in pregnancy (multiple abnormalities reported with prolonged treatment)

Itraconazole

- Rarely, severe hepatitis has been reported
- Avoid in heart failure and acute porphyria
- Avoid in pregnancy (toxicity at high doses in animal studies)

Topical antifungals

- Generally low systemic absorption so not contraindicated in pregnancy
  - Miconazole: toxicity in animals at high concentration
- Occasional local irritation/sensitisation to excipients

Oral metronidazole

- Gastrointestinal disturbance, metallic taste
- Neuropathy at high doses
- Not contraindicated in pregnancy but avoid 2-g single dose
- Metallic taste in breast milk: avoid large single doses

Clindamycin

- Pseudo-membranous colitis reported with oral and topical use
- Not contraindicated in pregnancy but one case of bloody diarrhoea reported in a breastfed infant

Bacterial vaginosis should be treated with metronidazole before termination of pregnancy to reduce the subsequent incidence of endometritis and pelvic inflammatory disease.

Recurrence

In some women the vaginal flora is in a dynamic state, with BV developing and remitting spontaneously. Symptomatic women with recurrent BV can become frustrated as although the condition responds rapidly to treatment with antibiotics, it but may quickly relapse. Our inability to alter this process reflects our current lack of knowledge of the factors that trigger bacterial vaginosis. Regular treatment with 0.75% metronidazole gel twice a week for 6 months reduces the rate of recurrence. Some women need simultaneous suppressive treatment for candida.

Trichomoniasis

This sexually transmissible infection can be carried for several months before causing symptoms. It is diagnosed in approximately 1% women attending GUM clinics, but prevalence is higher in many tropical countries, with rates of 10–20% in some settings. In men it is usually asymptomatic but may present as non-gonococcal urethritis.

Clinical features

- Vulvo-vaginitis, which can be severe, with inflammation sometimes extending out onto the labia majora and adjacent skin
- Purulent green or yellow discharge, sometimes offensive
- In many cases BV develops as well
- Punctate haemorrhages can occur on the cervix, giving the appearance of a 'strawberry cervix' (Figures 8.6 and 8.7)

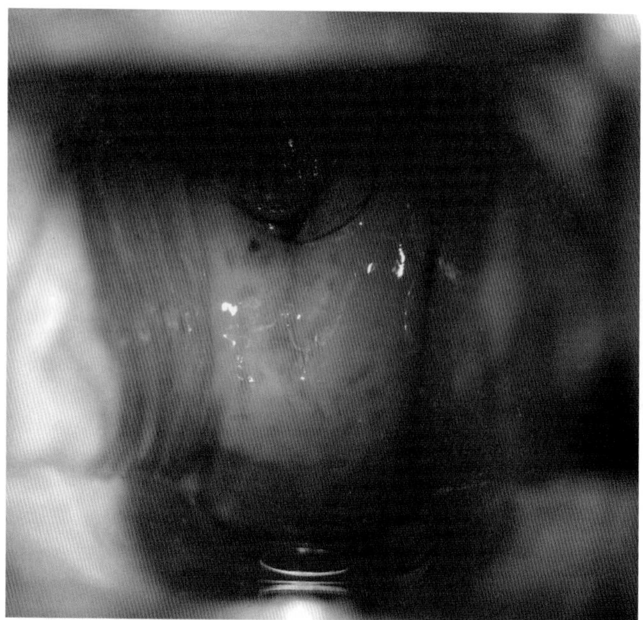

Figure 8.6 Strawberry cervix in a woman with trichomoniasis. Punctate haemorrhages are seen on the cervix. An IUCD thread is present.

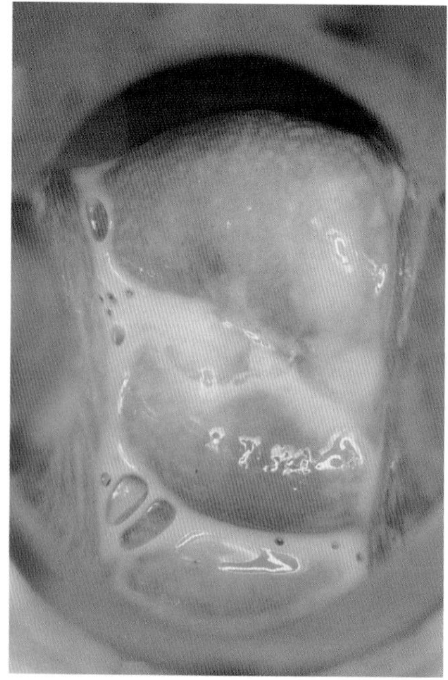

Figure 8.7 Trichomonal vaginitis – showing homogeneous off-white (or, classically, yellow–green) discharge. Courtesy of Peter Greenhouse.

The diagnosis is confirmed by microscopy of vaginal secretions mixed with saline, or culture, preferably in a specific medium such as Fineberg–Whittington. Numerous polymorphonuclear cells are seen and the motile organism is identified from its shape and four moving flagellae. Microscopy has a 60% sensitivity compared with culture. NAAT will become available in the next few years and promise a greater diagnostic sensitivity.

Management

Metronidazole either 2 g as a single dose or 400 mg twice a day for 5 days.

Partner notification is needed and the woman should not resume sexual intercourse until her sexual partner(s) has been treated. Tinidazole 2 g in a single dose is more expensive but occasionally works when metronidazole has failed.

Complications and pregnancy

Trichomonas has occasionally been identified in the upper genital tract of women with pelvic inflammatory disease but is probably not an important cause of upper genital tract pathology. It can be isolated from the bladder.

Although *Trichomonas* is a risk factor for preterm birth, treating asymptomatic infection has not been shown to improve outcome. Symptomatic women should be treated with a 5-day course of metronidazole.

Recurrence

Occasionally, persistent trichomoniasis is seen. This may be a result of poor compliance with medication, poor absorption, reinfection or, rarely, a resistant organism. The usual approach is to use higher doses of metronidazole, initially 400 mg three times a day, increasing to 1 g per rectum twice a day or intravenously. Neurological toxicity may be encountered with high doses. Some clinicians prescribe a broad-spectrum antibiotic such as co-amoxiclav to eliminate bacteria such as group B streptococci which might be metabolising metronidazole thereby diminishing its efficacy. Unfortunately, alternative treatments are limited, but include arsphenamine pessaries and clotrimazole, which has an inhibitory effect on *T. vaginalis*. Referral to a specialist is advised.

Gonorrhoea and chlamydia

Both gonorrhoea and chlamydial infection can cause a vaginal discharge, although they may both be aymptomatic. The discharge may be white, yellow, or green, and may be bloodstained and associated with intermenstrual and post-coital bleeding. Neither can be ruled out on history alone, and testing should be performed. On speculum examination a mucopurulent discharge may be seen coming from the cervix, and contact bleeding after swabbing is common. Endocervical swabs should be taken for chlamydia and gonorrhoea. NAATs that identify both organisms are becoming increasingly used in place of culture for gonorrhoea, so local guidelines should be followed.

Risk factors for presence of STIs

- Age under 25 years
- No condom use
- Symptoms developed after recent change of sexual partner or multiple contacts
- Recurrent or persistent symptoms
- Symptoms in partner
- Symptoms imply complications
- Partner's risk behaviour

Vaginal discharge in children

Vaginal infections are common in childhood, and mostly not related to sexual abuse. Causes include streptococcal infections and *Shigella*, which can cause a chronic haemorrhagic vaginitis, often with no history of diarrhoea. Recurrent vaginal infections should lead to suspicion of a foreign body. Pinworms (*Enterobius vermicularis*) migrate from the anus at night causing intense irritation and inevitably scratching. The clue to the diagnosis is the nocturnal pattern.

The cuboidal epithelium lining the vagina in children means that if sexual abuse occurs leading to infection with chlamydia or gonorrhoea, a generalised vaginitis occurs with purulent discharge.

Other conditions affecting the vagina

Atrophic vaginitis is common in post-menopausal women. This can lead to superficial dyspareunia and vaginal soreness. Oestrogen replacement with topical dienoestrol cream is effective.

Occasionally, a true bacterial vaginitis is encountered caused by a streptococcus or other organism. It responds to appropriate antibiotic therapy such as co-amoxiclav 375 mg three times a day for 7 days. Toxic shock syndrome is a rare condition associated with retention of tampons or foreign bodies in the vagina. An overgrowth of staphylococci producing a toxin causes systemic shock with fever, diarrhoea, vomiting, and an erythematous rash. More frequently, a foreign body or retained tampon merely causes an offensive discharge.

Self-help and over-the-counter treatments

Women should be advised to avoid douching and other washing practices that will disturb the endogenous flora. Use of over-the-counter candida treatments without confirmed diagnosis can lead to delays in receiving the correct diagnosis and treatment. Probiotics and lactic acid gels have not been evaluated sufficiently rigorously to allow a recommendation to be made, but some women derive symptomatic relief from them.

Further reading

American Centers for Disease Control (CDC) website with USA treatment guidelines. http://www.cdc.gov/std/treatment/

British Association for Sexual Health and HIV (BASHH). www.bashh.org.uk (Includes link to Clinical Effectiveness Group for latest guidelines.)

Duyebo OO, Anorlu RI, Ogunsola FT. The effects of antimicrobial therapy on bacterial vaginosis in non-pregnant women. *Cochrane Database Syst Rev* 2009;**3**:CD006055.

Forna F, Gülmezoglu AM. Interventions for treating trichomoniasis in women. *Cochrane Database Syst Rev* 2003;**2**:CD000218.

King K, Holmes P, Sparling F, Stamm WE, Piot P, Wasserheit JN, Corey L, Cohen M, eds. *Sexually Transmitted Diseases*, 4th edn. McGraw Hill, New York, 2007. (The most comprehensive reference source on STIs.)

Koumans EH, Markowitz LE, Hogan V. Indications for therapy and treatment recommendations for bacterial vaginosis in nonpregnant and pregnant women: a synthesis of data. *Clin Infect Dis* 2002;**35**(Suppl 2): S152–72.

McDonald HM, Brocklehurst P, Gordon A. Antibiotics for treating bacterial vaginosis in pregnancy. *Cochrane Database Syst Rev* 2007;**1**: CD000262.

Nurbhai M, Grimshaw J, Watson M, Bond CM, Mollison JA, Ludbrook A. Oral versus intra-vaginal imidazole and triazole anti-fungal treatment of uncomplicated vulvovaginal candidiasis (thrush). *Cochrane Database Syst Rev* 2007;**4**:CD002845.

Royal College of Obstetrics and Gynaecology (RCOG) web site. www.rcog.org.uk

Sobel JD, Ferris D, Schwebke J, Nyirjesy P, Wiesenfeld HC, Peipert J, *et al.* Suppressive antibacterial therapy with 0.75% metronidazole vaginal gel to prevent recurrent bacterial vaginosis. *Am J Obstet Gynecol* 2006;**194**(5):1283–9.

Sobel JD, Wiesenfeld HC, Martens M, Danna P, Hooton TM, Rompalo A, *et al.* Maintenance fluconazole therapy for recurrent vulvovaginal candidiasis. *N Engl J Med* 2004;**351**(9):876–83.

Young G, Jewell D. Topical treatment for vaginal candidiasis (thrush) in pregnancy. *Cochrane Database Syst Rev* 2001;**4**:CD000225.

CHAPTER 9

Pelvic Inflammatory Disease and Pelvic Pain

Jonathan D C Ross

Whittall Street Clinic, Birmingham, UK

OVERVIEW

- Pelvic inflammatory disease is a common condition among young women
- Gonorrhoea, chlamydia, and anaerobic bacteria are well-recognised causes, but in many women no pathogen is found
- Pelvic infection should be considered in any young sexually active woman who complains of lower abdominal pain
- Antibiotics are usually effective in controlling symptoms but a significant proportion of women go on to develop chronic pain or infertility
- Early diagnosis of chlamydia and prevention of reinfection can reduce the risk of long-term complications

Pelvic inflammatory disease (PID) occurs when infection spreads from the vagina through the cervix into the upper genital tract. The bacteria that cause PID are usually spread sexually, although in many cases no pathogen can be isolated. Gonorrhoea and chlamydia account for around 20% of cases in the UK, and it is likely that *Mycoplasma genitalium* and a variety of anaerobic bacteria are also involved in its pathogenesis.

Pelvic infection is a common cause of morbidity in young women and accounts for around 2% of consultations in primary care for this group. Over 17 000 women with PID are diagnosed each year in sexually transmitted infection clinics in England, which represents a doubling in the number of cases over the past 10 years.

Clinical diagnosis of PID

Many women with PID remain asymptomatic and may present for the first time with the complications of tubal damage such as infertility or chronic pelvic pain. In those with symptoms (Box 9.1; Figure 9.1) the most common presentations are with bilateral lower abdominal pain, dyspareunia, vaginal discharge, and intermenstrual bleeding. Women with severe PID may also have general malaise, fever, nausea, and vomiting. Around 10% of patients complain of right upper quadrant pain which occurs secondary to an associated inflammation of the liver capsule (Fitz-Hugh–Curtis syndrome) and occasionally this can dominate the clinical presentation (Figure 9.2).

Box 9.1 **Clinical diagnosis of PID**

Presenting symptoms

- Bilateral lower abdominal pain
- Abnormal vaginal discharge
- Intermenstrual and/or postcoital bleeding
- Dyspareunia

Clinical signs

- Bilateral lower abdominal tenderness
- Adnexal tenderness on vaginal examination
- Cervical motion tenderness on bimanual vaginal examination
- Fever

On examination women usually have lower abdominal tenderness associated with adnexal discomfort on bimanual vaginal examination, and cervical motion tenderness. The differential diagnosis (Box 9.2) includes appendicitis (the pain is usually unilateral and more likely to be associated with nausea and vomiting),

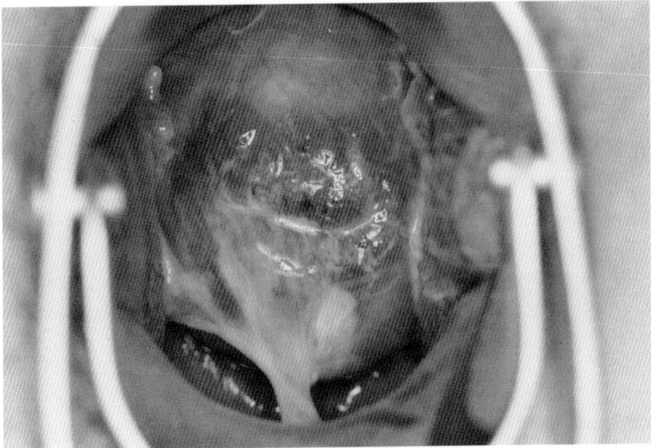

Figure 9.1 Mucopurulent cervicitis – caused by gonorrhoea or chlamydia. Courtesy of Peter Greenhouse.

ABC of Sexually Transmitted Infections, Sixth Edition.
Edited by Karen E. Rogstad.

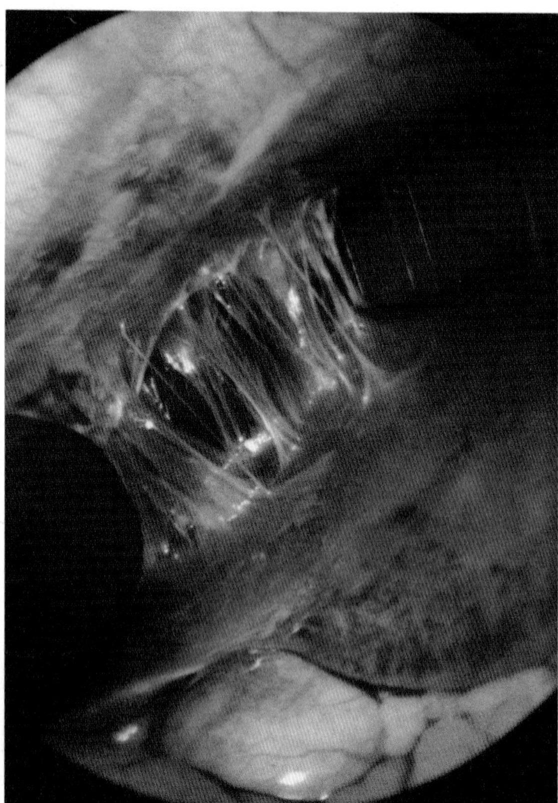

Figure 9.2 Chlamydial peri-hepatitis showing violin-string and bridal adhesions between liver surface and diaphragm. Courtesy of Peter Greenhouse.

ectopic pregnancy (often with a history of missed period), urinary tract infection (history of dysuria and frequency), ovarian cyst torsion or rupture (usually of sudden onset), endometriosis (often a more chronic history with symptoms sometimes linked to the menstrual cycle), and irritable bowel syndrome (sometimes associated with a change in bowel habit).

Box 9.2 **Differential diagnosis of lower abdominal pain**

- Ectopic pregnancy
- Appendicitis
- Urinary tract infection
- Ovarian cyst torsion or rupture
- Endometriosis
- Irritable bowel syndrome

Women who have a recent history of gynaecological surgery involving trans-cervical procedures are also at increased risk of developing pelvic infection (e.g. following endometrial biopsy, *in vitro* fertilization, or recent insertion of intra-uterine contraceptive device).

Investigations

All women with lower abdominal pain should have a pregnancy test performed to help exclude ectopic pregnancy. Women should be offered tests for gonorrhoea and chlamydia because the presence of these infections in the lower genital tract would make a diagnosis of PID more likely (specimens from the endocervix or self-taken vulvo-vaginal swabs should be sent for nucleic acid amplification tests). Microscopy, if available, can help with the diagnosis – the presence of gram-negative diplococci on a cervical smear indicates gonococcal infection, and the absence of neutrophils decreases the likelihood of PID.

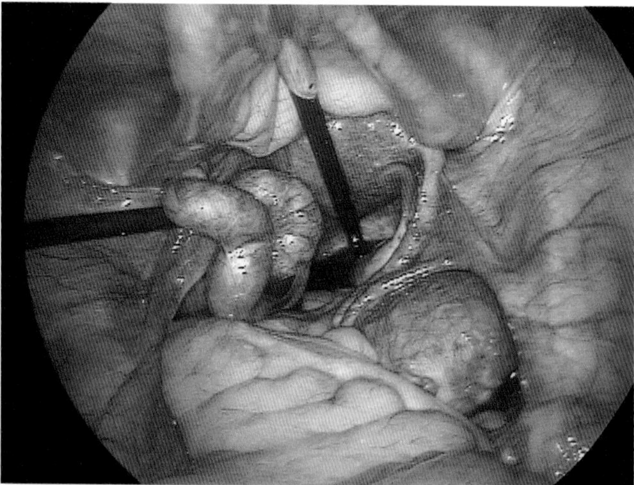

Figure 9.3 Blocked tube at laparoscopy.

Measuring the white blood count, or an inflammatory marker such as erythrocyte sedimentation rate (ESR) or C-reactive protein (CRP), is too non-specific to help make a diagnosis but may be useful in patients with severe disease to monitor the response to treatment.

Inflammation or blockage of the fallopian tubes can be seen directly during laparoscopy (Figure 9.3), but this procedure is not justified in the majority of women who have clinically mild disease. Laparoscopy is insensitive for mild PID when infection has not yet spread through the full thickness of the tube wall, and there is also substantial inter- and intra-observer variation in interpreting laparoscopy appearances. Trans-vaginal ultrasound can detect fluid collections in the pelvis such as a tubo-ovarian abscess or hydrosalpinx, but is unable to reliably identify uncomplicated tubal inflammation. An endometrial biopsy is a fairly simple procedure and the presence of histological endometritis is strongly associated with upper genital tract inflammation. Unfortunately, there is a risk of introducing infection into the upper genital tract while taking the biopsy and this, plus the delay in receiving histopathological results, limits its use in practice.

Treatment of acute PID

Most women with pelvic infection can be treated effectively as an outpatient (Box 9.3). Appropriate analgesia should be prescribed and the patient should be advised to avoid unprotected intercourse until they, and their partner, have completed treatment. They should be provided with a detailed explanation of what PID is, how it is acquired, what treatment is needed, and the risk of possible sequelae (a patient information leaflet is available at www.rcog.org).

Box 9.3 **Indications for hospital admission for women with acute PID**

- Surgical emergency cannot be excluded
- Clinically severe disease
- Presence of a tubo-ovarian abscess
- Pregnancy
- Lack of response to oral therapy
- Intolerance to oral therapy

A clinical diagnosis of PID is 65–90% sensitive but only 20–50% specific. Despite this, treatment for PID should be considered in all young, sexually active women complaining of bilateral lower abdominal pain who are found to have adnexal tenderness on examination. This is because the risks of missing a diagnosis of PID, with its associated sequelae, are generally considered to be greater than giving a short course of antibiotics to women who subsequently turn out not to have PID.

The choice of antibiotic regimen is made based on local antimicrobial sensitivity patterns and should cover *Neisseria gonorrhoeae*, *Chlamydia trachomatis*, and anaerobic infection (Boxes 9.4 and 9.5).

Box 9.4 **Outpatient treatment of PID**

- Ofloxacin 400 mg twice daily plus metronidazole 400 mg twice daily for 14 days
- Intramuscular ceftriaxone 250 mg single dose followed by oral doxycycline 100 mg twice daily plus metronidazole 400 mg twice daily for 14 days
- Moxifloxacin 400 mg once a day for 14 days*

*Because of evidence of an increased risk of liver reactions and other serious risks (such as QT interval prolongation), oral moxifloxacin should be used only when it is considered inappropriate to use the other antibacterial agents recommended for PID or when these have failed.

Box 9.5 **Inpatient treatment of PID**

- Intravenous cefoxitin (or ceftriaxone) plus intravenous doxycycline followed by oral doxycycline plus oral metronidazole to complete a 14-day course
- Intravenous clindamycin plus intravenous gentamicin followed by oral doxycycline plus oral metronidazole to complete a 14-day course

Some women are unable to tolerate metronidazole because of nausea and vomiting. If this occurs it is reasonable to stop the metronidazole but complete the other antibiotics in the regimen. Many areas in the world, including the UK, have reported increasing levels of quinolone-resistant *N. gonorrhoeae*. Ofloxacin and moxifloxacin should therefore be avoided in women who are at high risk of gonorrhoea (e.g. in clinically severe disease, where their partner is known to be infected with gonorrhoea, or if gram-negative diplococci are found on cervical microscopy). PID in pregnancy is fortunately rare but when it does occur can be treated with ceftriaxone, azithromycin, and metronidazole.

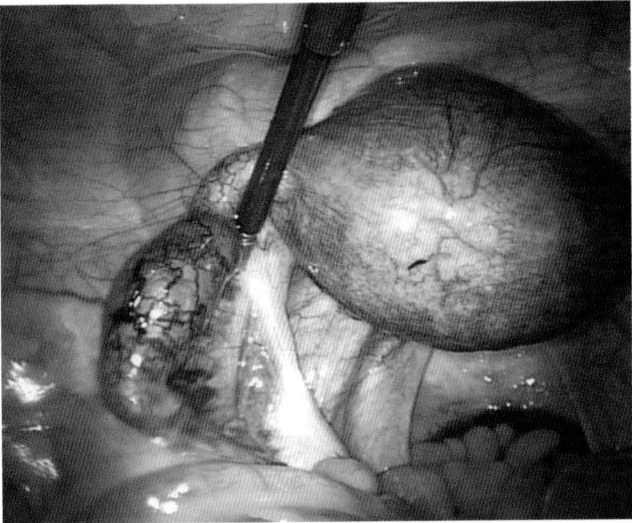

Figure 9.4 Laparoscopic view of ectopic pregnancy.

The presence of an intra-uterine contraceptive device (IUD) does not increase the risk of PID except for the initial few weeks after its insertion. However, if PID develops in a women who has an IUD *in situ* then its removal should be considered because this may improve the short-term resolution of symptoms. This decision needs to be balanced against the risk of pregnancy, and may be deferred in women with mild disease.

Antibiotic therapy for pelvic infection leads to the resolution of the symptoms and signs in over 90% of women. Despite this, around 40% will go on to develop chronic pelvic pain, 15% infertility, and 1% ectopic pregnancy (Figure 9.4). Women with repeated episodes of PID are at particularly high risk of long-term sequelae, the risk of infertility roughly doubling after each episode.

Further management

There is usually an improvement in symptoms within 2–3 days and if this does not occur then an alternative diagnosis should be considered. A further review after 4 weeks may be useful to ensure that the patient has completed the antibiotic course, to check that her partners have been treated, and to reinforce safe sex messages (e.g. use condoms, regular screening for sexually transmitted infections). Surgical intervention may occasionally be required to drain a pelvic abscess or perform adhesiolysis.

Partner notification

The male partners of women with PID should be offered screening for gonorrhoea and chlamydia, including the current partner and other contacts within the past 6 months (although this time limit may vary according to the sexual history). Sexual intercourse should be avoided until both the woman and her partner have been treated concurrently and it is appropriate to give the male partner empirical treatment to cover chlamydia while the results of tests are awaited (e.g. azithromycin 1 g single dose).

Prevention of pelvic infection

The early treatment of chlamydia has been shown to reduce the risk of pelvic inflammatory disease and this can be achieved through screening programmes directed at sexually active young women.

Women undergoing trans-cervical surgical procedures should also be screened for chlamydia and gonorrhoea, and offered prophylactic antibiotic cover if results of screening are not available at the time of the procedure (Box 9.6).

Box 9.6 **Opportunities for chlamydia screening to prevent pelvic infection**

All women and men

- Younger than 25 years
- Older than 25 years with a new sexual partner, or two or more partners in the previous year
- Of any age with symptoms
- Attending GUM clinics

All women

- Younger than 35 years before surgical uterine instrumentation (e.g. hysteroscopy)
- Before IUCD insertion
- Before termination of pregnancy

Pelvic pain

Chronic pelvic pain is defined as pain in the pelvis and lower abdomen lasting more than 6 months. It affects around 4% of women but its pathogenesis and optimal management remain uncertain. PID is one cause of chronic pelvic pain but endometriosis, pelvic adhesions, musculoskeletal disorders, interstitial cystitis, venous congestion, irritable bowel syndrome, and psychological disorders may also be implicated. Although laparoscopy is often performed, an underlying cause is not always identified and if investigations fail to identify a treatable cause then symptomatic therapy utilising effective pain control is essential.

Further reading

American College of Obstetricians and Gynecologists. Chronic pelvic pain. ACOG Practice Bulletin No. 51. *Obstet Gynecol* 2004;**103**:589–605.

BASHH PID treatment guidelines. Available at www.bashh.org

Ness RB, Sopper DE, Holley RL, Peiper TJ, Randell H, Sweet RL, *et al.* Effectiveness of in patient and out patient treatment strategies for women with pelvic inflammatory disease: results from the Pelvic Inflammatory Disease Evaluation in Clinical Health (PEACH Randomised Trial). *Am J Obstet Gynecol* 2002:**186**(5):929–37.

Royal College of Obstetrics and Gynaecology PID guidelines. Available at www.rcog.org (A patient information leaflet on PID is also available at this site.)

Templeton A, ed. *The Prevention of Pelvic Infection: Recommendations Arising from the 31st RCOG Study Group*. RCOG Press, London, 1996.

UK *Chlamydia* Screening Programme. Available at www.dh.gov.uk

CHAPTER 10

Vulval Diseases

Pat Munday

Watford Sexual Health Centre, West Herts Hospitals NHS Trust, Watford, UK

OVERVIEW

- Vulval disease is common and presents with itching, soreness, or a lesion
- History and examination will identify the majority of conditions
- Biopsy is required if the diagnosis is uncertain or there is suspicion of malignancy
- Most conditions respond well to appropriate treatment and advice about skin care
- Chronic vulval conditions can have a significant effect on a woman's self-esteem, sexuality, and relationships

Women with vulval problems present with a limited number of symptoms. Their evaluation requires attention to the detail of the history, examination in a good light, and sometimes repeated assessments before the diagnosis can be reached with confidence. Chronic vulval disease can have a profound impact on a woman's life leading to loss of self-esteem, sexual dysfunction, and relationship problems. In turn these may exacerbate the vulval symptoms. The doctor undertaking vulval work must therefore be empathetic and a skilled listener, picking up verbal and non-verbal cues. It is now recognised that the best model of care for women with chronic vulval disease is a multidisciplinary team which may include a genitourinary physician, dermatologist, gynaecologist, psychosexual therapist or psychologist, physiotherapist, and nurse specialists.

Chronic vulval disease may have a profound impact on a woman's life leading to loss of self-esteem, sexual dysfunction, and relationship problems. In turn, these may exacerbate vulval symptoms. Evaluation of psychosexual issues is a key aspect of management

Vulval symptoms

Vulval itching (pruritus) leading to a desire to scratch, should be distinguished from vulval soreness (Box 10.1). Vulval soreness/pain is described as throbbing, burning, or stabbing and may lead to superficial dyspareunia. Some women describe swelling and redness for which there may, or may not, be objective evidence. Women may notice lesions, rashes, lumps, and spots which may be symptomatic or asymptomatic. The clinician should ascertain the duration of symptoms, whether they are continuous or intermittent, and their localisation.

Box 10.1 **Common causes of vulval pruritus**

Dermatological conditions

- Lichen sclerosus
- Lichen planus
- Eczema/lichen simplex
- Psoriasis

Infections and infestations

- Candidiasis
- Trichomoniasis
- Prodrome of recurrent herpes simplex infection
- Genital warts
- Scabies
- Pediculosis pubis
- Threadworms

Other

- Pre-malignant and malignant lesions
- Diabetes
- Renal and hepatic disease
- Idiopathic

Vulval signs

The vulva should be examined in detail with a good light. The findings should be recorded in a detailed diagram, or a photograph, taken with the patient's consent. A full examination of the patient's skin and mucosal surfaces, and other systems when appropriate, should be undertaken (Box 10.2).

Investigations

The investigations will be determined by the differential diagnosis. Tests for sexually transmitted and other vaginal infections and

ABC of Sexually Transmitted Infections, Sixth Edition.
Edited by Karen E. Rogstad.

Box 10.2 **Features of the vulval examination**

- Loss of architecture (loss of labia minora; burying of clitoris, narrow introitus)
- Presence of lesions
  - Single or multiple
  - Papular or flat
  - Ulcerated
- Erythema or oedema: generalised or localised
- Skin texture: thickened or thinned
- Excoriation
- Localised tenderness
- Visible vaginal discharge

swabs from lesions for bacterial and/or viral culture, polymerase chain reaction (PCR) or other diagnostic test may be indicated. Skin biopsy and patch testing may be useful.

General principles of management

Patients should be given a detailed explanation of their condition with an information leaflet containing resources such as internet sites and support groups. Time spent carefully explaining the treatment regimen, especially when using topical steroids, is essential to obtain the best outcomes. Good skin care should be emphasized (Box 10.3).

Box 10.3 **General advice for skin conditions**

- Soap substitute (e.g. aqueous cream, emulsifying ointment)
- Emollient
- Avoid soaps, bubble baths, bath and shower additives, shampoo and hair conditioners and dyes
- Wear loose-fitting clothing avoiding nylon, lycra, etc.
- Wash after defaecation or wipe from front to back to avoid vulval contamination
- Avoid condoms with spermicide
- Avoid biological washing powders, fabric conditioners

Vulval dermatoses

Lichen sclerosus

This common chronic inflammatory condition is found most commonly in peri- and postmenopausal women–but may present in children (where it has been confused with lesions caused by sexual abuse), in women in their reproductive years and the elderly. Because the primary symptom is pruritus, both women and their clinicians often think first of thrush and unless an examination is undertaken, the woman may continue to use antifungal therapy without benefit. The condition is thought to be autoimmune and is associated with other autoimmune conditions such as hypothyroidism and vitiligo.

The physical appearances are characteristic. Early cases have white polygonal papules which coalesce and produce thickened white and crinkly skin (Figure 10.1), often in a 'figure of eight' distribution. There may be petechial haemorrhages and areas of atrophy. In advanced cases the vulval architecture is destroyed with adhesions leading to loss of the labia minora, burying of the clitoris and narrowing of the introitus leading to superficial dyspareunia and then apareunia (Figure 10.2).

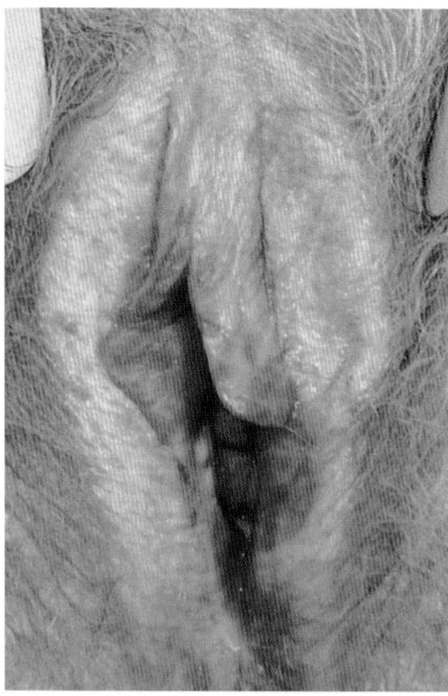

Figure 10.1 Lichen sclerosus with typical skin changes of the labia majora, including excoriation. Courtesy of Dr Frances Tatnall.

Biopsy is necessary when the diagnosis is uncertain. Treatment with highly potent topical steroids is very effective and in most cases the inflammatory process is switched off and the woman becomes largely symptom free. Mild recurrences may be treated with short courses of topical steroids. A small number of women have ongoing symptoms and require specialist dermatological management.

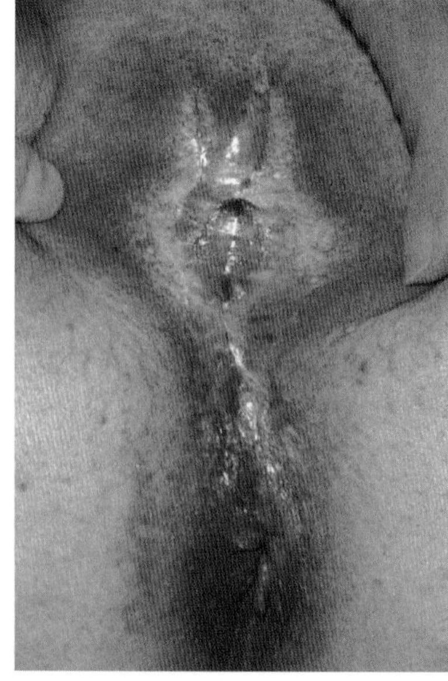

Figure 10.2 Late lichen sclerosus with loss of vulval architecture and narrowing of the introitus. Courtesy of Dr Frances Tatnall.

Women should be informed that the risk of squamous cell carcinoma (SCC) is increased and advised to have regular follow-up and practise self-examination.

Lichen planus

On the vulva, lichen planus can present in either the classic form or as an erosive condition of mucus membranes. Classic lichen planus appears as purplish, flat-topped, striated, polygonal papules (Figure 10.3). Itching may be treated with a moderate to potent topical steroid. Erosive lichen planus presents as vulval or introital soreness and dyspareunia (Figure 10.4). If the vagina is involved there may be adhesion formation. Similar lesions occur on the buccal mucosa. The differential diagnosis includes oestrogen deficiency, infective vulvo-vaginitis, Zoon's vulvitis, and bullous disorders such as pemphigus. A biopsy is usually required but may not be conclusive and response to topical steroids is often less satisfactory than for lichen sclerosus.

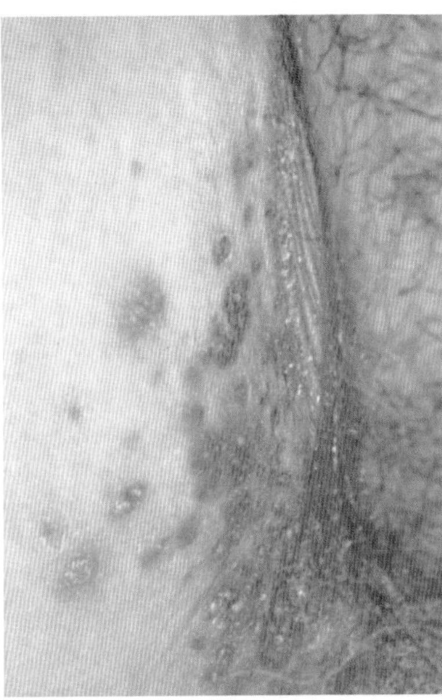

Figure 10.3 Classic lichen planus showing typical lesions. Courtesy of Dr Frances Tatnall.

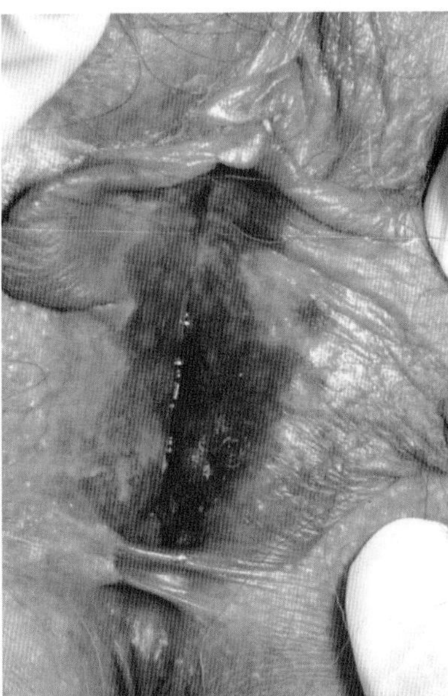

Figure 10.4 Erosive lichen planus showing introital erythema. Courtesy of Dr Frances Tatnall.

Psoriasis

Psoriasis, presenting with pruritus, may be found on the genital area but the lesions may differ from those found elsewhere as they may lack the shiny silvery appearance and may be smooth and erythematous. The well-defined edge is often a clue to the diagnosis. Perianal psoriasis is often missed (Figure 10.5). Careful examination of the elbows, knees, scalp, and nails may identify lesions elsewhere. Psoriasis responds to moderate and potent topical steroids but often relapses.

Eczema

Irritant and allergic eczema in response to topical medicaments and other products are common (Figure 10.6). The patient presents with itching and soreness and management involves removal of the offending product, good skin management, and a mild topical steroid. Patch testing may be helpful. Eczematous changes in atopic women also occur and present with itching and excoriation. Prolonged symptoms may lead to lichenification which exacerbates the itching. Seborrhoeic dermatitis occasionally affects the vulva and produces diffusely red lesions.

Idiopathic pruritus vulvae/ani

Itching that occurs in the absence of any dermatological abnormality may respond to emollients and oral antihistamines.

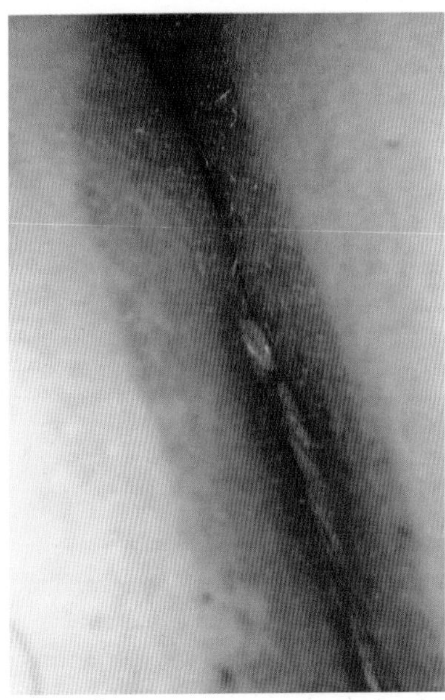

Figure 10.5 Perianal psoriasis showing erythema and well-defined edge.

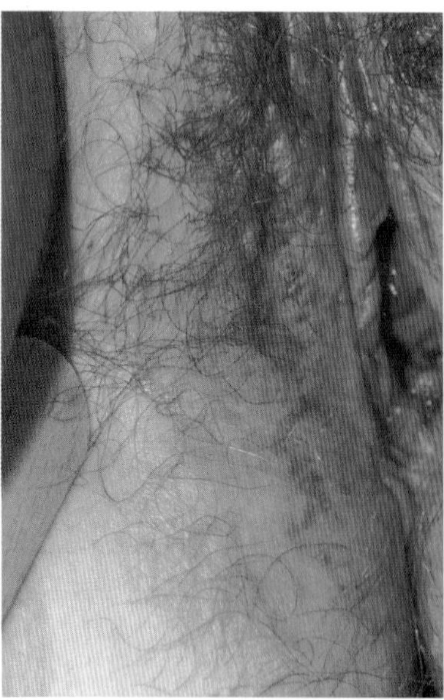

Figure 10.6 Eczema showing excoriation and some lichenification.

Pre-malignant and malignant conditions of the vulva

Vulval intra-epithelial neoplasia

This precursor lesion is almost always caused by oncogenic human papillomavirus (HPV). The natural history is not well understood but a proportion of patients develop invasive cancer. Almost all are smokers or former smokers. The lesions can be single or multifocal, and red, white, or pigmented (Figures 10.7 and 10.8). Clinicians should have a high index of suspicion and a low threshold for biopsy. Patients with vulval intra-epithelial neoplasia (VIN) may have intra-epithelial neoplasia elsewhere and careful examination of the cervix, vagina, and perianal area is required. Surgical and laser treatments are used but more recently there are reports of successful use of imiquimod cream.

Biopsy is required if the diagnosis is uncertain or if there is a suspicion of malignancy. An atypical response to treatment should provoke a review of the diagnosis and biopsy

Squamous cell carcinoma

This lesion accounts for 90% of vulval cancer and occurs either on a background of lichen sclerosus or VIN. Most patients are elderly but SCC in younger women is seen more frequently now, possibly as a result of the increased prevalence of HPV. Early biopsy of suspicious or persistent lesions is essential.

Basal cell carcinoma

This tumour, generally found in elderly women, is locally invasive but is rare on the vulva, accounting for about 2% of vulval malignancies, as it is usually caused by exposure to sunlight. Suspicious lesions should be referred for biopsy and/or wide local excision.

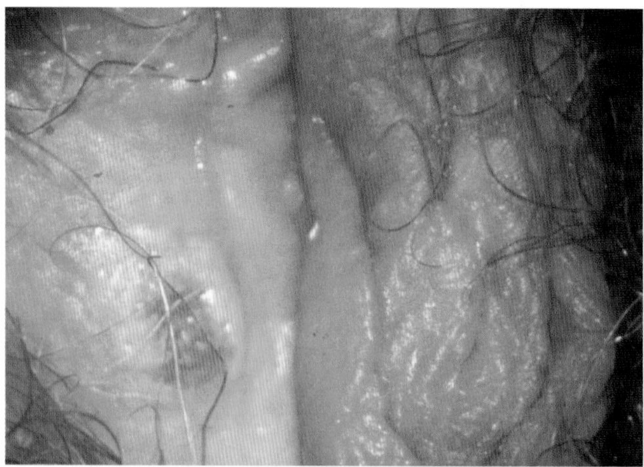

Figure 10.7 Vulval intra-epithelial neoplasia 3 (VIN-3) – single lesion.

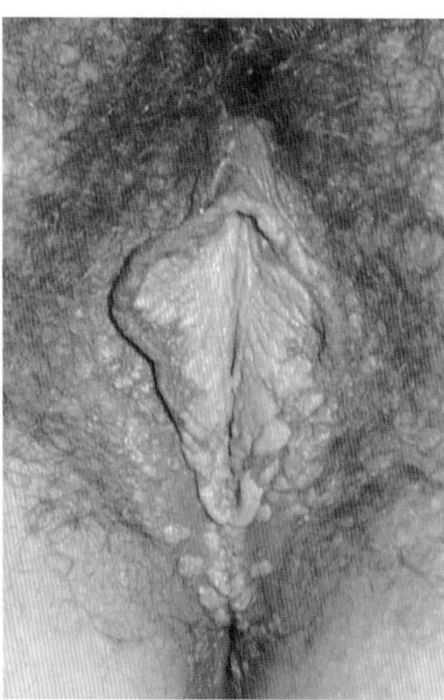

Figure 10.8 VIN-3 – multifocal disease.

Paget's disease

Extramammary Paget's disease may be found on the vulva and patients present with localised or widespread red, moist, or scaly lesions. Identification of Paget's disease should lead to a search for an underlying malignancy. Treatment is surgical.

Malignant melanoma

This tumour, which accounts for 10% of vulval cancers, may arise *de novo* or in an existing naevus (Figure 10.9). It is characterised by its irregular shape, pigmentation and edge and, most significantly, by recent change. Patients may complain of a lump or bleeding. Patients with any suspicious lesion should be referred urgently to a dermatologist.

Pigment changes

Pigmented lesions are common on the vulva and any suspicious lesions should be biopsied (Box 10.4).

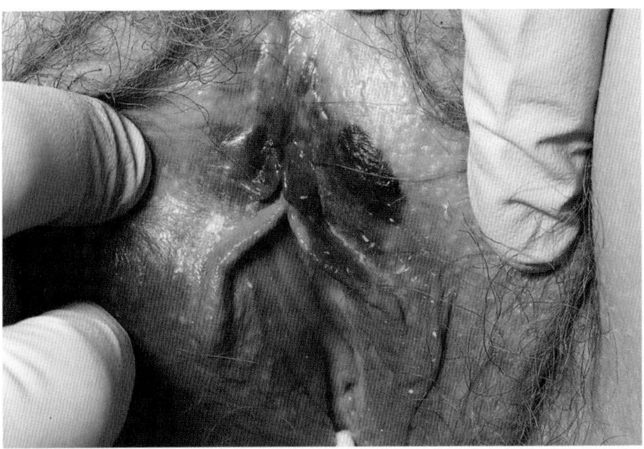

Figure 10.9 Malignant melanoma. Courtesy of Dr Frances Tatnall.

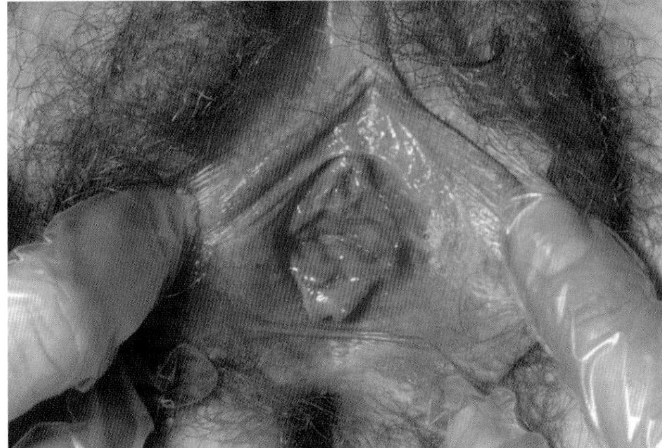

Figure 10.10 Provoked localised vulvodynia – small patches of erythema which are tender to pressure with a cotton-wool tipped swab.

Box 10.4 **Pigmentary changes of the vulva**

- Postinflammatory hyper- (or hypo-) pigmentation
- Benign moles (naevi)
- Pigmented warts
- Vitiligo
- VIN
- Malignant melanoma

Vulvodynia

This condition is defined by the International Society for the Study of Vulvovaginal Disease (ISSVD) as a complaint of chronic burning, soreness, or pain, associated with few, if any, physical signs and in which other infectious and dermatological conditions have been excluded. The recent classification of vulvodynia distinguishes between provoked vulvodynia, previously called vulval vestibulitis, which is localised to the introital area, and unprovoked vulvodynia, previously called essential or dysaesthetic vulvodynia, which is more generalised. Some patients have features of both types.

Provoked localised vulvodynia

This condition is found in young women who complain of vulval soreness, superficial dyspareunia, and sometimes pain inserting tampons. There may be a preceding infection or other condition and many women believe they have recurrent thrush, although there is no abnormal discharge or itching. On examination there may be subtle red patches in the introitus (Figure 10.10) which are tender to touch with a cotton-wool tipped swab. Women often go on to develop vaginismus, loss of libido, and loss of self-esteem. This then impacts on their relationship and exacerbates symptoms which may become generalised and not necessarily provoked by penetration. Often women have sought a diagnosis from many different clinicians and have been told that the problem is 'psychological'.

Unprovoked generalised vulvodynia

This condition is more common in the older woman and presents as generalised burning and soreness in the absence of an alternative diagnosis or any physical signs, not even introital tenderness. The diagnosis is made by recognising the typical history and the exclusion of dermatological and infective conditions. Many such women have dyspareunia, or have given up penetrative sex.

Management of both conditions is difficult and should begin with a careful explanation of the diagnosis and exploration of the patient's understanding and fears and the impact on her life. Young women often fear a sexually transmitted infection, impacting on fertility, and older women, cancer. In patients with long-standing symptoms there are inevitably effects on sexuality, relationships, and general well-being. Numerous treatments have been proposed and few evaluated in any rigorous way. A multidisciplinary approach is required to deal with both the condition itself and the sequelae.

Hormonal changes

Vulval and vaginal soreness may develop in postmenopausal women as a result of lack of oestrogen, and sometimes appear in breast-feeding women. Vulval and vaginal erythematous changes may be associated with a discharge. Treatment with topical oestrogen therapy or hormone replacement therapy is usually effective.

Bartholin's cyst and abscess

The ducts of Bartholin's glands have a narrow aperture which may become blocked leading to an accumulation of fluid within the duct and cyst formation. When the fluid becomes infected an abscess may develop. Bartholin's cysts are painless swellings, recognised by their typical site at the lower third of the introitus. An abscess is painful and red and may discharge pus (Figure 10.11). Asymptomatic Bartholin's cysts do not require treatment unless they interfere with intercourse. If a patient presents early with a Bartholin's abscess, it may respond to broad-spectrum antibiotics but surgical referral with marsupialisation of the abscess is often required. Bartholin's abscess may be caused by sexually transmitted organisms such as *Neisseria gonorrhoeae* and *Chlamydia trachomatis*, and appropriate

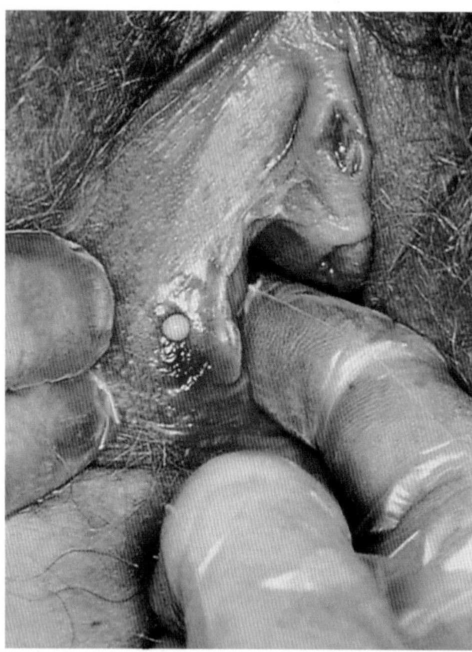

Figure 10.11 Discharging Bartholin's abscess. From King A, Nicol C. *Venereal Diseases*. Baillière Tindall, London, 1969.

swabs should be taken, but the majority of cases are caused by skin contaminants such as staphylococci.

Female sexual dysfunction

Female sexual dysfunction (FSD) is more common than male sexual dysfunction and can occur for many reasons, including as a result of having acquired an STI. Because the strongest associations with FSD relate to relationship and psychological rather than organic issues, health care workers may feel reluctant to ask women about their sexual functioning, fearing it may open up a 'can of worms'. One simple approach might be to ask if the woman has a sexual problem and if she does to ask an open ended question such as 'Would you like to tell me more about it?'

Patients may present to sexual health services with vulval pain or dyspareunia, or complaining of low libido. A full assessment should determine whether this is loss of desire, arousal, or problems with orgasm, although women often have more than one problem. Co-existent disease, hormonal imbalances (e.g. low testosterone or oestrogen), drugs, previous sexual abuse/violence, and depression are among the many causes. Treatments should be tailored to the underlying cause and include psycho-sexual and cognitive behavioural therapy. There is some evidence on drug therapy for hypoactive sexual desire disorder (HSSD) and arousal disorders – in particular from hormone replacement therapy such as tibolone, testosterone (Intrinsa), phosphodiesterase inhibitors such as sildenafil or newer agents which are currently under investigation. To obtain optimal results with medications they should be undertaken alongside psychological therapies.

Acknowledgement

The author would like to thank Dr David Goldmeier for the section on sexual dysfunction.

Further reading

Bachmann GA, Rosen R, Pinn VW, Utian WH, Ayers C, Basson R, *et al.* Vulvodynia: a state-of-the-art consensus on definition, diagnosis and management. *J Reprod Med* 2006;**51**:447–56.

Edwards L. *Genital Dermatology Atlas*. Lippincott Williams and Wilkins, Philadelphia, 2004.

Neill SM, Lewis FM. *Ridley's The Vulva*, 3rd edn. Wiley-Blackwell, Oxford, 2009.

www.bad.org.uk.

www.bashh.org/guidelines.

www.bssvd.org.

CHAPTER 11

Sexually Transmitted Infections and HIV in Pregnancy

Janet Wilson

Department of Genitourinary Medicine, The General Infirmary at Leeds, Leeds, UK

OVERVIEW

- As in non-pregnant women, STIs in pregnancy may be asymptomatic
- It is important to perform the normal risk assessment for STIs by taking a sexual history as part of the pregnancy management
- Most STIs, particularly if detected early, can be treated and cleared without any harm to the pregnancy or infant
- Antenatal HIV screening and interventions to prevent mother–child transmission have led to a dramatic fall in infected infants in the United Kingdom, with transmission rates of <2%

The discovery of a sexually transmitted infection (STI) in pregnancy may cause alarm to the woman and her clinician. The main concern is any potential harm to the unborn child. Most STIs, particularly if detected early, can be treated and cleared without any harm to the pregnancy or infant. Indeed, this is the principle behind antenatal screening (Box 11.1).

As in non-pregnant women, STIs may be asymptomatic. It is important to perform the normal risk assessment by taking a sexual history as part of the pregnancy management. The diagnostic tests used are the same as in non-pregnant women but treatments must be chosen carefully as some are contraindicated in pregnancy. Metabolism of some drugs may be altered, resulting in lower cure rates. Consequently, a test of cure may be recommended in pregnant women.

The infections can affect pregnancy in a number of ways. They can spread from the cervix or vagina into the uterine cavity causing chorioamnionitis leading to premature rupture of membranes, preterm delivery, and low birth weight. Some infections cross the placenta causing intrauterine infection of the fetus. Others are transmitted to the infant during delivery, and some can cause postpartum infection in the mother (Table 11.1).

ABC of Sexually Transmitted Infections, Sixth Edition.
Edited by Karen E. Rogstad.

Box 11.1 **Screening for infections in pregnancy**

Screening routinely recommended for all women in UK

- Serology for syphilis
- Serology for hepatitis B
- HIV antibody test

Screening recommended in certain circumstances

- Women <25 years should be directed to their local national chlamydia screening programme within England
- Screening for anti-hepatitis C virus (anti-HCV) antibodies should be performed in high risk groups, such as intravenous drug users and women who received organ transplant or blood transfusion before HCV screening commenced

Other STIs and infections

- Tests for gonorrhoea, chlamydia, *Trichimonas vaginalis*, candida and bacterial vaginosis should be performed in pregnant women with a current STI, or symptoms/signs suggestive of a STI and those who are HIV positive
- Evidence does not support routine antenatal screening for gonorrhoea, bacterial vaginosis, *Trichimonas vaginalis* and herpes (using type-specific antibody testing for herpes simplex viruses HSV-1 and HSV-2) in asymptomatic pregnant women.

Chlamydia

Mother

- Prevalence is about 10% in women aged <25 years including pregnant women. Chlamydia screening should be offered to pregnant women <25 years
- Other women should be tested if they have symptoms or signs suggestive of chlamydia
- Infection can spread from the cervix into the uterine cavity causing chorioamnionitis
- Chlamydia can cause premature rupture of membranes, preterm delivery, low birth weight, and postpartum infection

Treatment

Treatment is with azithromycin 1 g single dose or erythromycin 500 mg twice a day for 14 days. The safety of azithromycin in

Table 11.1 Routes of infection.

Ascending infections	Perinatal transmission
Chlamydia trachomatis	*Chlamydia trachomatis*
Neisseria gonorrhoeae	*Neisseria gonorrhoeae*
Trichomonas vaginalis	HIV
Bacterial vaginosis	Herpes
	Human papillomavirus
	Hepatitis B
	Hepatitis C
Transplacental spread	**Postpartum infections**
Syphilis	*Chlamydia trachomatis*
HIV	*Neisseria gonorrhoeae*
	Bacterial vaginosis

pregnancy is not yet fully assessed, although available data indicate it is safe. World Health Organization (WHO) and US guidelines recommend azithromycin to treat chlamydia in pregnancy. The British National Formulary (BNF) recommends use in pregnancy and lactation only if no alternative is available. Azithromycin has fewer side effects and significantly better compliance than erythromycin. Doxycycline and ofloxacin are contraindicated in pregnancy.

Partner notification is essential to prevent reinfection. Advise the woman to avoid sex (including oral sex) until she and her partner(s) have completed treatment, or for 7 days if azithromycin is used.

Because of reduced efficacy of treatment in pregnancy, a test of cure should be performed 5 weeks after completing therapy, or after 6 weeks if azithromycin is given.

Infant

- Perinatal transmission rate in babies born to untreated infected mothers is 50–70%
- The main presentation is conjunctivitis between days 5 and 12
- Nasopharynx is also a common site of infection, leading to otitis media or pneumonia in infants aged 4–12 weeks (Figure 11.1)
- Infants may develop vaginal infection
- Diagnosis is by culture or nucleic acid amplification test (NAAT) on a sample obtained from an everted eyelid

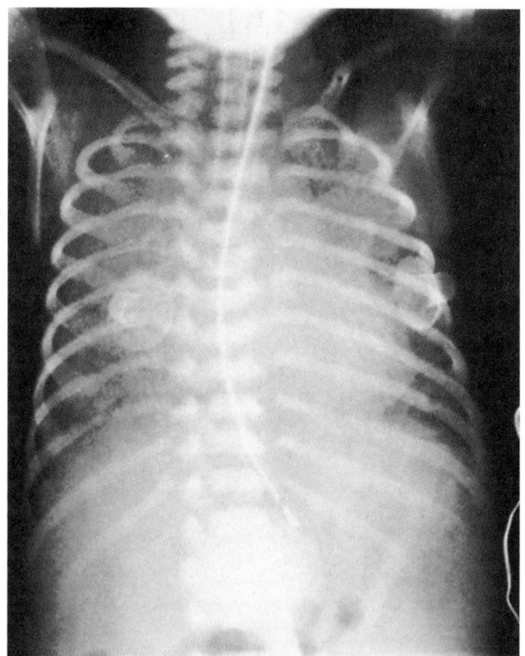

Figure 11.1 Chlamydial pneumonitis.

Gonorrhoea

Mother

- Gonorrhoea rates are much lower than chlamydia; usually <1% even in younger women
- Women should be tested if they have symptoms or signs suggestive of gonorrhoea
- Infection can spread from the cervix into the uterine cavity causing chorioamnionitis
- Gonorrhoea can cause premature rupture of membranes, preterm delivery, low birth weight, and postpartum infection
- Test for chlamydia in women with gonorrhoea; up to 40% will have both infections

Treatment

Treatment is with cefixime 400 mg single oral dose, cefriaxone 250 mg IM single dose, or spectinomycin 2 g IM single dose in those with penicillin and/or cephalosporin allergy. Tetracyclines and quinolones are contraindicated in pregnancy. Azithromycin 1 g single dose is often given at the same time in view of the high rate of co-infection with chlamydia.

Partner notification is essential to prevent reinfection. Advise the woman to avoid sex (including oral sex) until 7 days after she and her partner(s) have completed treatment.

If medication is taken, symptoms resolved, and there is no risk of reinfection, test of cure is not needed as pregnancy does not diminish gonorrhoea treatment efficacy.

Infant

- Perinatal transmission rate in babies born to untreated infected mothers is about 40%
- The main presentation is conjunctivitis 2–5 days after birth (Figure 11.2); may cause profuse purulent discharge, with oedema of the eyelids. If untreated it can lead to corneal ulceration and perforation causing blindness
- The infant may develop vaginal infection
- Diagnosis is by gram stain and culture of conjunctival sample

Trichomoniasis

Mother

- Prevalence of trichomoniasis is low in the United Kingdom but is the most common non-viral STI worldwide
- Women should be tested if they have symptoms or signs suggestive of infection
- Trichomoniasis can cause preterm delivery and low birth weight
- Perform screening for gonorrhoea and chlamydia as co-infection is common

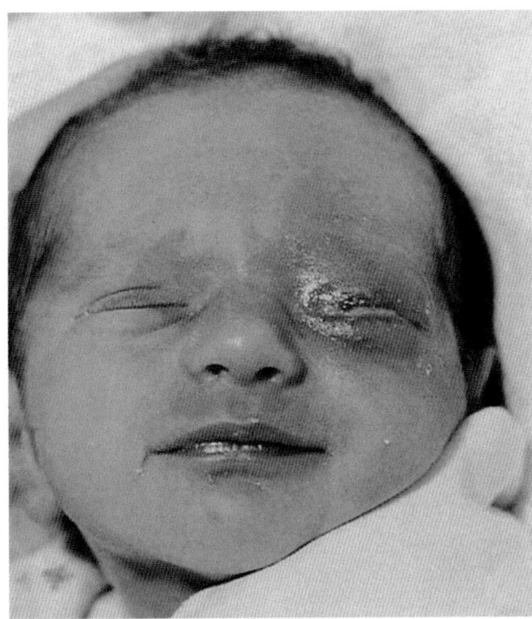

Figure 11.2 Ophthalmia neonatorum.

Treatment

Treatment is with metronidazole 400 mg twice daily for 5–7 days. There is no evidence of teratogenicity from metronidazole in the first trimester of pregnancy. The BNF advises against high dose regimens in pregnancy.

Partner notification is essential to prevent reinfection. Advise the woman to avoid sex until 7 days after she and her partner(s) have completed treatment.

Test of cure is only advised if symptoms remain or recur.

Infant

There are no direct infective complications to infants but they may develop vaginal infection.

Bacterial vaginosis

Mother

- Fifteen per cent of pregnant women have bacterial vaginosis (BV), half have no symptoms
- BV can cause late miscarriage, preterm birth, preterm premature rupture of membranes, and postpartum endometritis
- Screening for asymptomatic BV in pregnancy is not recommended. Women should be tested if they have symptoms and signs suggestive of BV

Treatment

Treatment is with metronidazole 400 mg twice daily for 5–7 days, metronidazole intravaginal gel (0.75%) once daily for 5 days, or clindamycin intravaginal cream (2%) once daily for 7 days. Test of cure is only advised if symptoms remain.

Infant

There are no direct infective complications to the infant.

Syphilis

Mother

- Syphilis is rare in the United Kingdom but there has been a recent rise in prevalence
- Worldwide, there is a high prevalence in some countries, causing high infant morbidity and mortality
- It can be transmitted transplacentally at any stage of pregnancy
- Syphilis can cause miscarriage, preterm labour, stillbirth, and congenital syphilis
- The risk of congenital syphilis is related to the stage of infection in the mother. High rates occur within first 2 years but transmission can still occur after 4 years
- Antenatal syphilis screening detects women with untreated syphilis in pregnancy. Treatment of the mother early in pregnancy treats the fetus, preventing congenital syphilis
- Women with syphilis should be screened for other STIs including HIV

Treatment

Treatment is with benzathine penicillin 2.4 MU IM weekly for up to three doses, or procaine penicillin 600 000 units IM daily for up to 17 days.

Partner notification is essential to prevent reinfection. Advise the woman to avoid sex (including oral sex) until the results of first follow-up serology test are known.

Follow-up syphilis serology should be performed, initially monthly. A fourfold drop in rapid plasma reagin/venereal disease research laboratory (RPR/VDRL) test results indicates an adequate response to treatment.

Infant

Many infected infants are asymptomatic at birth. The most common features of early congenital syphilis include:

- Rash (maculopapular, bullous, and desquamation)
- Hepatosplenomegaly
- Syphilitic snuffles (Figure 11.3)
- Periostitis

The features of late syphilis include:

- Interstitial keratitis
- Hutchinson's incisors (Figure 11.4), Moon's mulberry molars, rhagades
- Saddlenose deformity, frontal bossing
- Deafness

Infection is diagnosed by detection of *Treponema pallidum* from the infant's lesions/body fluids, and positive immunoglobulin M enzyme immunoassay (IgM EIA) serology.

Genital warts

Mother

- Genital warts may rapidly enlarge, especially in the last trimester
- Vaginal delivery should be planned; very rarely cause problems in pregnancy or labour

- Treat with cryotherapy, trichloroacetic acid, or excision. No treatment is an option
- Clearance may be difficult during pregnancy. Treatment aims to minimise wart numbers at delivery to reduce neonatal exposure to the virus
- During the postnatal period spontaneous regression often occurs
- Avoid podophyllotoxin because of possible teratogenic effects, imiquimod is not licensed in pregnancy

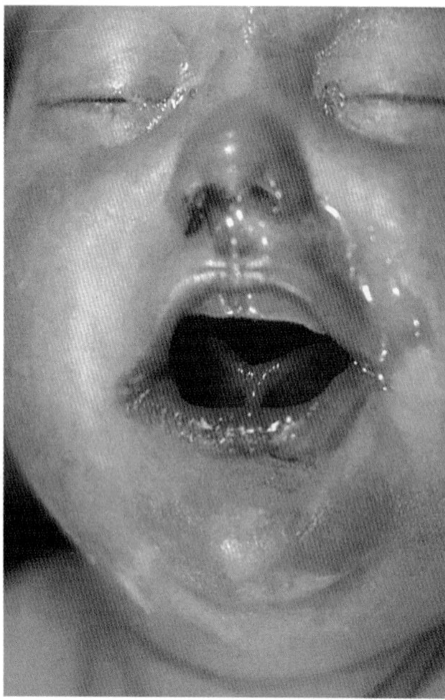

Figure 11.3 Congenital syphilis of infant. Courtesy of CDC/Dr Norman Cob.

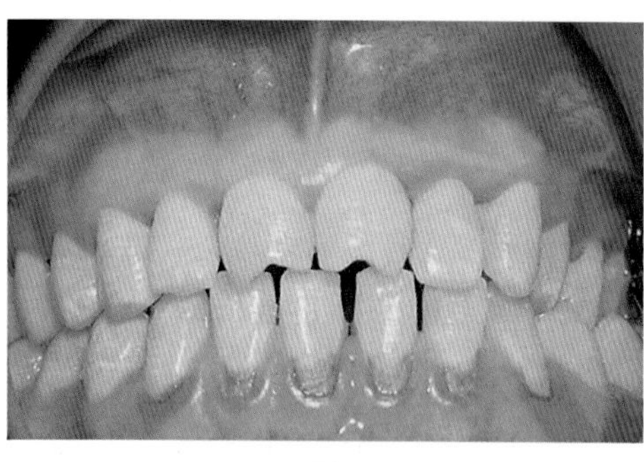

(a)

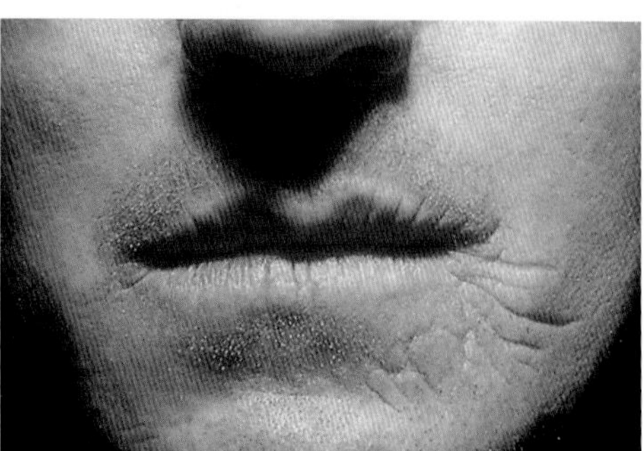

(b)

Figure 11.4 Congenital syphilis on: (a) teeth, and (b) mouth.

Infant

Laryngeal papillomatosis and genital warts may develop but both are rare.

Genital herpes

Mother

- The risk of vertical transmission of genital herpes depends whether it is the first episode or recurrent herpes
- It can be difficult to distinguish between recurrent and first episode genital herpes; type-specific herpes simplex virus (HSV) serology may be helpful

First episode

- Give oral or intravenous aciclovir depending on the clinical severity. (Aciclovir is not licensed for use in pregnancy but has been used extensively in pregnant women with no reported problems.)
- Vaginal delivery should be planned
- Daily suppressive aciclovir from 36 weeks reduces the likelihood of HSV lesions at term and the need to offer caesarean section (CS)
- The risk of transmission is greater (up to 40%) when the first episode occurs in the third trimester
- CS should be offered to all women with first episode at the time of delivery, or within 6 weeks of expected date of delivery (EDD) or onset of labour
- If vaginal delivery is unavoidable, aciclovir treatment of the mother and baby should be considered

Recurrent episodes

- Recurrences during pregnancy pose no threat to the pregnancy or fetus
- The risk of neonatal herpes with recurrent HSV at onset of labour is <1%. This suggests that passive immunity from maternal antibodies is protective to the infant
- Avoid fetal scalp monitors as they can be a site of inoculation of virus and increase transmission risk
- CS can be considered for women with recurrent HSV at the onset of labour; risk of transmission with vaginal delivery is small so needs to be weighed against the risks of CS to the mother
- Daily suppressive aciclovir from 36 weeks reduces recurrent clinical HSV and viral detection at the time of delivery and the need to offer CS

Infant

- HSV-1 and HSV-2 can cause neonatal herpes
- Incidence is 1 in 60 000 live births in the United Kingdom; this is lower than other European countries and the United States. Most cases are from direct contact with infected maternal genital secretion but postnatal transmission can occur from nosocomial or community-acquired herpes infection

- Neonatal herpes is almost always symptomatic and frequently fatal
- There are three categories of infection: localised to the site of viral entry (skin, eye, or mouth); encephalitis; and disseminated infection. Disseminated infection has the worst prognosis
- Diagnosis needs a high index of suspicion. Vesicular fluid can be sent for electron microscopy and HSV polymerase chain reaction (PCR)

HIV infection

Mother

- In 2008, 0.21% of women giving birth in England and Scotland were HIV-infected
- HIV prevalence among pregnant women in London has been stable at 0.37% since 2004
- Prevalence in pregnant women outside London has increased fivefold in the past decade but remains relatively low at 0.15% in 2008 (Figure 11.5)
- Sub-Saharan African-born pregnant women outside London have significantly higher HIV prevalence (3.1%) than those living inside London (2.3%)
- Prevalence in United Kingdom-born women was low in 2008 (0.05%) but there has been a statistically significant increase since 2000. Detection of HIV in pregnant women in the United Kingdom remains high; >90% are diagnosed before delivery
- Screening for STIs and genital infections should be performed early in the pregnancy
- HIV probably has little effect on pregnancy outcome but highly active antiretroviral therapy (HAART) appears to increase preterm birth
- HIV can be transmitted to the infant *in utero*, at delivery, and by breastfeeding; the majority of cases occur during delivery
- Risk of transmission depends on maternal HIV viral load; higher viral loads are associated with increased risk
- Prior to the routine use of HAART, the transmission rate was 13% in Europe in non-breastfeeding women. Breastfeeding adds about a further 15% transmission rate

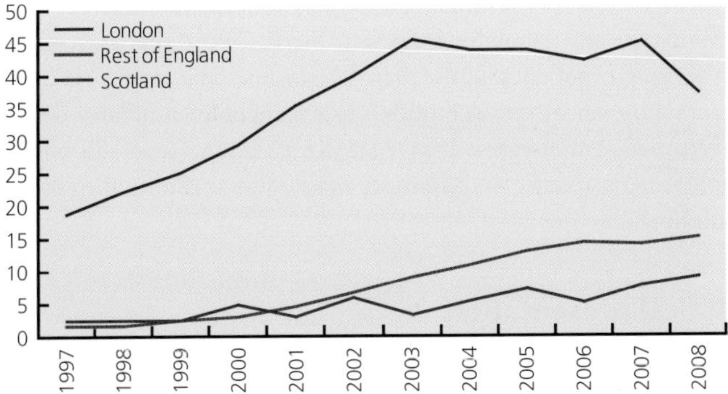

Figure 11.5 Rates of HIV prevalence in pregnant women from 1997 to 2007. (Data from unlinked anonymous survey of newborn infant dried blood spots.)

- With HAART and/or elective CS, transmission rate can be reduced to <2%

Interventions to prevent mother–child transmission

Women not already taking HAART should commence standard HAART during the second trimester in order to achieve undetectable viral load by 36 weeks allowing vaginal delivery. Some mothers who achieve an undetectable viral load still prefer a planned CS at 39 weeks. Women receiving no HAART, or those unable to achieve undetectable viral load, should have a planned CS at 38 weeks.

Infants should be given postexposure prophylaxis with antiretroviral therapy for 4 weeks and breastfeeding should be avoided.

Infant

- Antenatal HIV screening and interventions to prevent mother–child transmission (MTCT) led to a dramatic fall in infected infants in the United Kingdom
- The MTCT rate in 1993, when interventions were virtually non-existent, was 25.6%
- Between 2000 and 2002, the MTCT rate fell to 1.6%; 2003–2006 to 1.0%. Now MTCT rates are 0.7% among mothers on HAART
- No significant difference between mode of delivery (planned CS versus vaginal delivery) is seen in mothers on HAART
- There is no evidence of congenital abnormalities with exposure to HAART, even in the first trimester
- Infants are routinely given postexposure prophylaxis with antiretroviral therapy for 4 weeks
- Strict formula feeding only
- HIV DNA PCR on peripheral blood lymphocytes should be performed at 1 day, 6 weeks, and 12 weeks of age
- If all tests are negative, and the infant is not being breastfed, the parents can be informed that the infant is not HIV infected
- Loss of the maternal HIV antibodies should be confirmed at 18 months

Further reading

de Ruiter A, Mercey D, Anderson J, Chakraborty R, Clayden P, Foster G, *et al.* British HIV Association and Children's HIV Association guidelines for the management of HIV infection in pregnant women 2008. *HIV Med* 2008;**9**:452–502.

Giraudon I, Forde J, Maguire H, Arnold J, Permalloo N. Antenatal screening and prevalence of infection: surveillance in London, 2000–2007. *Euro Surveill* 2009;**14**(9):8–12. Available online at http://www.eurosurveillance.org/ViewArticle.aspx?ArticleId = 19134.

Goh BT, Thornton AC. Antenatal screening for syphilis. *Sex Transm Inf* 2007;**83**:345–6.

National Institute for Health and Clinical Excellence. *Antenatal Care: Routine Care for the Healthy Pregnant Woman.* NICE, March 2008.

Royal College of Obstetricians and Gynaecologists. *Green-top Guideline no 30: Management of Genital Herpes in Pregnancy.* RCOG, September 2007.

CHAPTER 12

Genital Ulcer Disease

Raj Patel [1] *and Nadi Gupta* [2]

[1] Royal South Hants Hospital, Southampton, UK
[2] Sheffield Teaching Hospitals NHS Foundation Trust, Sheffield, UK

OVERVIEW

Genital herpes

- Genital herpes is the most common cause of sexually acquired genital ulceration in the UK
- HSV-1 infection is the most common cause of first episode genital ulceration in young people
- Most patients with HSV-2 infection will have recurrent disease
- Effective strategies exist to diminish transmission risk

Lymphogranuloma venereum

- LGV outbreaks continue to arise in men who have sex with men
- Diagnosis should be suspected in patients presenting with anorectal symptoms

Chancroid and donovanosis

- These tropical STIs are both rare in the UK

Genital ulcer disease represents one of the more complex clinical problems in sexual health care. Genital ulceration may be caused by sexually transmitted infections (STIs), other infectious agents, dermatological conditions, or trauma. The list of differential diagnoses is extensive and can be divided into those that are painful or painless and whether the ulcer is solitary or multiple (Figure 12.1), although exceptions do exist. Sexual history-taking can establish or exclude particular risk factors for many of the rarer causes such as tropical STIs. Although many dermatological causes can occur, most have typical manifestations in non-genital sites. The most common STI causes of genital ulceration in the developed world are genital herpes, primary syphilis (see Chapter 13), and lymphogranuloma venereum. Cases of donovanosis and chancroid tend to only be seen as imported STIs in travellers, although epidemics in closed communities occasionally occur.

Genital herpes

Genital herpes is a common infection caused by herpes simplex virus type 1 (HSV-1) or type 2 (HSV-2). These viruses are closely related and cause clinically indistinguishable illnesses when first acquired. Historically, most HSV-1 infections were acquired in childhood causing oropharyngeal HSV infection and recurrent cold sores. However, this is no longer the case and most teenagers are susceptible to HSV-1 at sexual debut. HSV-1, acquired through orogenital contact, is now the most common cause of first episode genital herpes in young men and women in the United Kingdom.

Natural history

The incubation period of HSV infection is usually 5–14 days. Less than half of those infected develop any signs or symptoms during initial acquisition. The virus enters into the distal axonal processes of the sensory neuron and travels to the sensory (dorsal root) ganglion where it remains in a latent state. The virus periodically reactivates, travelling down the axon and into the basal skin layers. Some of these episodes will result in symptoms and signs while others will be asymptomatic (Figure 12.2). Infected patients who are asymptomatic and therefore unaware of their infection can transmit the infection to a sexual partner.

Because of the variability in severity, and the atypical nature of any clinical illness, only a minority of those infected with genital HSV ever recognise their illness or have a correct diagnosis made.

The prevalence of HSV-2 infection in the UK population is around 9.%. Higher rates occur in commercial sex workers and men who have sex with men (MSM).

Genital HSV-2 infection recurs more frequently than HSV-1. HSV-2 typically recurs four times in the first year after infection (10% may experience more than 10 episodes per year). HSV-1 recurs about once every 18 months. Approximately 4% of those with severe recurrent disease will have HSV-1 infection. Generally, both symptomatic disease and asymptomatic viral shedding diminish with time.

Clinical presentation

First episode genital herpes

The ‘first episode’ is defined as the first time a person has clinical features of genital herpes (Table 12.1). The first episode of genital herpes may occur following initial acquisition of virus or it may occur some time later. Typical lesions start as vesicles which then become superficial exquisitely painful ulcers (Figure 12.3). Ulcers can coalesce to form larger superficial lesions with characteristic

ABC of Sexually Transmitted Infections, Sixth Edition.
Edited by Karen E. Rogstad.

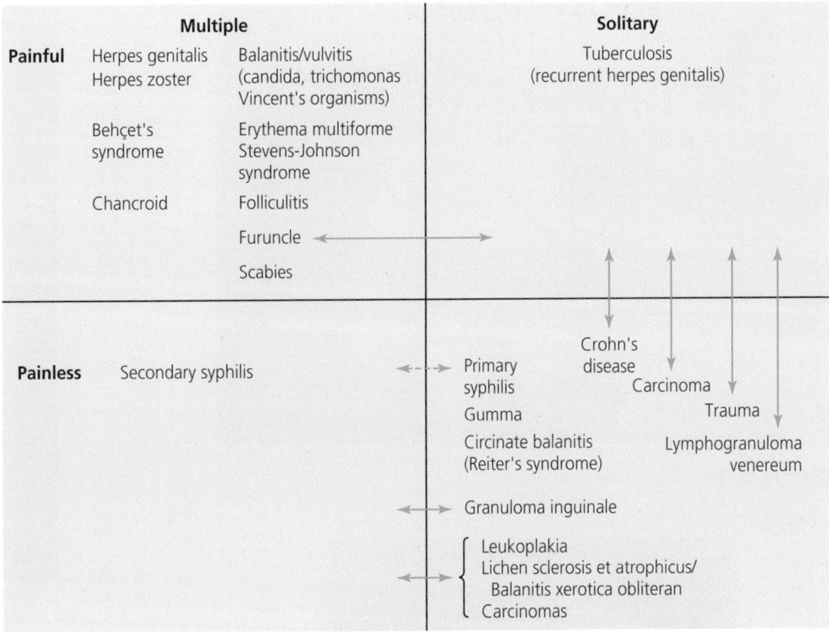

Figure 12.1 Causes of genital ulceration and erosions. Courtesy of Dr F. Cowan.

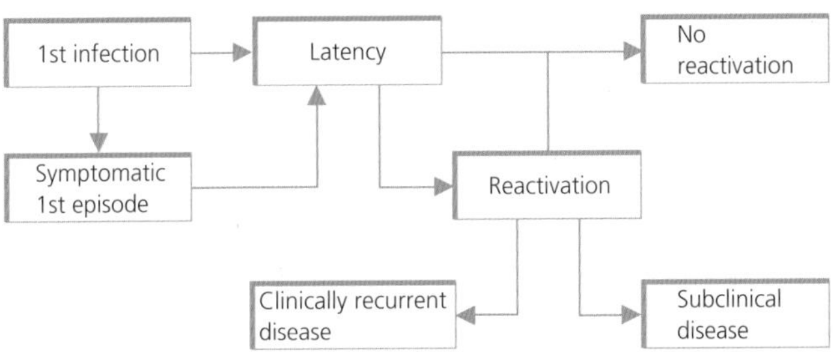

Figure 12.2 Natural history of herpes simplex virus (HSV) infection.

Table 12.1 Clinical features and frequency of symptoms.

Clinical presentation of first episode genital herpes						
Site	**Symptoms**					
	Pain	**Dysuria**	**Retention**	**Constipation**	**Discharge**	**None**
Penis (glans, coronal sulcus and shaft)	+					±
Urethra (male)	++	+	+		+	+
Anus/rectum	+		±	+	+	+
Buttocks/ thighs/ scrotum	+					
Vulva/urethra	++	+	±		±	±
Vagina	+				+	±
Cervix	+				++	+

Source: Courtesy of Dr F. Cowan.

serpiginous edges (Figures 12.4–12.6). There is often an associated local tender lymphadenopathy. Muscle aches involving the lower limbs are frequently reported. Systemic features of headache, malaise, and photophobia are present in 10% of patients.

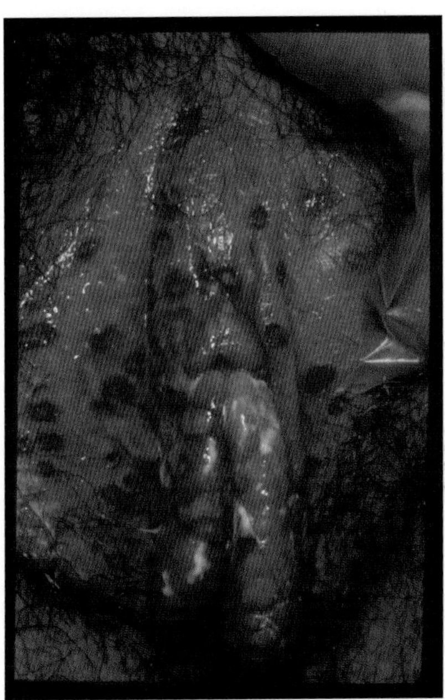

Figure 12.3 First episode herpes simplex virus. Courtesy of Dr D Rowen.

Many patients have other features such as fissures, erythema, and dysuria. It is common for patients presenting with dysuria to be misdiagnosed as having a urinary tract infection if they are not examined. Healing without scarring is usual. A typical episode lasts for 3 weeks (Figure 12.7). The most common complications include superinfection of lesions and adhesion formation. Dysuria when severe can lead to urinary retention. A range of complications can occur (Table 12.2).

Recurrent episodes

Recurrent episodes occur when latent virus is reactivated. Many patients notice prodromal symptoms of localised tingling and itch

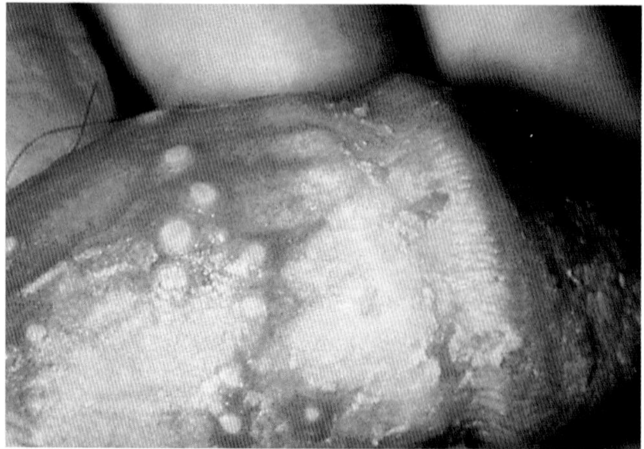

Figure 12.4 First episode genital herpes.

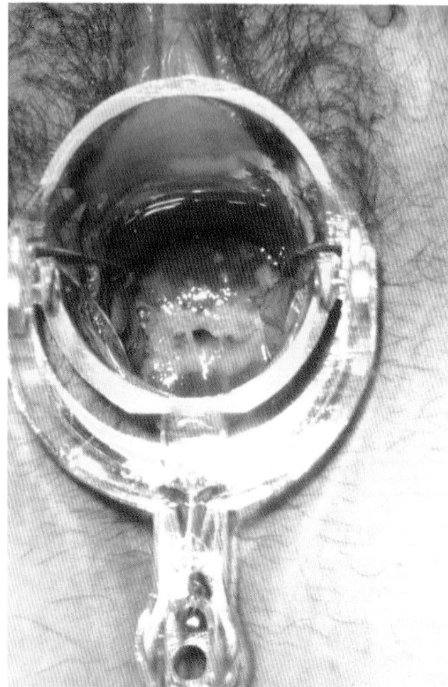

Figure 12.5 Herpes of the cervix. Courtesy of Dr Colm O'Mahoney.

Table 12.2 Complications of herpes simplex virus (HSV) infection.

Local	Superinfection of lesions with streptococci and/or staphylococci, adhesion formation, vaginal candidal infection exacerbating symptoms
	External dysuria – may be severe enough to precipitate retention of urine
Distant	Myalgia, dissemination (rare outside the neonate and pregnancy)
	Autoinoculation to distant sites
	Erythema multiforme
Neurological	Headaches, encephalitis, radiculitis, transverse myelitis, autonomic neuropathy
Psychological	Anxiety, depression

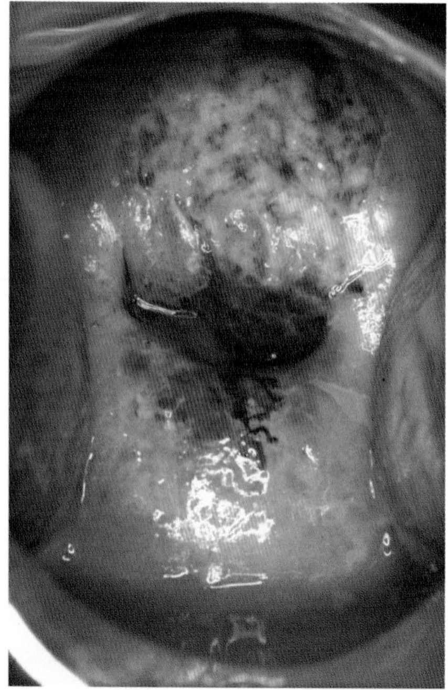

Figure 12.6 Herpetic necrotic cervicitis. This severe eroded lesion resembles a cervical carcinoma and is accompanied by copious clear serous fluid discharge. Courtesy of Peter Greenhouse.

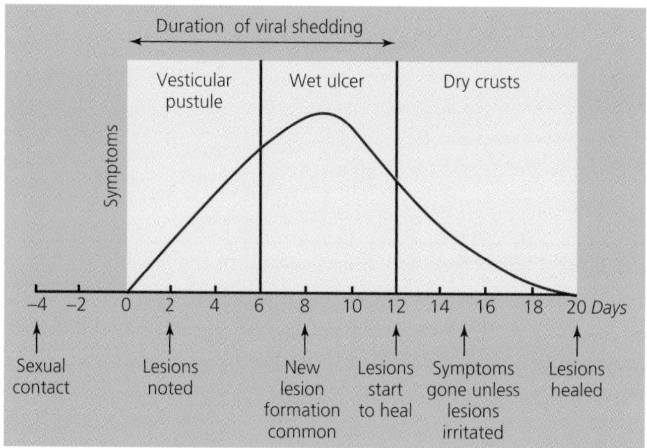

Figure 12.7 Course of first episode genital herpes. Courtesy of Dr L. Corey.

that occur prior to the development of lesions. However, false prodromes, when no lesions occur, are frequently described. There are usually no precipitating factors although localised trauma and ultraviolet irradiation in the affected dermatome have both been shown to be effective triggers. Recurrences are generally short lived and milder than acquisition episodes (Figure 12.8). The site and features of genital HSV recurrences will often settle into a pattern. Recurrences can occur anywhere in the dermatome involved and may involve the perianal, buttock, and thigh areas. There are certain factors associated with increased frequency of symptomatic recurrence (Box 12.1).

> Box 12.1 **Factors associated with increased risk of frequent symptomatic recurrent disease**
>
> - Genital HSV-2 infection
> - No previous infection with other HSV type
> - Gender (male > female)
> - First year following infection
> - A symptomatic acquisition episode
> - A prolonged acquisition episode
> - Damaged immune system

Diagnosis

Diagnosis of genital herpes is made by polymerase chain reaction (PCR), culture, or antigen detection directly from genital lesions with PCR being the most accurate. Viral typing is of benefit because it provides some prognostic value. Serological tests are available that can identify the presence of antibodies to HSV-1 or HSV-2. Such tests can be valuable in excluding HSV infection. Other STIs need to be excluded.

Treatment

First episode

All currently licensed antivirals (aciclovir, famciclovir, and valaciclovir) are equally effective in reducing the severity and duration of the episode (Table 12.3). Patients presenting with first episode genital herpes should be offered treatment with oral antivirals, particularly in the early stages of illness (first 5 days), if new lesions are still appearing, and in the presence of systemic symptoms. Treatment should be offered even if disease appears relatively mild because progression can be rapid.

Treatment should be given for a minimum of 5 days and may need to be extended to 10 days if the patient remains systemically unwell, if new lesions continue to appear, or if complications are present.

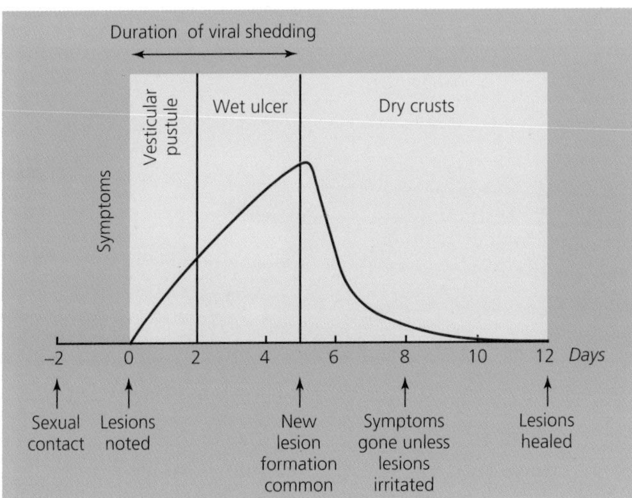

Figure 12.8 Course of recurrent genital herpes. Courtesy of Dr L. Corey.

Table 12.3 Treatment options.

Treatment of first episode (all for 5–10 days)	Aciclovir 400 mg three times a day or 200 mg five times a day Valaciclovir 500 mg twice a day Famciclovir 250 mg three times a day
Episodic treatment	Aciclovir 800 mg three times a day for 2 days or 200 mg five times a day for 5 days Valaciclovir 500 mg twice daily for 3–5 days Famciclovir 1 g twice daily for 1 day or 125 mg twice daily for 5 days
Suppressive therapy	Aciclovir 400 mg twice daily Valaciclovir 500 mg – 1 g once daily Reassessment of ongoing need should be carried out regularly and at least annually

Patients with severe dysuria may find urinating in a warm salt bath helpful. Short-term use of topical anaesthetic gels such as lidocaine may also ease micturition. Oral analgesics should be considered.

Recurrent episodes

Most patient's find that their recurrences are mild, infrequent, and short lived. They neither request nor require any specific therapy. However, where disease is problematic a range of therapeutic options are available.

Taking a short course of treatment early in a recurrence during the prodrome or in the first 24–48 hours as a lesion is developing has been shown to abort lesions and hasten healing. This strategy of episodic treatment does not work for all patients and is not suitable for those who have frequent disease or evidence of psychosexual impact.

For patients with severe, frequent, or complicated disease or with specific concerns around managing transmission risk, continuous daily suppressive therapy is likely to be more beneficial. Patients need to be aware that this does not alter the underlying natural history and that transmission, although significantly reduced, may still occur while on therapy.

Counselling

There are many lay misconceptions regarding genital herpes. It is of paramount importance that care is taken when providing the putative diagnosis and to aim to 'normalise' the condition. Appropriate psychological support should be offered when necessary (Box 12.2).

Transmission occurs when HSV present on the skin is inoculated on to broken skin or mucous membranes, usually by close physical contact. Viral shedding can occur in the absence of any genital symptoms or signs. Patients with genital herpes need to be aware that there is a small but definite risk of transmission to their sexual partners despite the absence of any genital symptoms. Transmission is easier from men to women than from women to men and appears to be greater in the earlier phases of relationships.

Taking continuous suppressive therapy with any antiviral is associated with a significant reduction in recurrence rate and

Box 12.2 **HSV counselling**

- Possible source of infection
- Possible duration of infection
- Natural course of illness – must include risks of asymptomatic shedding
- Future treatment options
- Options for reducing transmission to sexual partners
- Reassurance around risks of transmission to a fetus in pregnancy – advisability of informing midwife and obstetric team
- Importance for men to avoid new transmissions to partners during pregnancy
- Role and value of partner notification

asymptomatic shedding. A large study using daily valaciclovir showed that transmission rates can be halved on therapy.

Condoms, although they do not cover all the potential sites of genital shedding or inoculation, have been shown to reduce transmission. Other risk reduction strategies include avoiding sex when lesions or prodromes are present (Box 12.3).

Box 12.3 **Managing transmission anxiety**

- Reducing risk of transmission
- Avoid sex when symptoms or signs suggestive of HSV infection present
- Use condoms (reduces transmission by 50%)
- Suppressive antivirals will reduce transmission by up to 50% (this effect has only been looked for with one antiviral to date)
- Sharing a diagnosis with a partner allows the couple to work together to avoid transmission

Transmissions in pregnancy should be avoided if at all possible. Acquisition of HSV infection in the third trimester of pregnancy is associated with an unacceptable high risk of HSV transmission to the neonate if vaginal delivery is attempted. Disease acquired prior to the third trimester is associated with much less risk but may still require special precautions during delivery.

Lymphogranuloma venereum

Aetiology

Lymphogranuloma venereum (LGV) is also known as tropical or climatic bubo, and lymphogranuloma inguinale. It is an STI caused by *Chlamydia trachomatis*, serovars L1, L2, and L3. Unlike the oculogenital strains of *C. trachomatis* (serovars A–K) which cause mucosal disease, these organisms invade and destroy lymphatic tissue.

Epidemiology

Lymphogranuloma venereum has long been recognised to be prevalent in many tropical countries, particularly in parts of Africa, Asia, the Caribbean, Central and South America. Classic LGV (seen in tropical countries) is usually acquired heterosexually. Until 2003, LGV had been rare in the developed world for several decades. Since 2003, there have been a series of LGV outbreaks (L2 serovar) in Europe and North America among men who have sex with men (MSM) who principally present with anorectal syndromes of proctitis or proctocolitis (see Chapters 6 and 20).

Clinical features

The clinical course of LGV infection may be divided into three stages: primary (transient genital ulceration), secondary (inguinal or anorectal syndrome), and tertiary (genito-anorectal syndrome).

The primary stage occurs about 3–30 days after infection and is characterised by transient papules or ulcers at the site of inoculation. The lesion is usually a single non-indurated ulcer, occasionally painful, and heals rapidly without scarring.

The secondary stage occurs on average 2–6 weeks after the primary stage, manifesting with either inguinal or anorectal sympyoms. The typical presentation (seen in the tropics) of LGV is as an inguinal syndrome consisting of unilateral inguinal and/or femoral lymphadenopathy and the formation of buboes (enlarged tender painful glands in the groin). About one-third of patients may have the characteristic 'groove sign' – a groove-like depression caused by femoral and inguinal lymph node enlargement above and below the inguinal ligament (Figure 12.9). Inguinal buboes may suppurate and rupture. In women, inguinal and/or femoral lymphadenopathy is less common than in men probably because primary involvement is usually in the vagina, cervix, posterior urethra, or rectum, which drain into the deep iliac or perirectal lymph nodes. The secondary stage may also present as an anorectal syndrome in those engaging in anal intercourse (see Chapters 6 and 20).

The tertiary stage follows chronic untreated infection and may occur any number of years after infection. The resultant fibrosis leads to lymphatic obstruction and genital lymphoedema. Women may develop oedema (elephantiasis) of the vulva with formation of polypoid growths, fistulae, ulceration, and scarring (esthiomene). Elephantiasis may affect the male genitalia leading to oedema and deformity of the penis. Late complications include rectal strictures,

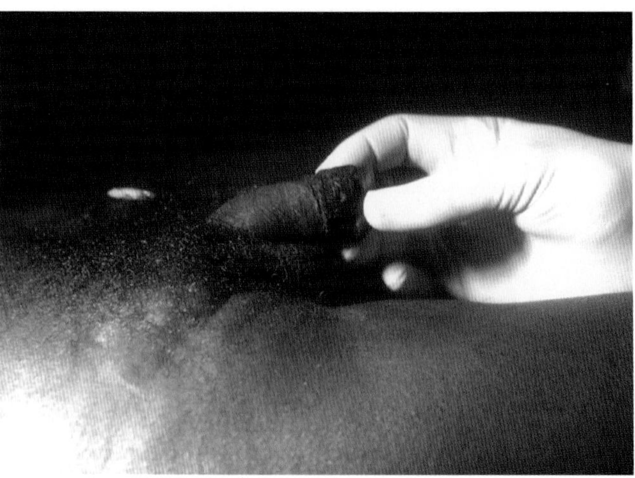

Figure 12.9 Lymphogranuloma venereum, with groove sign. Courtesy of Dr Colm O'Mahoney.

proctitis, colitis, perianal abscess, perineal fistulae, rectovaginal fistulae, and urethral fistulae. Intestinal obstruction may result from stricture formation.

Diagnosis

Lymphogranuloma venereum must be considered in anyone presenting with genital ulceration, regional lymphadenopathy, and/or anorectal manifestations. Diagnosis is confirmed by detecting the L serovar of *C. trachomatis* by PCR from lesional samples.

Management

Patients should be advised to avoid sexual intercourse until they and their partner(s) have finished treatment.

Accepted first-line treatment is doxycycline 100 mg twice daily or erythromycin 500 mg four times daily – both should be given for 3 weeks. Buboes may require repeated aspiration even after appropriate antimicrobial therapy. Patients with long-term complications such as fibrosis and fistulae require surgical intervention.

Chancroid

Chancroid is caused by *Haemophilus ducreyi*. It has a high incidence in tropical countries such as Africa, Asia, South America and the Caribbean. The incubation period is 3–10 days.

The main clinical features are single or multiple non-indurated ('soft sore') painful anogenital ulcers with a purulent base with contact bleeding, painful – mostly unilateral – inguinal lymphadenopathy (Figure 12.10). Complications are tissue destruction (phagedenic ulceration), inguinal abscess formation (bubo), and chronic suppurative sinuses.

Diagnosis is by microscopy/culture but both are poorly sensitive. PCR is the most sensitive test but not widely available. A swab is taken for microscopy from a cleaned ulcer or bubo by rolling the swab through 180 degrees on the slide (reveals typical bacilli running in parallel in a 'shoal of fish' formation).

Treatment is with azithromycin 1 g single dose, ceftriaxone 250 mg IM single dose, ciprofloxacin 500 mg orally twice daily for 3 days, or erythromycin 500 mg orally four times daily for 7 days. Needle aspiration or incision and drainage of fluctuant buboes should be performed.

Donovanosis (granuloma inguinale)

Donovanosis is caused by *Klebsiella* (*Calymmatobacterium*) *granulomatis*. It occurs in localised areas of Papua New Guinea, India, Brazil, South Africa, and Aboriginal Australia.

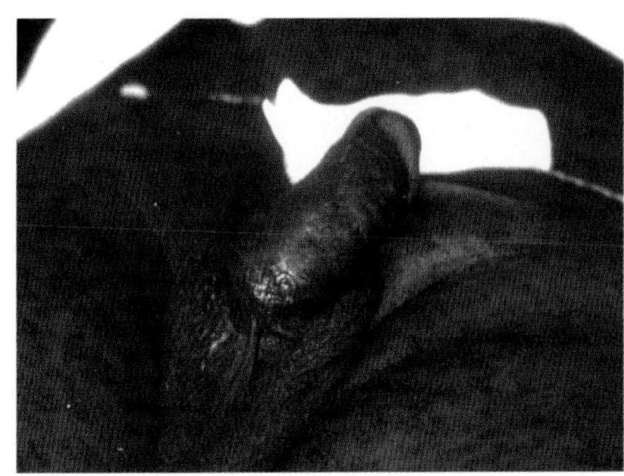

Figure 12.10 Chancroid ulcer. Courtesy of Dr Colm O'Mahoney.

The incubation period is uncertain, probably around 50 days. The main clinical features are slow-growing painless friable genital and inguinal lesions which are typically granulomatous, beefy-red, and haemorrhagic. Complications are destruction of genital tissue, genital lymphoedema (elephantiasis), and stenosis (anus, urethra, vagina).

Diagnosis is by demonstration of intracellular Donovan bodies (bipolar 'closed safety pin'-like organisms) from either cellular material obtained from scraping/impression smear/swab/crushing pinched off tissue fragment or biopsy.

Treatment is with azithromycin 1 g weekly daily, ceftriaxone 1 g daily IM, co-trimoxazole 960 mg twice daily, doxycycline 100 mg twice daily, or erythromycin 500 mg four times a day, all for a minimum of 3 weeks or until the lesions are healing.

Further reading

Corey L, Wald A. Genital herpes. In Holmes KK, Sparling PF, Stamm WE, Piot P, Wasserheit JN, Corey L, *et al. Sexually Transmistted Diseases*, 4th edn. McGraw Hill, New York, 2008, pp. 399–438.

Corey L, Wald A, Patel R, Sacks SL, Tyring SK, Warren T, *et al.* Once-daily valacyclovir to reduce the risk of transmission of genital herpes. *N Engl J Med* 2004;**350**(1):11–20.

National Guideline for the Management of Genital Herpes, LGV, Chancroid, Donovanosis. Available at www.bashh.org/guidelines.

Patel R. Educational interventions and the prevention of herpes simplex virus transmission. *Herpes* 2004;**11**(Suppl 3):155A–60A.

Wald A. Genital herpes. *Clin Evid* 2002;**8**:1608–19. (Update in *Clin Evid* 2003;**9**:1729–40.)

CHAPTER 13

Syphilis: Clinical Features, Diagnosis, and Management

Patrick French

Camden Primary Care Trust, London, UK

> **OVERVIEW**
>
> - Syphilis remains an important infection worldwide: it facilitates HIV transmission and it is a significant cause of perinatal morbidity and mortality
> - It is vital to consider a diagnosis of syphilis in a wide range of clinical syndromes
> - Syphilis is often asymptomatic, so screening populations at risk of syphilis acquisition or where preventing syphilis transmission is particularly harmful (e.g. pregnancy and blood donation) is essential
> - The cornerstone of syphilis diagnosis remains serological tests. Diagnostic algorithms for syphilis testing are available
> - Parenteral penicillin remains the treatment of choice for all stages of syphilis

Syphilis is a bacterial infection caused by *Treponema pallidum subsp pallidum* (abbreviated to *T. pallidum* in this chapter) which is either sexually transmitted or transmitted from mother to child during pregnancy (Figure 13.1; Box 13.1).

> Box 13.1 **Characteristics of *Treponema pallidum*: the cause of syphilis**
>
> - Coiled motile spirochaete bacterium
> - Humans are the only natural host
> - Genome sequenced, very small, circular
> - Obligate parasite (severely limited metabolic capabilities)
> - No *in vitro* culture

The introduction of penicillin had a dramatic impact on early syphilis in the 1940s. In the United Kingdom, syphilis decreased substantially from the peak during the Second World War and between 1985 and 1998 transmission of syphilis within the United Kingdom was extremely rare (Figure 13.2). Since 1999 there has been a sustained outbreak in the United Kingdom particularly amongst men who have sex with men with a parallel but less marked increase in heterosexual men and women. It remains a major cause of morbidity and mortality worldwide with an estimated 12–14 million new infections per year.

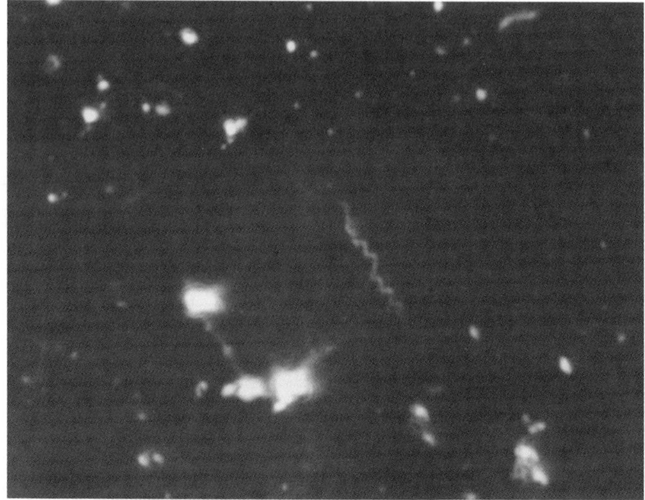

Figure 13.1 *Treponema pallidum*: the cause of syphilis, dark ground microscopy. Courtesy of CDC, VDRL Department.

The ulcerative lesions of primary and secondary syphilis are an important facilitator of HIV transmission in many parts of the world and it is estimated that 0.75–1.3 million babies are born with congenital syphilis every year.

Stages and natural history of syphilis

Syphilis has a natural history of usually distinct but occasionally overlapping 'stages' (Table 13.1).

Primary syphilis

The incubation period for primary syphilis is 9–90 days (usually 14–21 days). Lesions are found at the site of inoculation. This is usually in the genital or perianal areas but may be extragenital, with the mouth being the most common extragenital site.

The lesion is normally solitary and painless (Figure 13.3a, b), but can be multiple and painful (Figure 13.3c). It first develops as a red macule which progresses to a papule and finally ulcerates.

ABC of Sexually Transmitted Infections, Sixth Edition.
Edited by Karen E. Rogstad.

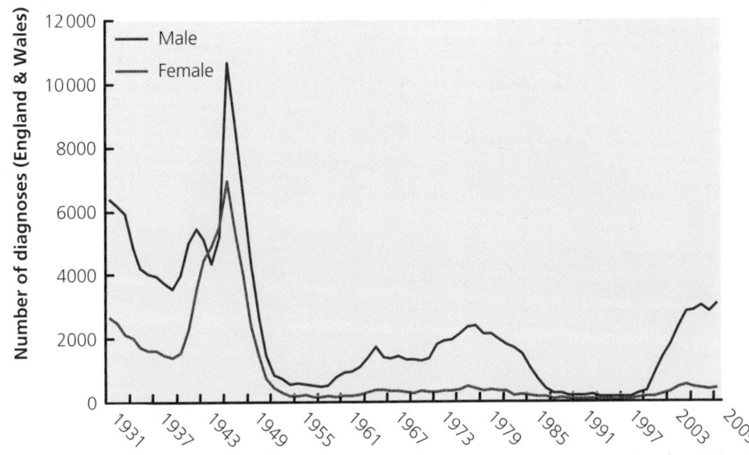

Figure 13.2 Infectious syphilis in England & Wales 1931–2009. Courtesy of the Health Protection Agency.

Table 13.1 Stages of syphilis and natural history.

Stage	Time after exposure
Early infectious	
Primary	9–90 days (usually 14–21 days)
Secondary	6 weeks to 6 months (4–8 weeks after primary infection)
Latent (early)–asymptomatic	Less than 2 years
Late non-infectious	
Latent (late) – asymptomatic	>2 years
Neurosyphilis	3–20 years
Cardiovascular syphilis	>10–40 years
Gummatous syphilis	3–12 years

This ulcer is usually round and clean with an indurated base and defined edges. Local inguinal lymph nodes are moderately enlarged, rubbery, painless, and discrete.

The primary lesions heal within 3–10 weeks and may go unnoticed by the patient, particularly lesions on the cervix, rectum, anal canal and margin.

Secondary syphilis

The lesions of secondary syphilis usually occur 4–8 weeks after appearance of the primary lesion. In about one-third of cases the primary lesion is still present. The lesions are generalised, affecting both skin and mucous membranes (Table 13.2).

Table 13.2 Clinical features of secondary syphilis.

Skin lesions	75–80%
Generalised lymphadenopathy	50–60%
Mucous membrane lesions	30%
Malaise, fevers	15%
Hepatitis	Rare (<10%)
Glomerulonephritis and nephritic syndrome	Rare (<10%)
Iridocyclitis and choroidoretinitis	Rare (<10%)
Neurological disease (meningitis and cranial nerve palsies)	Rare (<10%)
Alopecia	Rare (<10%)
Lesions of secondary syphilis	
Skin	Macular or papular Condylomata lata Papulosquamous Pustular
Mucous membranes	Erosions

The skin lesions are usually symmetrical and non-itchy. They can be macular, papular, papulosquamous, and, very rarely, pustular. The macular lesions (0.5–1 cm in diameter) appear on the trunk and arms. The papular lesions are coppery red and are the same size as the macules. They may occur on the trunk, palms, arms, legs, soles, face, and genitalia. Skin lesions are commonly a mixture of macular and papular lesions (maculopapular; Figures 13.4 and 13.5a).

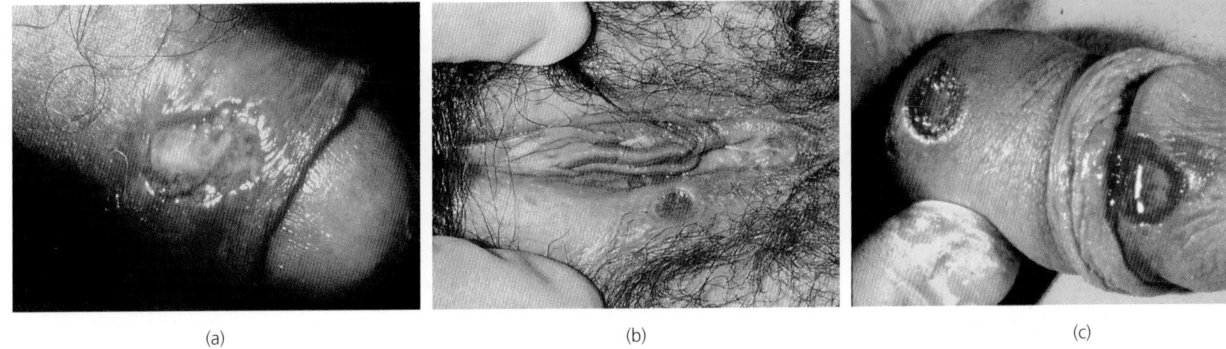

Figure 13.3 Primary syphilis: (a) chancre of penis; (b) chancre of vulva; (c) "kissing" ulcers of the penis.

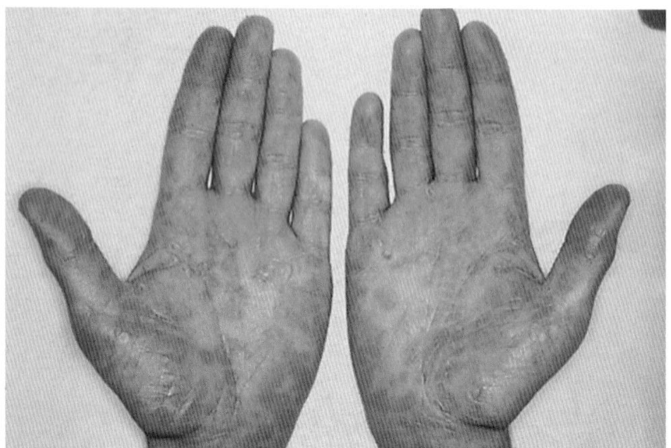

Figure 13.4 Secondary syphilis: maculopapular rash on hands.

In warm, opposed areas of the body, such as the anus and labia, papular lesions can become large and coalese to form large fleshy masses (condylomata lata) (Figure 13.5b). The papulosquamous lesions are found when scaling of the papules occurs and can be seen in association with straightforward papular lesions. If papulosquamous lesions occur on the palms or soles they are sometimes described as psoriasiform.

Pustular lesions are rare and occur when the papular lesions undergo central necrosis. Mucous membrane lesions are shallow painless erosions which are usually found in association with papular skin lesions and affect the mucous surface of the lips, cheeks, tongue, face, pharynx, larynx, nose, vulva, vagina, glans penis, prepuce, and cervix. They have a greyish appearance and are sometimes described as 'snail track' ulcers.

Non-specific constitutional symptoms of malaise, fever, anorexia, and generalised lymphadenopathy may be present. The secondary stage is one of bacteraemia, and any organ may show evidence of this, for example hepatitis, iritis, meningitis, and optic neuritis with papilloedema.

Without treatment, the symptoms and signs resolve. About one-quarter of untreated patients have recurrent episodes of secondary syphilis but this is rare after the first year of infection.

Latent syphilis

People with untreated syphilis but no symptoms or signs of infection have latent syphilis. This latent period is divided into an early stage, in which the disease has been present for less than 2 years, and a late stage, in which the disease has been present for more than 2 years.

Acquired syphilis has been classified traditionally as either early infectious or late non-infectious syphilis. The arbitrary cut-off point between these stages is defined as 2 years in the United Kingdom and World Health Organization guidelines but 1 year according to the European and Centers for Disease Control (CDC, United States) guidelines

Natural history studies of syphilis during the early part of the twentieth century found that 10% of patients develop neurological lesions, 10% cardiovascular lesions, and 15% gummatous lesions (Table 13.1). It is uncertain whether the natural history of syphilis remains the same and it is extremely rare to see late syphilis in the developed world. This may be because of the decline in infectious syphilis, improved clinics and treatment facilities, and perhaps a widespread use of antibiotics that may inadvertently treat syphilis.

Neurosyphilis

Neurosyphilis is classified as asymptomatic, meningovascular, or parenchymatous (general paresis and tabes dorsalis).

Meningovascular syphilis

This can be present in the early and late stages of syphilis. Patients can present with acute meningeal involvement during the secondary

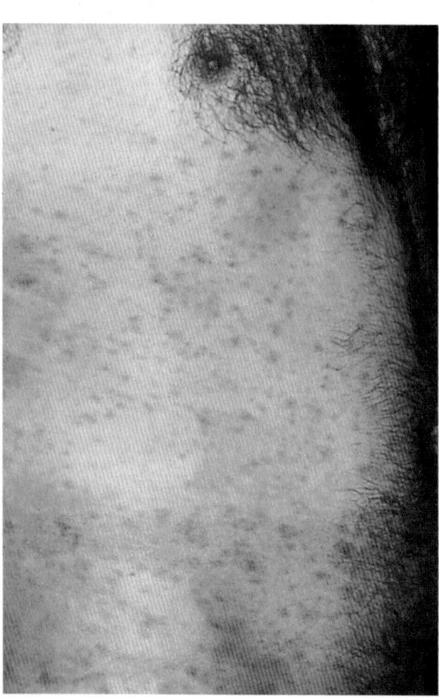

(a)

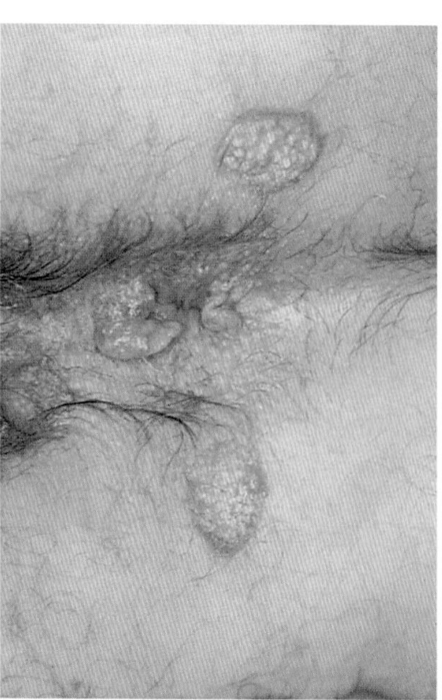

(b)

Figure 13.5 Secondary syphilis: (a): maculopapular rash on chest; (b) condylomata lata – perianal.

stages of the disease, which often coincides with the development of skin lesions. Headache is the main symptom.

Signs of meningitis are found with third, sixth, and eighth cranial nerve involvement, papilloedema, and, rarely homonymous hemianopia or hemiplegia. Late meningovascular syphilis presents less acutely but headaches may still be a presenting symptom. Cranial nerve palsies (third, sixth, seventh, and eighth) and papillary abnormalities are seen. The pupils are small and unequal in size and react to accommodation but not light (Argyll Robertson pupils). Cerebral and spinal cord (anterior spinal artery) vessels may be affected.

Parenchymatous neurosyphilis

This may present as general paresis, tabes dorsalis, or, rarely, as a combination of the two. General paresis with resulting cerebral atrophy occurs 10–20 years after the original primary infection (Box 13.2).

Box 13.2 **General paresis**

Symptoms

Early

- Irritability
- Fatigability
- Personality changes
- Headaches
- Impaired memory
- Tremors

Late

- Lack of insight
- Depression or euphoria
- Confusion and disorientation
- Delusions
- Seizures
- Transient paralysis and aphasia

Signs

- Expressionless facies
- Tremor of lips, tongue, and hands
- Dysarthria
- Impairment of handwriting
- Hyperactive tendon reflexes
- Pupillary abnormalities
- Optic atrophy
- Convulsions
- Extensor plantar responses

Tabes dorsalis is characterised by increasing ataxia, failing vision, sphincter disturbances, and attacks of severe pain (Box 13.3). These pains are described as 'lightening' because they occur as acute stabbing pain mostly in the legs. The signs of tabes dorsalis are largely caused by degeneration of the posterior columns: absent ankle and knee reflexes (rarely, biceps and triceps), impaired vibration and position sense, and a positive Romberg's sign.

Asymptomatic neurosyphilis

As the name implies, no neurological symptoms or signs are detected in asymptomatic neurosyphilis and the diagnosis is based entirely on positive test results in serum and cerebrospinal fluid.

Box 13.3 **Tabes dorsalis**

Symptoms

- Lightening pains
- Ataxia
- Bladder disturbance
- Paraesthesiae
- Tabetic crises
- Visual loss
- Rectal incontinence
- Deafness
- Impotence

Signs

- Argyll Robertson pupils
- Absent ankle reflexes
- Absent knee reflexes
- Absent biceps and triceps reflexes
- Romberg's signs
- Impaired vibration sense
- Impaired position sense
- Impaired sense of touch and pain
- Optic atrophy
- Ocular palsies
- Charcot's joints

Cardiovascular syphilis

This most commonly occurs in large vessels, particularly the aorta, but medium and small sized vessels may also be affected. The aorta is affected by an aortitis (with or without coronary ostial stenosis), aneurysm of the ascending part, and aortic incompetence. The symptoms of an aneurysm affecting the arch usually result from the pressure on structures within the superior mediastinum (Figure 13.6).

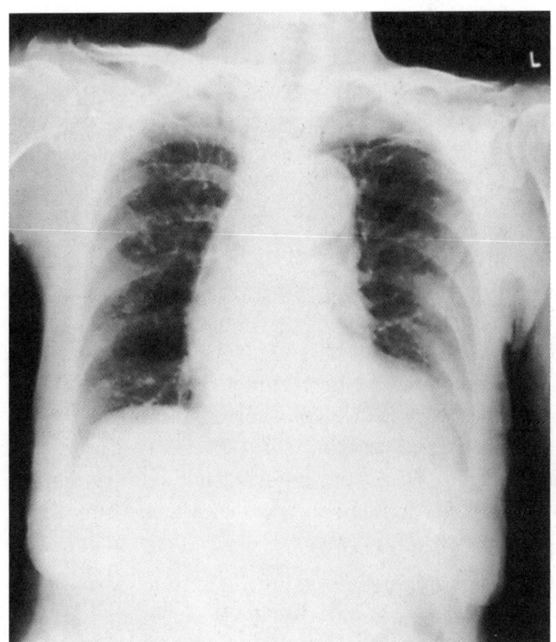

Figure 13.6 Chest X-ray, cardiovascular syphilis – aortic aneurysm and cardiomegaly.

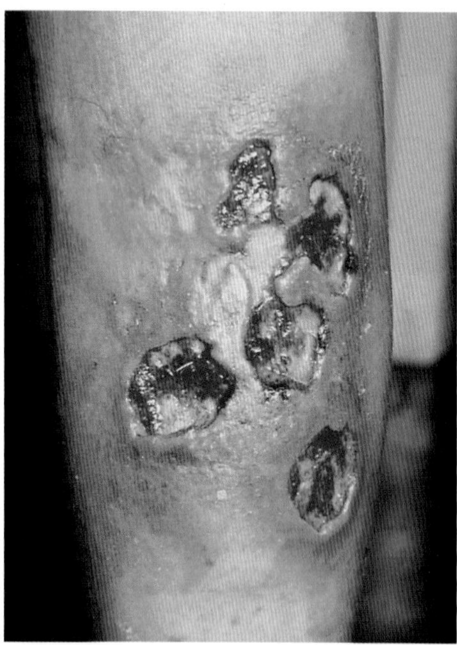

Figure 13.7 Gummata of the leg.

Gummata

These are granulomatous lesions that develop 3–12 years after the primary infection. Gummata may occur on the skin or mucous membranes and in bone or viscera. Skin lesions are usually nodular. They can occur anywhere on the skin and are found as small groups of painless lesions that are indolent, firm, coppery red, and about 0.5–1 cm in diameter (Figure 13.7).

Diagnosis and management

Establishing a diagnosis of syphilis is usually straightforward but sometimes can be difficult and it is reasonable for all suspected cases to be referred to or discussed with an STI specialist. The diagnosis can be confirmed by history, physical examination, and one or all of *T. pallidum* polymerase chain reaction (PCR) or dark ground microscopy, serology, examination of cerebrospinal fluid, and radiology. The application and interpretation of these investigations depend on the clinical stage of the syphilis.

History and examination

Assessment of an individual suspected to have syphilis should include a careful history of previous syphilis screening and previous diagnosis of syphilis. If a diagnosis of syphilis has been made in the past, then it is important to attempt to determine the stage of disease, the treatment given, and the serological response to treatment, particularly the rapid plasma reagin (RPR) or venereal disease research laboratory (VDRL) test. History-taking and examination should assess for possible symptoms and signs of early and late syphilis.

The tests for syphilis

Treponema pallidum cannot be cultured and diagnostic tests for syphilis depend on direct identification of *T. pallidum* or serological tests.

Direct tests

Dark ground microscopy

This test can be used to establish the diagnosis from the lesions of primary and secondary syphilis or occasionally from material obtained by puncture of the inguinal nodes (especially if a topical antiseptic has been applied or if lesions are healed or concealed) (Figure 13.1). The presence of oral commensal treponaemes makes microscopy unreliable for mouth lesions.

Three separate specimens from the lesion(s) should be examined by dark ground microscopy initially and, if necessary, on three consecutive days. This is done by cleaning the lesion with a gauze swab soaked in normal saline and squeezing it to encourage a serum exudate. The serum is then scraped off the lesion and placed on the three slides.

In the past, dark ground microscopy was a vital test in primary syphilis because it might be the only means of establishing a positive diagnosis. However, considerable experience is required to recognise *T. pallidum* and it is a test usually confined to specialist centres. The treponaeme is bluish-white, closely coiled (8–24 coils), and 6–20 μm long (Figure 13.1). It has three characteristic movements: watch spring, corkscrew, and angular.

T. pallidum nucleic acid amplification testing

Increasingly, *T. pallidum* nucleic acid amplification tests (NAATs) are being used to diagnose early syphilis. These tests have excellent sensitivity and specificity compared with dark ground microscopy and eliminate the observer variability problems that make it difficult to use dark ground microscopy in non-specialist settings. It is likely that *T. pallidum* NAATs will become increasingly established in clinical settings.

Serological tests

The serological tests used to diagnose syphilis are either non-specific (non-treponemal) or specific (treponemal) (Table 13.3; Box 13.4). These tests have different and complimentary characteristics and in combination within an algorithm can be used to screen for and confirm a diagnosis of syphilis (Figure 13.8). Specific tests for syphilis are useful for confirming the diagnosis particularly at first presentation; however, these tests usually remain positive throughout a patient's life even after successful treatment. Non-specific tests are useful for monitoring the response to treatment and the diagnosis of reinfection of syphilis. However, they may also give false positive results in a variety of conditions.

Non-specific tests

The most widely used non-specific test is the RPR test (some centres use the VDRL test). These tests depend on the appearance of cardiolipin antibody (reagin) in the serum and usually become positive 3–5 weeks after the patient has contracted the infection. They are both quantitative tests and can be useful in assessing the stage and activity of the disease. Decreasing titres are associated with treatment response and increasing titres are associated with treatment failure and reinfection. However, VDRL and RPR titres also decay naturally without treatment, so untreated patients may have active disease despite low titre or negative RPR and VDRL results.

Both tests may yield biological false positive reactions to acute infections (such as herpes viruses, measles, and mumps) or after

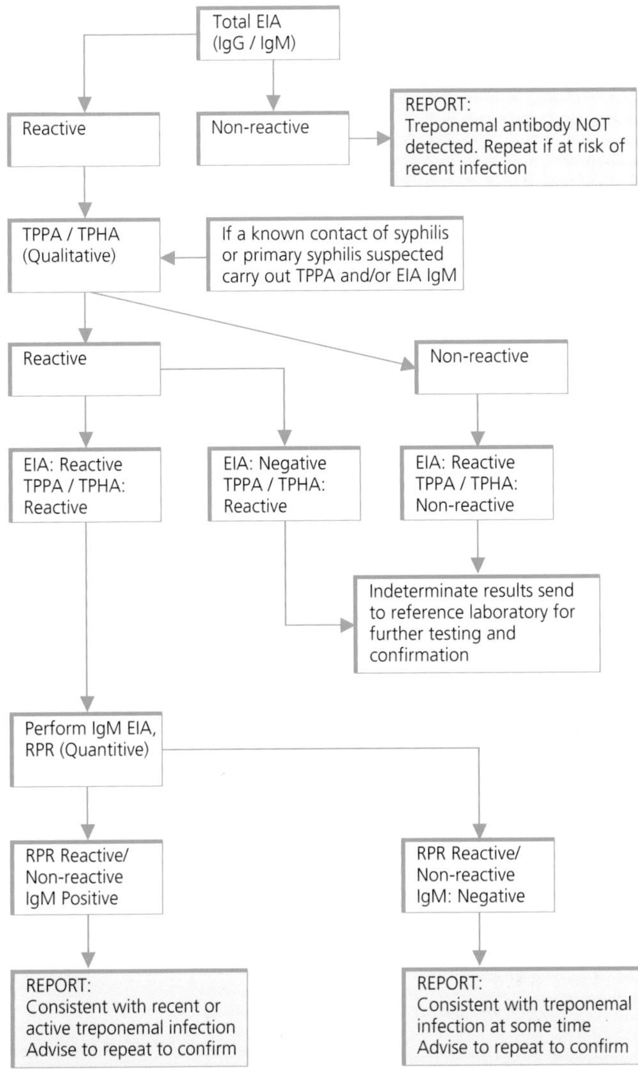

Figure 13.8 Syphilis testing algorithm. Adapted from Serological Diagnosis of Syphilis, Standards Unit, Evaluation and Standards Laboratory, 2007. Health Protection Agency, UK.

Box 13.4 **Serological tests**

Non-specific

- Rapid plasma reagin (RPR)
- Venereal disease reference laboratory (VDRL)

Specific

- *T. pallidum* enzyme immunoassay (EIA)
- *T. pallidum* particle agglutination assay (TPPA)
- Chemiluminescent microparticle immunoassay (CMIA)
- Absorbed fluorescent treponemal antibody (FTA)
- *T. pallidum* haemagglutination assay (TPHA)

immunisation against typhoid or yellow fever. Chronic causes of biological false positive reactions include autoimmune diseases and rheumatoid arthritis.

Table 13.3 Diagnosis and serological interpretation.

Results positive	Diagnosis
None	Syphilis not present or very early primary syphilis
All	Untreated, recently treated, or latent syphilis
EIA and RPR only	Primary syphilis (if ulcer present)
EIA and TPPA	Treated syphilis or untreated late latent or late syphilis
EIA only	Early primary syphilis (or false positive EIA)
VDRL/RPR only	False positive

EIA, enzyme immunoassay; RPR, rapid plasma reagin; TPPA, *T. pallidum* particle agglutination assay; VDRL, venereal disease reference laboratory.

Specific tests

The specific tests include the *Treponema pallidum* enzyme immunoassay (EIA) tests which are replacing the fluorescent treponemal antibody test (FTA) and *T. pallidum* haemagglutination assay (TPHA) test as the specific test of choice for syphilis screening. The *T. pallidum* particle agglutination assay (TPPA) is more often used in preference to the TPHA to confirm a positive EIA test. The EIA tests have the advantage of becoming positive early on in the course of infection and are easier to automate. The combined IgG/IgM EIA test is usually the first to become positive – 2–4 weeks after infection. These tests are positive in 85–90% of cases of primary syphilis. In early syphilis they may be the only positive serological tests.

Specific and non-specific tests are also positive in other treponemal conditions that are similar to syphilis, such as yaws, bejel, and pinta. Bejel and pinta are unusual conditions; however, yaws remains endemic in a number of countries around the world. Yaws is caused by the spirochaete *Treponema pallidum subsp pertenue*. It is usually an infection acquired in childhood and is characterised by skin ulceration, usually of the lower limbs.

Cerebrospinal fluid tests

Abnormalities of the cerebrospinal fluid (CSF) may be found at any stage of syphilis and are common in early syphilis (particularly the secondary stage). Lumbar puncture is not routinely required in early syphilis or in asymptomatic late syphilis; however, it is important that all patients with suspected neurosyphilis have a full neurological examination and CSF assessment. Some specialists also recommend that all patients with HIV infection and syphilis for more than 2 years should have a lumbar puncture to assess possible neurological involvement (see below).

Most patients with neurosyphilis will have a CSF white cell count $>5 \times 10^6$/L and a protein level >40 g/L. Provided that the CSF is not contaminated with macroscopic blood, the treponemal and non-treponemal tests are useful to diagnose neurosyphilis. Most patients with positive CSF RPR or VDRL tests will have neurosyphilis, although some people with probable neurosyphilis may have negative non-specific tests but a raised white cell count. Although many individuals with positive treponemal serum tests have positive EIA or TPPA in the CSF, negative tests virtually rule out neurosyphilis.

Table 13.4 Treatment of syphilis.

Stage	Standard treatment	Alternatives*
Primary, secondary and early latent syphilis (less than 2 years)	Benzathine penicillin 2.4 mega units IM as a single dose or aqueous procaine penicillin 600 000 units IM per day for 10 days	Doxycycline 100 mg orally twice a day for 14 days
Late latent syphilis (more than 2 years) Cardiovascular syphilis Gummatous syphilis	Benzathine penicillin 2.4 mega units IM weekly over 2 weeks (three injections) Aqueous procaine penicillin 600 000 units IM per day for 17 days	Doxycycline 100 mg orally twice a day for 28 days
Neurosyphilis	Aqueous procaine penicillin 1.8–2.4 mega units IM per day for 17 days combined with probenecid 500 mg four times per day	Doxycycline 200 mg orally twice daily for 28 days†

*Many specialists recommend that pregnant patients who are allergic to penicillin should be offered penicillin desensitisation.
†Some specialists recommend that patients with neurosyphilis who are allergic to penicillin should be offered penicillin desensitisation.

Chest X-ray

Chest radiography (posterior and anterior and left lateral) to show the arch of the aorta and to screen for aortic dilatation should be performed on those who may have had infection for more than 20 years.

Treatment and prognosis

Penicillin remains the treatment of choice. In primary, secondary, and early latent syphilis treatment can be given in a form of benzathine pencillin as a single injection or 10 days of procaine penicillin. Patients with penicillin allergy or patients who decline parenteral treatment can be prescribed doxycycline therapy (Table 13.4). Further advice on treatment options is available from the web sites of specialist organisations and the CDC in the United States.

The prognosis of treated syphilis depends on the stage of the disease and the degree of tissue damage in cardiovascular and neurological syphilis. Adequate treatment of primary, secondary, and latent syphilis will always halt the progression of the disease. The prognosis in symptomatic neurosyphilis is variable. Although, in general, the inflammatory process is arrested by adequate treatment, tissue damage may be too great to give any improvement. In cardiovascular disease, the onset of symptoms usually indicates established aortic medial necrosis that is not reversed by treatment.

All patients who are being treated for syphilis should be warned of potential treatment reactions including antibiotic allergy, the procaine reaction, and the Jarisch–Herxheimer reaction.

The Jarisch–Herxheimer reaction is common in primary and secondary syphilis and patients must be warned that fever and 'flu like symptoms may occur 3–12 hours after the first injection of penicillin; occasionally, the chancre or skin lesions enlarge or become more widespread. Reassurance and antipyretics such as paracetamol and non-steroidal anti-inflammatory agents are all that is required.

For a patient with early infectious syphilis, contact tracing must be carried out on all sexual contacts in the previous 3–6 months. In late syphilis when a patient is no longer infectious, serological testing is usually only practicable in the patient's regular partner(s). If late syphilis is diagnosed in a mother it may be necessary to test her children (see Chapter 11).

Overview of syphilis

Cause
- *T. pallidum subsp pallidum* a spirochaete bacterium

Initial site of infection
- Site of exposure, usually genitals, perianal area, or mouth

Incubation period
- Usually 2–3 weeks (range 9–90 days) to primary syphilis

Primary syphilis
- Ulceration at site of exposure

Secondary syphilis
- Systemic illness 2–3 months (range 1–6 months) after primary syphilis

Early latent syphilis
- Asymptomatic syphilis of less than 2 years' duration

Late latent syphilis
- Asymptomatic syphilis of more than 2 years' duration

Gummata
- Necrotic nodules or plaques
- 3–12 years after primary infection

Neurosyphilis
- General paresis: 10–20 years after primary infection
- Tabes dorsalis (dorsal column impairment) 10–20 years after primary infection

Meningovascular syphilis
- Early (part of secondary syphilis)
- Late (2–20 years)

Cardiovascular syphilis
- Aortic regurgitation, angina, and aortic aneurysm
- 10–40 years after primary infection

Diagnosis
- Identification of *T. pallidum* in lesions of early syphilis (dark ground microscopy or PCR tests)
- Serology (specific or non-specific)
- Identification of complications of late syphilis

Treatment
- Parenteral pencillin (see text)
- Alternative – doxycycline

Syphilis and pregnancy

All pregnant women should have antenatal screening for syphilis. Syphilis remains an important cause of neonatal morbidity and mortality worldwide and continues to occur in the United Kingdom. The risk of transmission to the baby is particularly high in the early stages of infection (see Chapter 11).

Box 13.5 **Syphilis and HIV co-infection**

- Primary syphilis: larger, painful, multiple ulcers
- Secondary syphilis: genital ulcers (slow healing of primary ulcers). Higher titres of RPR/VDRL tests
- Possibly more rapid progression to neurosyphilis

HIV infection and syphilis

The clinical presentation, serological tests, and treatment response of early syphilis are usually identical in patients with and without HIV infection (Box 13.5). However, some differences have been recognised in prospective studies. There is a suggestion that HIV-positive individuals with syphilis have a more rapid progression to neurosyphilis and other forms of late syphilis; however, this observation has been confined to case reports. All patients with syphilis should have HIV testing and all individuals with HIV infection should have regular tests for syphilis.

Further reading

Centers for Disease Control. STI Guidelines 2006. www.cdc.gov/STD/treatment/2006/toc.htm.

European Guidelines for STIs. www.iusti.org/regions/europe/default.htm.

Holmes KK, Sparling PF, Stamm WE, Piot P, Wasserheit JN, Corey L, *et al. Sexually Transmistted Diseases*, 4th edn. McGraw Hill, New York, 2008.

Microscopy for sexually transmitted infections: an educational DVD for health care professionals. Available from www.bashh.org.

UK National Guidelines for STI. www.bashh.org/guidelines.

CHAPTER 14

Genital Growths and Infestations

Clare L N Woodward and Angela J Robinson

Department of Genitounrinary Medicine, Mortimer Market Centre, London, UK

OVERVIEW

- To know the differential diagnosis of genital growths
- To diagnose and manage anogenital warts
- To diagnose and manage molluscum contagiosum
- To manage genital infestations
- To counsel patients about genital growths and infestations

Genital warts

Genital warts are the most common viral sexually acquired infection. In the UK population the number of cases reported from genitourinary medicine clinics has continuously risen since records began in 1971. Warts are caused by the human papilloma virus (HPV), a small DNA virus that infects cutaneous or mucosal epithelium (Figure 14.1). Over 100 HPV genotypes have been described, of which at least 40 primarily infect genital epithelium. These are subdivided into low and high risk according to their association with neoplasia. The majority of visible genital warts are caused by low risk genotypes HPV-6 and HPV-11. High and low risk types can coexist.

Transmission and incubation period

Genital warts are spread by direct skin to skin contact with an infected person. The virus can therefore be passed on without penetrative sex or when using a condom, as condoms do not cover all the genital skin. Auto-inoculation from other sites is very rare in adults, as HPV is site-specific, although the prepubertal genital mucosa can support the growth of some hand wart types such as type 2.

The median incubation period for warts is 3 months, with a range of 2 weeks to 9 months but this can be much longer. Many people (one estimate suggests 99%) infected with genital HPV will never develop visible warts but can still transmit the virus. It is therefore not possible to identify the source of infection in most cases. It may be more likely that HPV is transmitted if warts are present and the viral load of whole virions shed is greater. Less is known about passing subclinical HPV to sex partners, but the virus can be transmitted even when there are no visible signs.

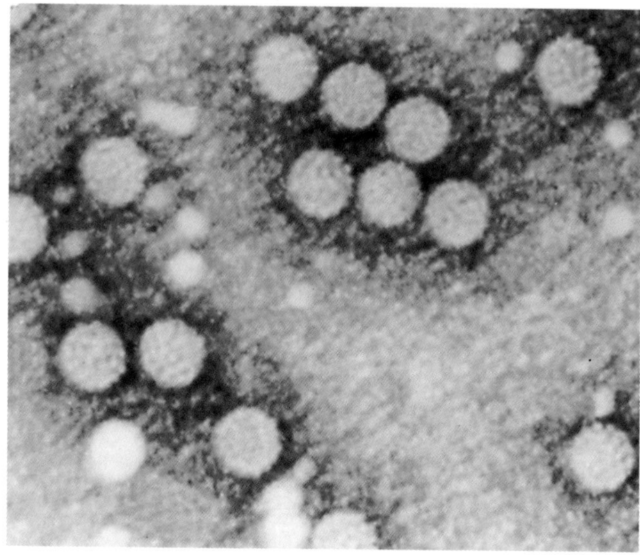

Figure 14.1 Papillomavirus.

Features

Most patients present after finding lumps around their genital area. Usually, these are asymptomatic, but they can be associated with a mild itch or irritation. Lesions may be single or multiple and tend to occur in areas that are traumatised during sexual intercourse but they may occur anywhere on genital skin. Perianal warts do not necessarily imply anal intercourse, but intra-anal warts are seen predominantly in patients who have had receptive anal sex. Warts have a variety of appearances (Figures 14.2–14.5; Box 14.1).

Diagnosis

Diagnosis is usually made by visual inspection with a bright light. The differential diagnosis is wide (Box 14.2). A biopsy should be considered when the diagnosis is uncertain; when warts are pigmented, indurated, or fixed; if lesions do not respond or worsen with treatment; or if there is persistent ulceration or bleeding. With immunocompromised patients more vigilance is required to ensure recognition of pre-malignant lesions.

ABC of Sexually Transmitted Infections, Sixth Edition.
Edited by Karen E. Rogstad.

Box 14.1 **Appearance of genital warts**

Condylomata acuminata

- Cauliflower-like appearance
- Skin-coloured, pink, or hyperpigmented
- Generally non-keratinised on mucosal surfaces; may be keratotic on skin

Smooth papules

- Usually dome-shaped and skin-coloured

Flat papules

- Macular to slightly raised
- Flesh-coloured, with smooth surface
- More commonly found on internal structures (e.g. cervix), but also occur on external genitalia

Keratotic warts

- Thick horny layer that can resemble common warts or seborrheic keratosis

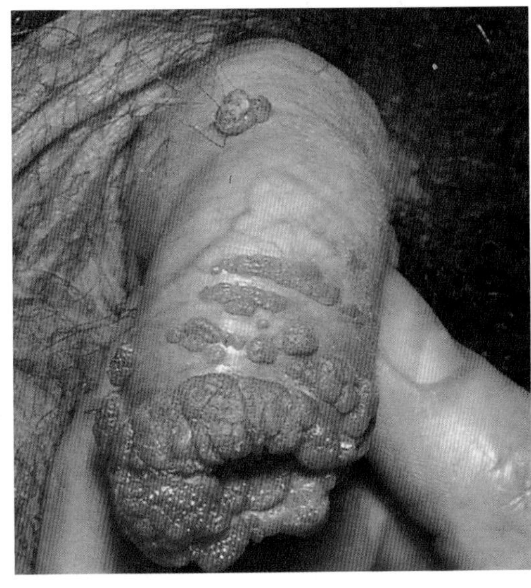

Figure 14.3 Penile warts.

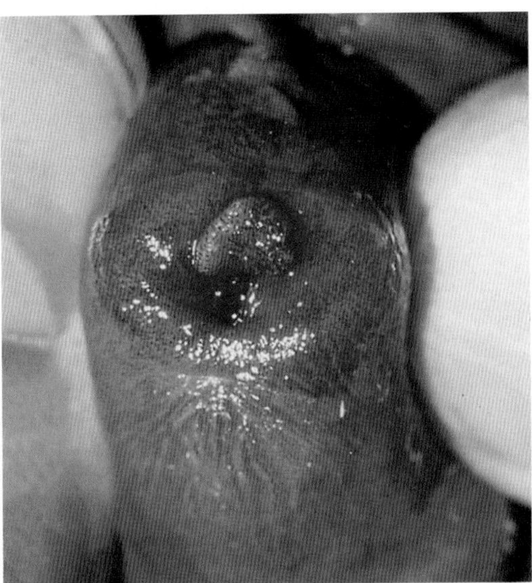

Figure 14.2 Intrameatal wart.

Box 14.2 **Differential diagnosis of genital warts**

Other infections

- Molluscum contagiosum
- Condylomata lata of syphilis

Acquired dermatological conditions

- Seborrheic keratosis
- Lichen planus
- Fibro-epithelial polyp, adenoma
- Melanocytic naevus
- Neoplastic lesions

Normal anatomical variants

- Pearly penile papules/coronal papillae
- Fordyce spots
- Vestibular papillae (micropapillomatosis labialis)
- Skin tags (acrochordons)

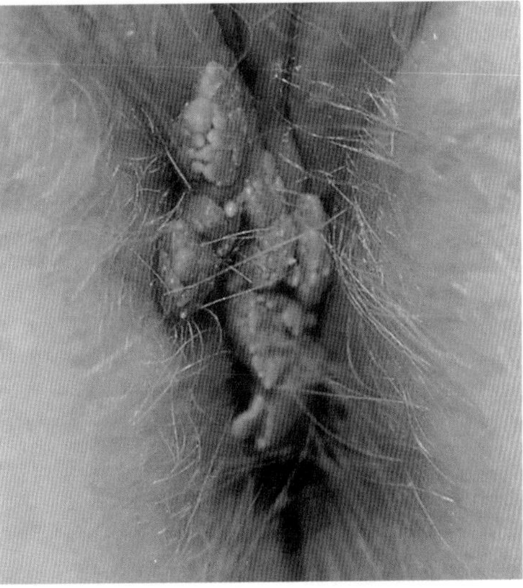

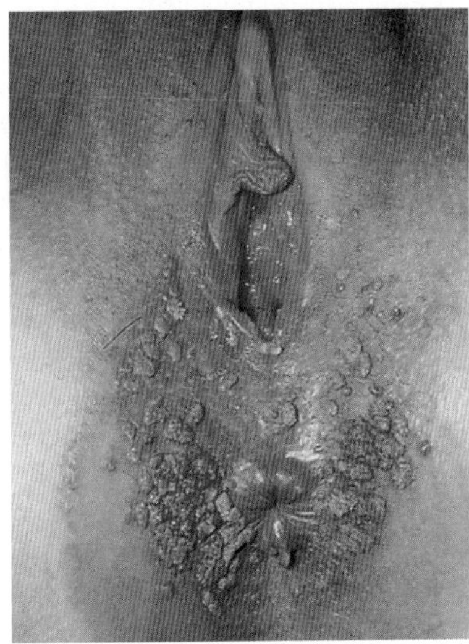

Figure 14.4 Vulval (left) and perianal (right) warts.

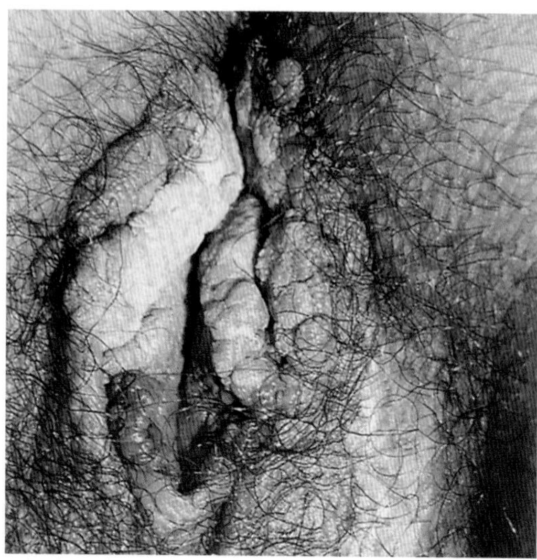

Figure 14.5 Massive warts in pregnancy.

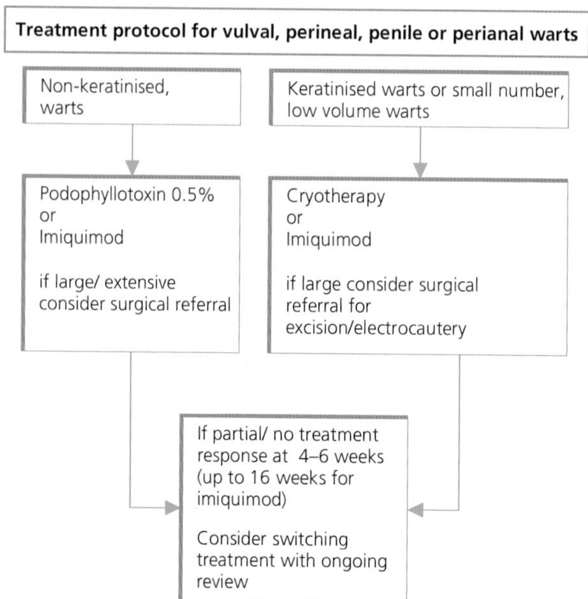

Figure 14.6 Treatment protocol for vulval, perineal, penile, or perianal warts.

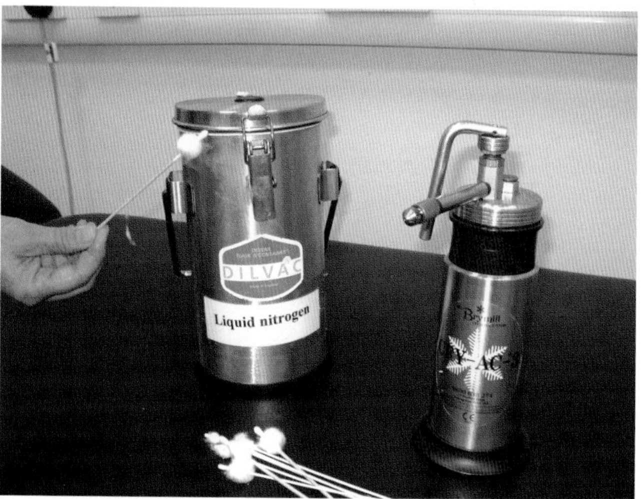

Figure 14.7 Liquid nitrogen for treatment of genital warts.

Management

Patients should be informed of the diagnosis, mode of transmission, and management options. Clear and accurate written information should be provided. They should also be offered a full sexually transmitted infection (STI) screen, to exclude concurrent STIs. There is evidence that using condoms and stopping smoking may improve HPV clearance. Tracing of previous sexual partners is not recommended, although current partner(s) may benefit from assessment to exclude undetected STI. No change is required in the screening intervals for cervical cytology for women with genital warts.

A multitude of treatment options is available for the management of warts. However, it is important to note that the available treatments have limited impact on viral clearance and infectivity and that most warts are treated for aesthetic reasons or symptomatic relief. The patient should be warned they may recur. Without treatment warts may disappear (5–30% at 3 months), stay the same (20%), or grow larger in size or number (50% at 3 months). Spontaneous resolution of genital warts is more common in children. No single treatment is ideal for all patients or all warts, and all treatments have significant failure rates. There is no definitive evidence from randomised trials to suggest that any of the available treatments is superior to any other.

Treatment choice depends on the morphology, number, and distribution of warts and patient preference. The risk of scarring and pigment change should be discussed before embarking on any treatment. Clinical outcome is improved by using a treatment protocol, with guidelines on treatment choice and follow-up (Figure 14.6).

Treatment can be subdivided into chemical applications, either cytotoxic or immune stimulant, and physical ablation. Commonly used chemical applications are podophyllotoxin 0.5% or imiquimod which is an α-interferon stimulant; occasionally trichloroacetic acid (TCA) is applied. 5-Fluorouracil, interferon injections, and podophyllin are no longer recommended in the routine management of genital warts. Soft non-keratinised warts often respond well to topical treatments. Cryotherapy is the most accessible ablative therapy (Figure 14.7); however, excision, electrosurgery, and laser treatment are options for more persistent warts. Keratinised warts are better treated by ablation, although imiquimod can be successful.

The majority of genital warts respond within 2–3 months of treatment but 30–60% of patients will experience a recurrence within 3 months. Most HPV infections will clear within 2 years in immunocompetent patients, leaving approximately 10% with subclinical HPV. Some special circumstances are considered in Table 14.1. Despite physical treatments being available, the negative psychological implications for patients receiving a diagnosis of genital warts should not be underestimated or trivialised. Genital warts have been associated with a significant detriment to quality of life including low self-esteem, clinical depression, increased stress, and negative impact on relationships. Patients need good and appropriate counselling to help manage these consequences.

Table 14.1 Special considerations.

Intravaginal warts	Treatment not often necessary. Cryotherapy, electrosurgery and TCA can be used
Cervical warts	None, or cryotherapy, electrosurgery, laser ablation, excision or TCA. Consider colposcopy if clinical concern or diagnostic uncertainty
Urethral meatal warts	If base of lesion seen: cryotherapy, electrosurgery, laser ablation, podophyllotoxin 0.5% or imiquimod If lesion deeper in urethra: none, or surgical ablation under direct vision
Intra-anal warts	None, cryotherapy, electrosurgery, laser ablation, TCA (with care), podophyllotoxin, imiquimod (see Chapter 20)
Pregnancy and immunosuppressed patients	See Chapter 11

TCA, trichloroacetic acid.

Prevention of warts and HPV-related cervical carcinoma with the HPV vaccine is discussed in Chapter 22.

Molluscum contagiosum

Molluscum contagiosum is caused by a pox virus, a large DNA virus that replicates in the cytoplasm of epithelial cells. It is transmitted by direct skin-to-skin contact, and when found on the genitals is most commonly secondary to sexual transmission (Figure 14.8). However, molluscum contagiosum is a common cutaneous infection of childhood transmitted through social contact and can be found in children on hands, faces, arms, and trunk. In immunocompromised patients lesions can also be found extragenitally, particularly on the face. The incubation period is usually 3–12 weeks, but can be up to 6 months.

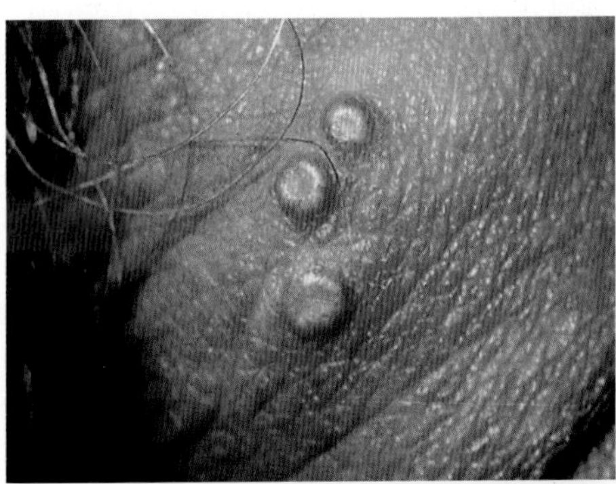

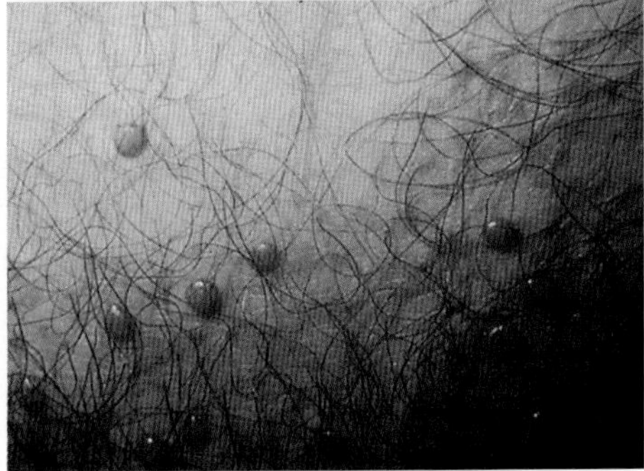

Figure 14.8 Molluscum contagiosum.

In genital infection, papules are found in the pubic hair, and on the thighs, buttocks, and lower abdomen but tend to spare mucous membranes. Clinically, lesions are multiple small (1–3 mm) smooth pearly coloured papules which often resemble fluid-filled vesicles but are in fact solid. Each papule develops a central umbilication as it reaches a few millimetres in diameter. Diagnosis is made by visual inspection and recognition of the typical lesions. If in doubt the central punctum can be extracted and poxvirus-like particles viewed under an electron microscope, or histology will reveal enlarged epithelial cells with intracytoplasmic molluscum bodies. A full STI screen should be offered.

Spontaneous resolution is common within 3 months, although up to 35% of patients experience a recurrence within 8–24 months. Treatment is offered for cosmetic reasons. Cryotherapy, extraction of the central core, and piercing with an orange stick that has been dipped in tincture of iodine or phenol are all recommended treatments for the genital area. Use of podophyllotoxin cream (0.5%) and imiquimod may help, but data on these remain limited. Partner notification is not required.

Scabies

Scabies is an infestation of the skin by the parasitic mite, *Sarcoptes scabiei* (Figure 14.9). It is transmitted by direct prolonged skin-to-skin contact. The mites can be transferred after about 20 minutes and can penetrate the epidermis after 30 minutes. Scabies can be sexually transmitted but also affects those who are not sexually active. Outbreaks are often seen when overcrowding occurs, for example in institutions and schools.

On first infection, symptoms, which are caused by a hypersensitivity reaction, generated by the absorption of mite excrement into skin capillaries, may take 4–6 weeks to develop. With reinfection, symptoms develop within 24–48 hours because of the previous sensitisation. The main symptom caused by this hypersensitivity is intense itching, which occurs especially at night.

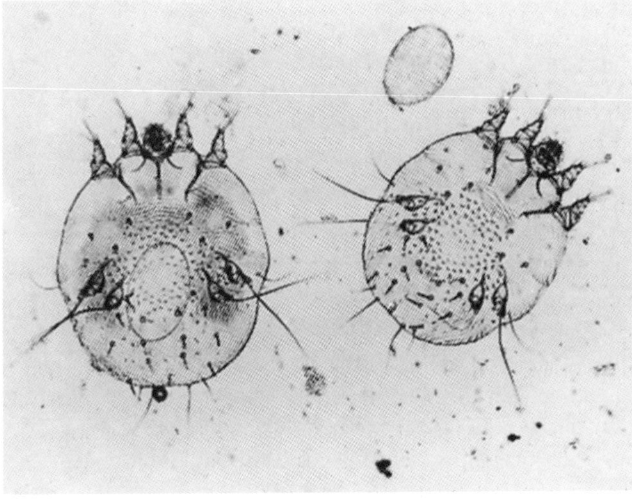

Figure 14.9 Scabei.

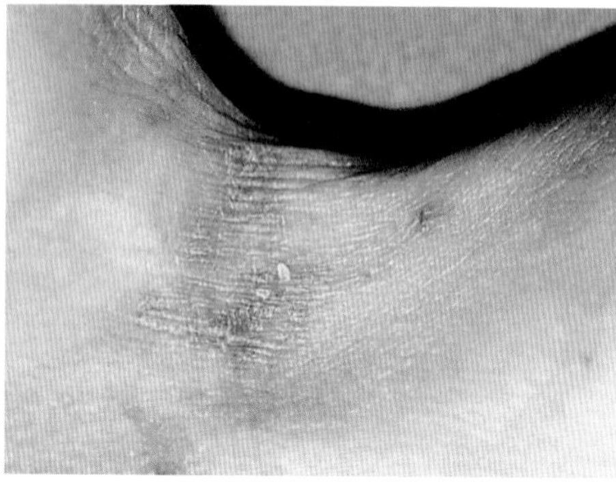

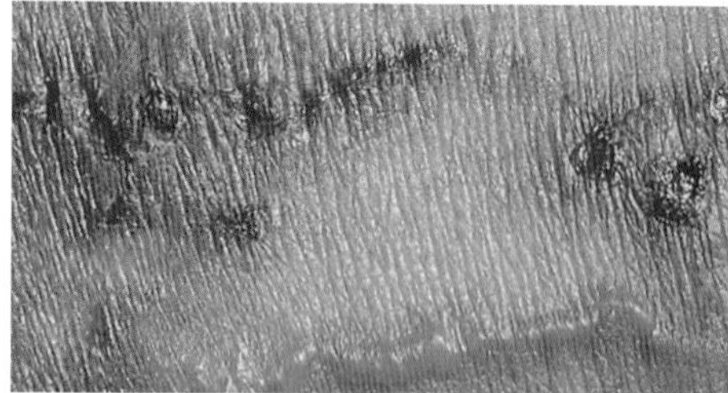

Figure 14.10 Finger cleft, burrow.

Scabies leads to a polymorphic and symmetrical rash which has a predilection for certain sites: the interdigital spaces of the hands, flexor surface of the wrists, extensor aspect of the elbows, anterior axillary folds, buttocks, and genitalia in males, and the periumbilical region (Figures 14.10 and 14.11). The rash can take a variety of forms but the pathognomonic lesion of scabies is the burrow, a small raised greyish wavy channel on the skin surface extending from an erythematous papule. Reddish-brown pruritic nodules are also seen and tend to affect the scrotum, penis, and groins. Sometimes an urticarial papular rash in the axillae and on the upper abdomen and upper thighs occurs. Excoriation and secondary bacterial infection can alter the appearance of lesions.

Diagnosis is usually based on the classic appearance and distribution of the rash and the presence of burrows. Confirmation, by demonstrating the presence of the mite, eggs, or faecal excrement, can be performed from skin scrapings, curettage, or shave biopsy with identification under a microscope.

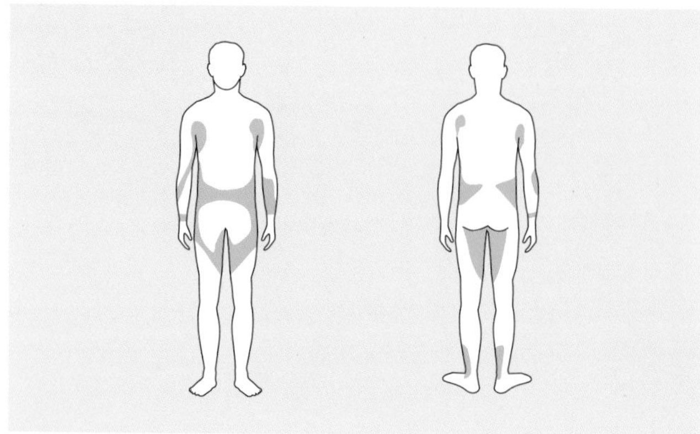

Figure 14.11 Areas infected by scabies infestation.

General advice should be given about avoiding close body contact until the patient and their partner(s) have completed treatment. A full screen for other STIs should be offered. Topical treatment is recommended, either permethrin 5% cream or malthion 0.5% aqueous lotion. These should be applied to the whole body from the neck downwards and washed off after 12 hours. The most convenient way is to apply, leave overnight, and wash off the next day. Patients should be warned that itch may persist for several weeks following treatment. This does not imply treatment failure, but is an effect of the antigenic material in the skin; antihistamines may help. Nodules may also persist long after treatment. Contaminated clothes and bed linen should be washed at 50°C.

Norwegian scabies is a crusted form of scabies that can occur in immunocompromised patients and the elderly. It manifests with crusted lesions with thick scales and may be widespread, but the itch is mild. Treatment is usually with ivermectin.

Pediculosis pubis

Pediculosis pubis is caused by the pubic louse, *Phthiris pubis*, and is commonly known as 'crabs' (Figure 14.12). It infests the hairs of the pubic and perianal areas, as well as other hairy areas that have the same diameter hair shaft. The grasp of the pubic louse's hook-like claw matches the diameter of hairs on thighs, abdomen, axillae, eyebrows, and eyelashes, allowing successful infestation. In contrast, the head louse grasp is uniquely adapted to the diameter of scalp hair which makes it difficult to transplant head lice to other areas of the body. Crabs are transmitted by direct skin-to-skin contact. The incubation period is between 5 days and several weeks. The main symptom is itch, dependent on individual sensitisation to the lice. Some patients present after seeing a louse moving or noting rust-coloured spots (louse faecal matter) on their underwear.

Diagnosis can be made with the naked eye, by observation of the lice or their eggs. There may be louse bites, which appear as bluish macules (maculae caeruleae). If necessary, examination under a light microscope can confirm morphology.

When pediculosis pubis is diagnosed, general advice should be given about avoiding close body contact until the patient and their

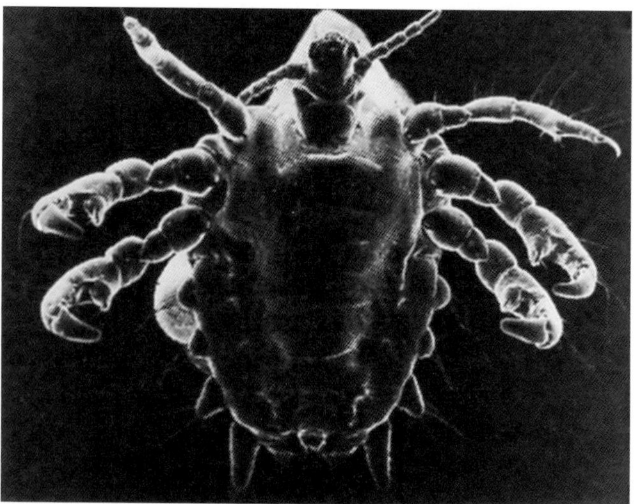

Figure 14.12 Pediculosis pubis.

Table 14.2 Recommended treatments for pediculosis pubis.

Recommended treatment	Application
Malthion 0.5% aqueous lotion	Apply to dry hair and wash out after at least 2, and preferably 12 hours
Permethrin 1% cream rinse	Apply to damp hair and wash out after 10 minutes; lotion can be used on eyelashes
Phenothrin 0.2%	Apply to dry hair and wash out after 2 hours
Carbaryl 0.5 and 1% (unlicensed indication)	Apply to dry hair and wash out 12 hours later
Simple eye ointment BP	For eyelashes, apply twice daily for 8–10 days (this method avoids eye irritation by topical insecticide)

partner(s) have completed treatment, and a full STI screen offered. Topical treatments recommended are shown in Table 14.2; a second application after 3–7 days is advised. Dead eggs may continue to adhere to hairs following treatment and these can be removed with a fine tooth comb.

Further reading

Centers for Disease Control and Prevention. Sexually Transmitted Disease Treatment Guidelines 2010. http://www.cdc.gov/std/treatment/2010/

Koutsky LA. Epidemiology of genital human papillomavirus infection. *Am J Med* 1997;**102**:3–8.

United Kingdom national guidelines on the management of anogenital warts, molluscum contagiosum, scabies infestation and *Phthirus pubis* infestation, 2007. Clinical Effectiveness Group, British Association of Sexual Health and HIV. Available from www.bashh.org.

CHAPTER 15

Viral Hepatitis

M Gary Brook

North West London Hospitals NHS Foundation Trust, London, UK

OVERVIEW

- Hepatitis types A, B, C, and D can be sexually transmitted
- The incidence of acute hepatitis C has risen steadily in HIV-positive men who have sex with men (MSM) over the last 10 years and most cases seem to be sexually transmitted
- Hepatitis B, C, and D are major causes of cirrhosis and liver cancer
- Hepatitis types A, B, and D are preventable by vaccine. Safer sex and condom use can reduce or prevent sexual transmision for all
- Chronic hepatitis B and C can be cured in a significant proportion of cases with appropriate treatment

Several viruses can cause hepatitis (Table 15.1). Of the five recognised pathogenic hepatitis viruses (types A–E), only types A–D have been shown to be sexually transmitted. There are other so-called hepatitis viruses that may also be sexually transmitted (G, GB, and TT) but there is no evidence that these organisms cause disease. The Epstein–Barr virus and cytomegalovirus (causes of glandular fever) can also cause hepatitis and are sometimes sexually transmitted.

Table 15.1 Comparison of hepatitis types A–D.

Hepatitis type	Incubation period	Transmission routes	Carrier state
A	2–6 weeks	Faeco-oral Sexual in MSM	No
B	Usually 8–12 weeks	Vertical, parenteral, sexual (MSM and heterosexual)	5–10% adults 90% infants
C	Usually 4–8 weeks	Vertical, parenteral Sexual (MSM and uncommonly heterosexual)	60–70%
D	6–8 weeks	Parenteral. Co-infection with hepatitis B Sexual (MSM and heterosexual)	2–5% as acute infection 70–80% in super-infection of chronic hepatitis B

MSM, men who have sex with men.

ABC of Sexually Transmitted Infections, Sixth Edition.
Edited by Karen E. Rogstad.

Hepatitis A virus

Epidemiology

Hepatitis A virus (HAV) is found throughout most of the world. The World Health Organization (WHO) recognises five patterns of distribution (Tables 15.2 and 15.3). Improving levels of sanitation in some countries have led to a fall in childhood infection, paradoxically resulting in a rise in adults susceptible to infection and thus symptomatic disease. Parenteral spread is also recognised in injecting drug users, men with haemophilia, and other users of blood products.

Sexual transmission

Sexually transmitted HAV occurs in men who have sex with men (MSM) linked to sex with anonymous partners, especially in the setting of saunas and 'darkrooms', group sex, oro-anal,

Table 15.2 World Health Organization-defined patterns of hepatitis A virus (HAV) endemicity.

HAV endemicity	Epidemiological patterns by region	Average age of patients (years)	Usual routes of transmission
Very high	Africa, parts of South America, the Middle East, and of South-East Asia	Under 5	Person-to-person Contaminated food and water
High	Brazil's Amazon basin, China, and Latin America	5–14	Person-to-person Contaminated food and water Outbreaks
Intermediate	Southern and Eastern Europe, some regions of the Middle East	5–24	Person-to-person Contaminated food and water Outbreaks
Low	Australia, USA, Western Europe	5–40	Common source outbreaks
Very low	Northern Europe and Japan	Over 20	Exposure during travel to high endemicity areas Uncommon source outbreaks

Table 15.3 Worldwide prevalence of hepatitis B, C, and D carriage.

Hepatitis type	Worldwide prevalence	Highest prevalence areas	Major routes of transmission worldwide
B	2 billion have been infected at some time in their life Currently 350 million chronic carriers	Africa, Asia, Alaska, and South America >8%. China and Taiwan 10–20%	Mother-to-infant (vertical) Child-to-child Sexual
C	170 million carriers	Far East, Mediterranean, parts of Africa and Eastern Europe	Parenteral: injecting drug use, reusable medical equipment, tattooing, traditional scarification and circumcision practices, blood products
D	10 million carriers	Russia, Romania, Southern Italy and other Mediterranean countries, parts of Africa and South America	Parenteral: injecting drug users, horizontal, non-sexual, intra-familial spread (exact mechanism unknown)

and digital–rectal intercourse. Outbreaks have been reported from large urban areas including London and Brighton. Seroprevalence studies show that MSM and heterosexual men attending STI clinics have similar rates of past exposure suggesting that only a minority of MSM are at increased risk. There is no evidence for spread through heterosexual sex.

Sexually transmitted HAV occurs in men who have sex with men (MSM) linked to sex with anonymous partners, especially in the setting of saunas and 'darkrooms', group sex, oro-anal, and digital–rectal intercourse

Clinical presentation

Symptoms of acute hepatitis start with a 'flu-like prodromal illness lasting up to 2 weeks (Figure 15.1). This is normally followed by icteric hepatitis (jaundice) for a few weeks which rarely lasts longer than 3 months. However, illness from HAV is very much age-related. Only 5–20% of children under 5 years old show symptoms, whereas clinical hepatitis occurs in 75–90% of adults, although the mortality is generally very low at around 0.3% of cases. There is a higher mortality in patients over 40 years or those with chronic liver disease such as that from hepatitis B, C, or alcohol. HIV does not influence the course of the illness.

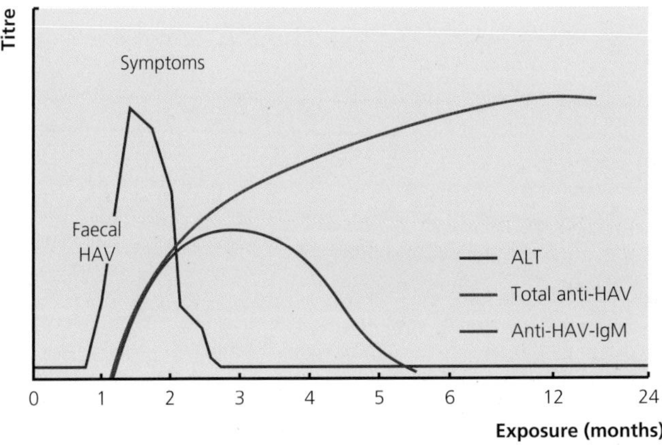

Figure 15.1 Hepatitis A: typical serological course. ALT, alanine aminotransferase; HAV, hepatitis A virus; IgM, immunoglobulin M.

Symptoms of acute hepatitis start with a 'flu-like prodromal illness lasting up to 2 weeks. This is normally followed by icteric hepatitis (jaundice) for a few weeks which rarely lasts longer than 3 months

Diagnosis and management

Acute hepatitis A cannot be distinguished clinically from types B, C, D, or E and liver function test abnormalities are similar for all (Table 15.4). The diagnosis is confirmed by serum antibody tests (Figures 15.1; Table 15.5).

Most patients with acute hepatitis will recover uneventfully with symptom control, rest, and hydration, and many can be kept at home. Isolation may be required to prevent spread to others, such as in patients with faecal incontinence, or during the time of infectivity in the prodromal illness and the first 2 weeks of jaundice.

Prevention

HAV vaccine is highly effective (>90%) at preventing infection and should be offered to MSM with an at-risk lifestyle, non-immune travellers to endemic countries, men with haemophilia, injecting drug users, patients with chronic liver disease, and sewage workers (Table 15.6). If a non-immune person has been exposed to someone in the infectious period of HAV infection they should be offered vaccination. Human normal immunoglobulin (HNIG) with anti-HAV activity is in short supply in the United Kingdom but can

Table 15.4 Biochemical features of acute viral hepatitis.

Test	Results
Serum amino-transferases (ALT)	Typically peaks at 500–10 000 IU/L. in the first few weeks. Higher in acute fulminant hepatitis
Serum bilirubin	30–100 μmol/L. Mixed conjugated/unconjugated with bilirubinuria
Serum alkaline phosphatase	Usually normal or only mildly raised (<300 IU/L) except in the uncommon cholestatic variant of acute viral hepatitis
Prothrombin time	May be slightly prolonged by 1–5 seconds. Prolongation >5 seconds (INR >1.5) suggests impending hepatic failure

INR, international normalised ratio.

Table 15.5 Confirmatory serum tests for viral hepatitis (common patterns).

Virus type	Acute infection	Chronic infection	Recovered/immune
Hepatitis A	IgM anti-HAV-positive	Does not occur	Total anti-HAV positive IgM anti-HAV-negative
Hepatitis B	IgM anti-HBc-positive HBsAg-positive, HBeAg-positive HBV-DNA-positive	IgM anti-HBc-negative (positive low titre in flares) HBsAg-positive, HBeAg-positive or negative HBV-DNA-positive or negative	IgG anti-HBc-positive, IgG anti-HBs-positive (may become negative) HBsAg-negative
Hepatitis C	IgG anti-HCV-positive by EIA (but may take up to 3 months or more) HCV-RNA-positive by PCR	As for acute infection	Antibody negative or IgG anti-HCV-positive by EIA HCV-RNA-negative by PCR
Hepatitis D	IgG and IgM anti-HDV-positive HDAg-positive, HDV-RNA-positive With markers of acute/chronic hepatitis B infection	As for acute infection	Antibody, antigen and RNA tests become negative within months of recovery

EIA, enzyme immunoassay; HAV, hepatitis A virus; HBc, hepatitis B core; HBeAg, hepatitis B e antigen; HBsAg, hepatitis B surface antigen; HBV, hepatitis B virus; HCV, hepatitis C virus; HDAg, hepatitis D antigen; HDV, hepatitis D virus; Ig, immunoglobulin; PCR, polymerase chain reaction.

Table 15.6 Vaccine schedules.

Vaccine	Schedule	Advantages
Hepatitis B	0, 1, 6 months 0, 1, 2, 12 months 0, 1, 3 weeks, 12 months	90% or more response May get a response within 3 months May get a response within 1 month
Hepatitis A+B	As hepatitis B	As hepatitis B
Hepatitis A	0, 6 months	Fewer doses than the A+B vaccine

be given within 1 week of exposure in patients with particular risk (e.g. immunosuppression).

HAV vaccine is highly effective (>90%) at preventing infection and should be offered to MSM with an at-risk lifestyle, non-immune travellers to endemic countries, men with haemophilia, injecting drug users, patients with chronic liver disease, and sewage workers

Hepatitis B virus

Epidemiology

For epidemiology of hepatitis B virus (HBV) see Tables 15.1 and 15.3. HBV infection is endemic in many parts of the world with very high carriage rates (up to 20%) seen in South and East Asia. High carriage rates (up to 10%) are also found in some regions of Central and South America, Africa and parts of Asia. Chronic carriage in the general population in Northern and Western Europe occurs in 0.1–2%. However, much higher carriage rates are found in certain sub-groups including injecting drug users, homosexual men, female sex workers and immigrants from high endemicity countries.

Sexual transmission

Heterosexual transmission through vaginal sex is approximately 40% efficient from someone with acute or HBeAg-positive hepatitis B. HBV infection in MSM is also transmitted readily and correlates with number of partners, oro-anal and genito-anal sexual contact. Despite the availability of an effective vaccine, HBV infection continues to be a significant problem in MSM in developed countries.

Heterosexual transmission through vaginal sex is approximately 40% efficient from people with acute or HBeAg-positive hepatitis B

Clinical presentation

As with HAV, acute infection of children with HBV is largely asymptomatic. In adulthood, 50–70% of acute infections are symptomatic and tend to be more severe than acute HAV infection. In immunocompromised patients, including those who are HIV-positive, asymptomatic acute infection is more common (20–40%).

HBV infection (Figures 15.2 and 15.3) can cause acute liver failure, chronic hepatitis, liver cirrhosis, and liver cancer.

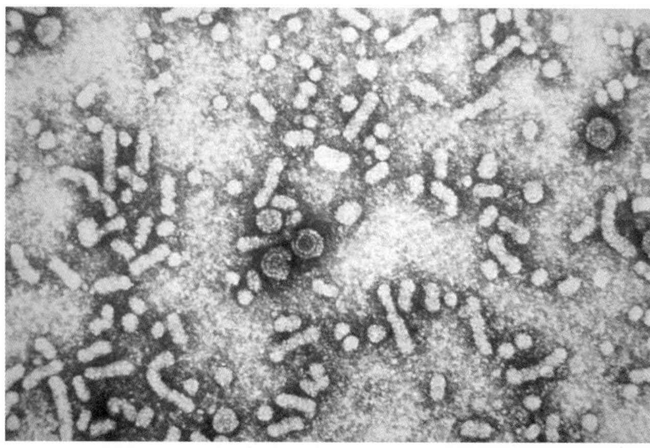

Figure 15.2 Electron micrograph of hepatitis B virus. Courtesy of CDC.

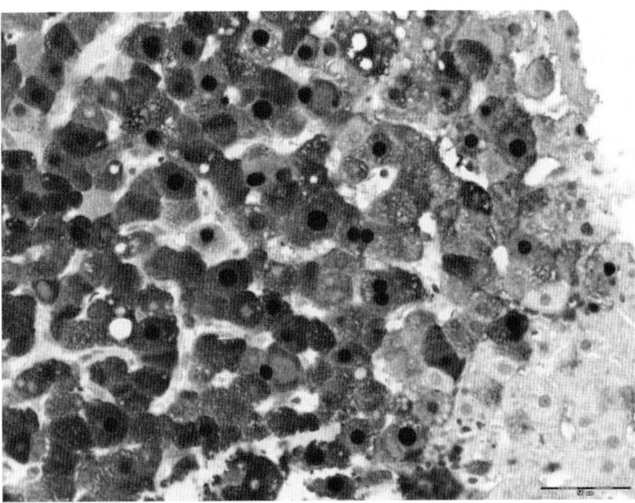

Figure 15.3 A liver biopsy showing nuclear and diffuse cytoplasmic staining pattern of HBV core antigen. Courtesy of Dr Paul Tadrous, Northwick Park Hospital.

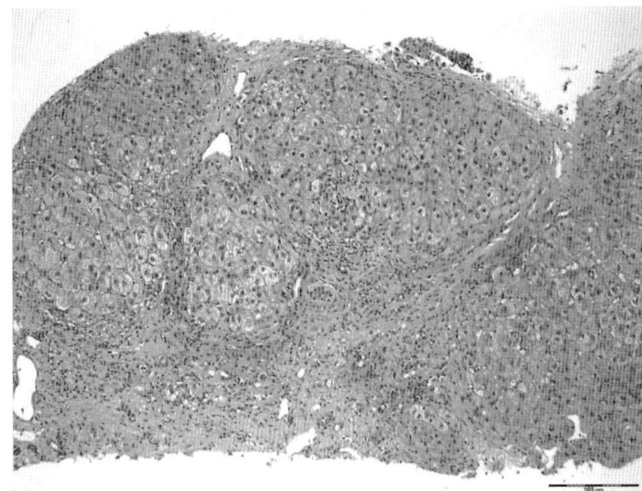

Figure 15.5 Cirrhosis of liver. Courtesy of Dr Paul Tadrous, Northwick Park Hospital.

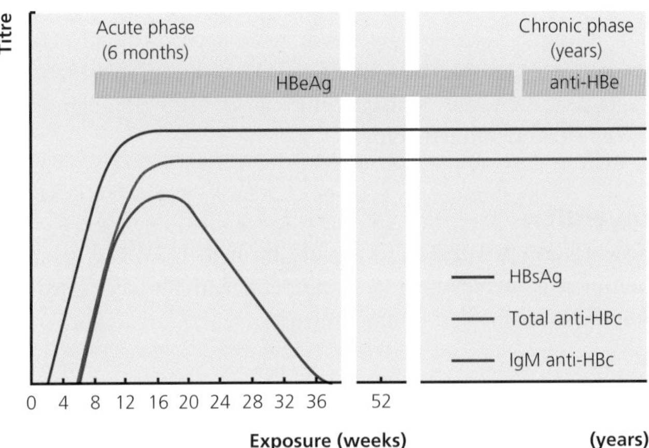

Figure 15.4 Hepatitis B: typical serological course of chronic infection. HBc, hepatitis B core; HBe, hepatitis B'e'; HBeAg, hepatitis B'e' antigen; HBsAg, hepatitis B surface antigen; IgM, immunoglobulin M.

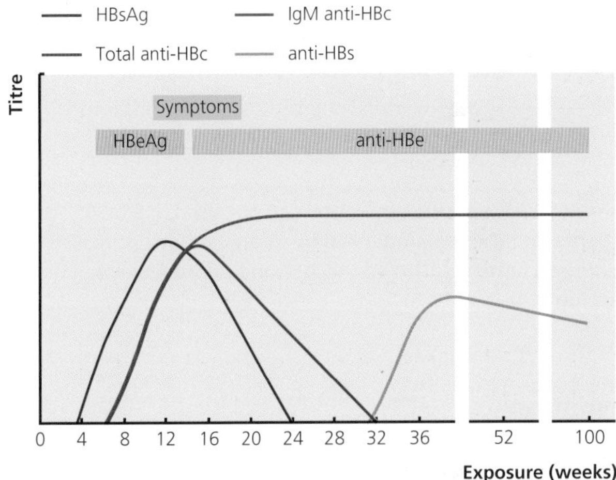

Figure 15.6 Hepatitis B: typical serological course of resolving acute infection. Anti-HBs, antibody to hepatitis B surface antigen; HBc, hepatitis B core; HBe, hepatitis Be; HBeAg, hepatitis Be antigen; HBsAg, hepatitis B surface antigen; IgM, immunoglobulin M.

Approximately 1% of those with acute symptomatic infection will develop liver failure, leading to death in up to 50%.

The majority of people with chronic infection (Figure 15.4) have no symptoms until cirrhosis and decompensated liver disease ensues, when they develop ascites, jaundice, bleeding oesophageal varices, and ultimately confusion, cachexia, and death. Complications occur more rapidly when there is associated hepatitis A, C, or D or HIV. Those with cirrhosis develop liver cancer at a rate of 3% per year, presenting with liver enlargement, weight loss, and rapid progression to death. Without treatment, about 25% of chronically infected children will eventually die of cirrhosis or liver cancer in adulthood, usually around the fourth decade of life, and as a result about a million people die annually worldwide from HBV.

Diagnosis and management

Acute infection cannot be distinguished clinically from other types. In chronic hepatitis, liver function tests (LFT) may only show a mildly raised serum alanine aminotransferase (ALT) level, although when cirrhosis or cancer (Figure 15.5) develop the LFT and serum prothrombin time become progressively more abnormal. These changes can be seen on liver biopsy and the large amounts of virus can be demonstrated on electron microscopy (Figures 15.2, 15.3 and 15.7). Diagnosis of HBV infection is by serum antibodies and antigens and if negative in HIV-positive patients, by viral DNA testing (Figure 15.6; Table 15.5).

The management of acute hepatitis is as for hepatitis A although antivirals are given for acute fulminant HBV infection. Chronic HBeAg-positive infection can be cured in 30–50% of patients with drugs such as pegylated interferon-α, lamivudine, entecavir, adefovir and tenofovir. The remainder can be virologically suppressed leading to normalisation of the ALT and improved liver histology. HIV co-infection with HBV complicates management as therapy is less effective at inducing HBeAg seroconversion, except in those with a high $CD4^+$ lymphocyte count. Although the prognosis of liver disease in untreated HIV/HBV co-infection may be worse,

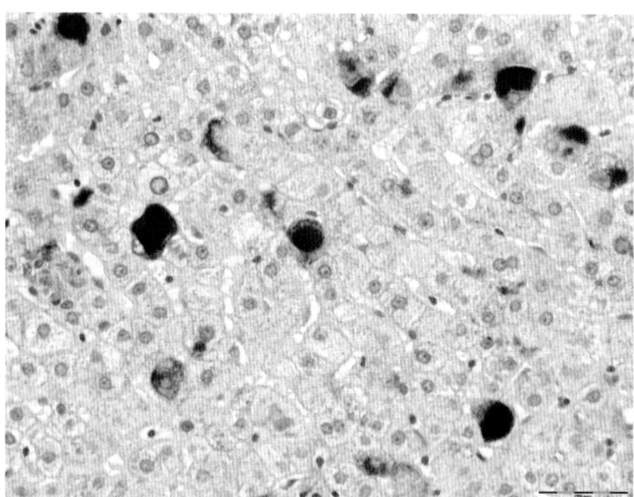

Figure 15.7 Liver biopsy showing scattered cells with strong cytoplasmic positivity for hepatitis B surface antigen. Courtesy of Dr Paul Tadrous, Northwick Park Hospital.

this can be ameliorated by giving tenofovir and either lamivudine or emtricitabine as part of the antiretroviral regimen. Liver transplantation and chemotherapy are required for decompensated cirrhosis or liver cancer (Figure 15.5).

Chronic HBeAg-positive infection can be cured in 30–50% of patients and the remainder can be virologically suppressed leading to normalisation of the ALT and improved liver histology

Prevention

Vaccination and consistent condom use will prevent most cases of sexually transmitted hepatitis B infection. Vaccination should be offered to MSM, sex workers, or injecting drug users. Universal vaccination is advocated by the WHO. The vaccine is also used as primary prophylaxis, after possible exposure, as early as possible. Hepatitis B immunoglobulin works as secondary prophylaxis if given within a week of exposure.

Vaccination and consistent condom use will prevent most cases of sexually transmitted hepatitis B if advised to those at risk such as MSM, sex workers, or injecting drug users

Hepatitis D (delta virus)

Epidemiology

This RNA virus can only exist as a co-infection with hepatitis B but its geographical distribution is not uniformly identical to HBV (Table 15.3).

Sexual transmission

Heterosexual and homosexual sexual transmission of delta virus is recognised both in endemic areas and in partners of injecting drug users in low prevalence countries.

Clinical presentation

Delta virus (HDV) can be acquired concurrently with HBV infection or as a super-infection of chronic HBV carriage. In acute co-infection, there may be two bouts of clinical hepatitis from each virus. Fulminant hepatitis is 10 times more likely than with other types of viral hepatitis with an 80% rate of fatality. HDV super-infection in a HBV carrier causes acute severe hepatitis with a high rate of fulminant disease and a 80% rate of chronicity. Up to 70% of chronic carriers develop cirrhosis which is more rapid in onset than with HBV, at 40% in 6 years. The incidence of liver cancer in HDV carriers with cirrhosis is three times higher than in HBV alone.

In acute HBV/HDV co-infection, there may be two bouts of clinical hepatitis from each virus. Fulminant hepatitis is 10 times more likely in HDV infection than with other types of viral hepatitis with an 80% fatality rate

Diagnosis and management

HDV infection is marked by severe acute hepatitis (Table 15.3). Laboratory diagnosis is by a serum anti-HDV test (Table 15.5), or antigen and RNA tests. Management is as for HBV although there is no effective antiviral therapy.

Prevention

This infection is largely preventable through HBV vaccination, condom use, sterile medical equipment, and the avoidance of equipment sharing in injecting drug users.

Hepatitis C virus (HCV)

Epidemiology

Hepatitis C virus (HCV) is predominantly parenterally transmitted (Table 15.1). Vertical transmission is seen at a rate of about 1% in HIV-negative women but is >9% in HIV co-infection.

Sexual transmission

HCV can be transmitted through unprotected vaginal sex at a rate approximating to 0.5–2% per year of a relationship. Transmission is higher if the source patient is also HIV-positive. Risk factors in MSM include traumatic anal sex, concurrent ulcerative STIs (herpes, lymphogranuloma venereum (LGV), syphilis), and the use of recreational drugs.

There has been a recent rise in homosexual spread of hepatitis C, especially in HIV-positive men. Risk factors include traumatic anal sex, concurrent ulcerative STIs (herpes, LGV, syphilis), and the use of recreational drugs

Clinical presentation

Jaundice occurs in only 20% of acute infections, the rest being asymptomatic. Fulminant hepatitis is rare except for hepatitis A super-infection of chronic HCV disease. However, 60–80% of patients develop chronic (>6 months) infection. Symptoms are mild and non-specific until cirrhosis intervenes, which is seen in 20% after 20 years. Five per cent of carriers develop liver cancer which is always related to cirrhosis. Cirrhosis is more frequent and develops more rapidly if there is a high alcohol intake, HIV, or HBV co-infection.

Diagnosis and management

Diagnosis is by serum antibodies (and, if negative in HIV-positive patients, by viral RNA testing) and most are positive within 3 months if a third-generation tests is used, although it can take up to 9 months. A polymerase chain reaction (PCR) assay is then used to determine if the patient is an HCV carrier (Table 15.5). Pegylated interferon and ribavirin for 6 months cures 50–90% of carriers depending on the viral genotype. The cure rate is lower if the patient is also HIV-positive.

Pegylated interferon and ribavirin for 6 months cures 50–90% of HCV carriers depending on viral genotype. The cure rate is lower if the patient is also HIV-positive

Prevention

There is no effective vaccine. Preventative interventions include non-reusable medical equipment, education on safer drug use, testing of donated blood, and safer sex including condoms. HCV carriers should be immunised against hepatitis A and B to prevent the severe consequences of co-infection.

Further reading

Brook MG, Nelson M, Bhagani S. Clinical Effectiveness Group, British Association of Sexual Health and HIV. United Kingdom national guideline on the treatment of the viral hepatitides A, B and C, 2008. Available at http://www.bashh.org/documents/1927.

British HIV Association. Guidelines for the management of co-infection with HIV-1 and chronic hepatitis B or C, 2009. Available at http://www.bhiva.org/cms1191540.asp.

Department of Health. Immunisation against infectious disease 'The Green Book'. Available at http://www.dh.gov.uk/en/Publichealth/Healthprotection/Immunisation/Greenbook/DH_4097254.

National Institute for Health and Clinical Excellence. Peginterferon alfa and ribavirin. Available at http://www.nice.org.uk/TA106.

World Health Organization. Hepatitis. Available at http://www.who.int/csr/disease/hepatitis/en/.

CHAPTER 16

Systemic Manifestations of STIs

Elizabeth Carlin

Sherwood Forest Hospitals NHS Foundation Trust and Nottingham University Hospitals NHS Trust, Nottinghamshire, UK

OVERVIEW

- Most infections remain at the initial site of infection or spread locally
- Systemic manifestations of STIs, apart from HIV infection, are relatively uncommon
- Symptoms and signs may involve several different systems
- Considering an underlying STI if systemic signs are present is key to making the diagnosis

In most individuals with a sexually transmitted infection (STI) the infection remains localised to the site of initial infection either in the ano-genital area or the pharynx. In some cases the infection may spread locally, for example *Chlamydia trachomatis* infection spreading from the cervix to the fallopian tubes to cause salpingitis, or from the male urethra to the epididymis and testes to cause epididymo-orchitis. In others the infection may be transferred to another site on the body by the person themselves. This is known as auto-inoculation. An example of this is conjunctival infection following the transfer of *C. trachomatis* and *Neisseria gonorrhoeae* from the genital area to the eye by hand.

Systemic manifestations of STIs occur when the infection spreads to distant sites, usually by a haematogenous or lymphatic route, causing symptoms and signs remote from the genital tract. The STIs that most commonly have systemic features are HIV, syphilis, and hepatitis A, B, and C. In most other STIs systemic manifestations only occur in a minority of individuals but if they do occur they can be serious (Box 16.1).

Box 16.1 **Systemic manifestations of STIs**

- Sexually acquired reactive arthritis (SARA)
- Disseminated gonococcal infection (DGI)
- Fitz-Hugh–Curtis syndrome
- Syphilis, either secondary or tertiary
- Herpetic meningitis
- Donavanosis, liver or bone involvement

ABC of Sexually Transmitted Infections, Sixth Edition.
Edited by Karen E. Rogstad.

Sexually acquired reactive arthritis

Reactive arthritis is a sterile inflammation of the synovial membrane, tendons, and fascia triggered by an infection at a distant site, usually gastrointestinal or genital. When the triggering infection is an STI the reactive arthritis is known as sexually acquired reactive arthritis (SARA). This includes the condition previously described as sexually acquired Reiter's syndrome, consisting of urethritis, arthritis, and conjunctivitis.

SARA is relatively rare but is most frequently associated with urethritis or cervicitis and has been reported in 0.8–4% of cases. It is most commonly linked to *C. trachomatis*, which is detected in about three-quarters of cases, but also with *N. gonorrhoeae*. It is unclear why SARA develops in certain individuals but it is likely that having persistent and viable organisms in the joint is an important factor. SARA is identified much more commonly in men and in those who are HLA-B27-positive or who have a family history of spondyloarthritis or iritis.

Clinical presentation

Most individuals with SARA give a history of sexual intercourse within 3 months of the onset of arthritis. This is usually with a new partner and in over 80% of cases the arthritis develops within 30 days of intercourse (Figure 16.1).

The majority of men give a recent history of urethral discharge and/or dysuria and the mean interval between the onset of genital symptoms and arthritis is 14 days. The timeframe is less clear with women as most have no genital symptoms.

Other systemic manifestations such as cutaneous or mucous membrane lesions, uveitis, and, rarely, cardiac or neurological involvement may be present.

Joint, tendon, and fascia

The arthritis is manifest by pain, with or without swelling and stiffness, at one or more joints, usually less than six, in an asymmetrical distribution. The affected joints tend to be in the lower limbs such as the knees, ankles, and feet.

Pain, tenderness, stiffness, and sometimes swelling may occur in up to 40% of individuals at the sites of tendon or fascial attachments at entheses, especially the heel, which may cause problems in walking. Similarly, dactylitis and tenosynovitis may

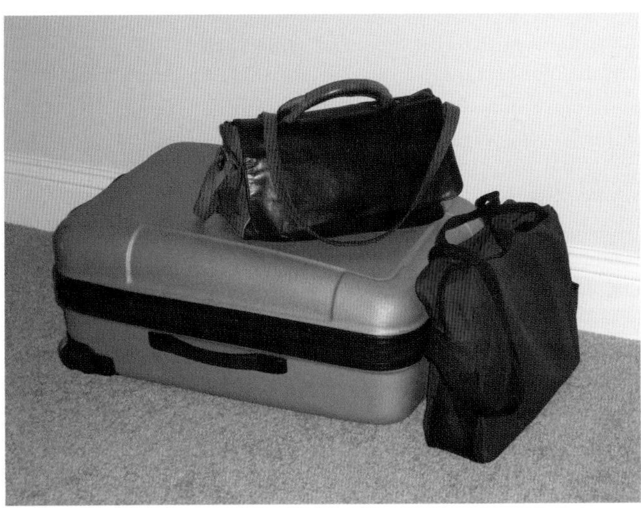

Figure 16.1 Check the recent travel history and for gastrointestinal symptoms so that a gastrointestinal infective trigger is not missed.

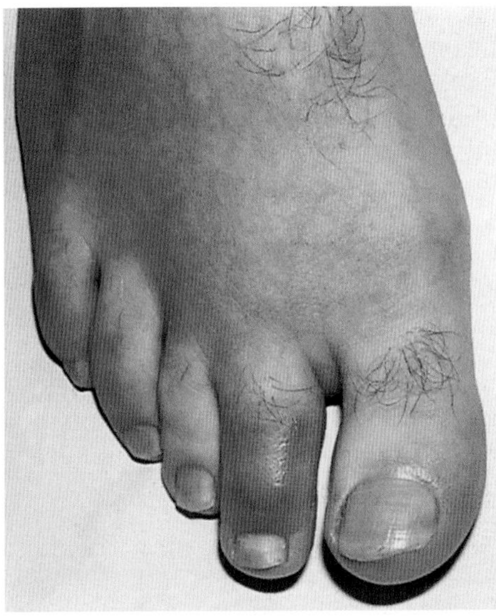

Figure 16.2 Dactylitis. Reproduced with permission from *ABC of Rheumatology*, A. Adebajo, Wiley-Blackwell, 2010.

cause pain and restrict movement of the hands and feet. Dactylitis usually presents with a swollen finger or toe and tenosynovitis presents with tenderness, with or without swelling, over the tendon sheath and crepitus on movement (Figure 16.2).

Low back pain and stiffness is common in the acute episode with sacro-iliitis occurring in some individuals. It is important to distinguish this from other pathology such as lumbosacral disc disease.

Conjunctiva and iris

Many experience irritability in the eyes and photophobia and up to 50% develop conjunctivitis with pain and redness of the conjunctiva (Figure 16.3). The conjunctivitis is often bilateral and precedes the arthritis by a few days. Iritis is much less common but it is important to recognise it as without appropriate treatment

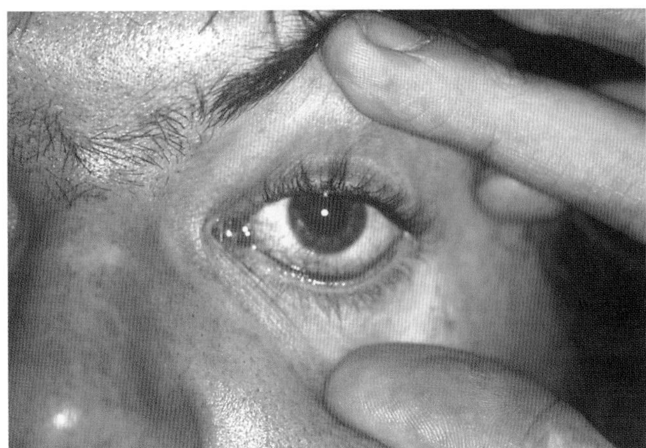

Figure 16.3 Conjunctivitis. Courtesy of CDC/Joe Miller.

it can result in permanent blindness. Slit lamp examination is needed to differentiate between conjunctivits and iritis. Other eye manifestations are rare.

Genital infection

Urethritis, epididymo-orchitis, mucopurulent cervicitis, proctitis, or abdominal pain due to pelvic inflammatory disease may be seen. However, genital infection may be asymptomatic, particularly in women or with rectal infection.

Skin manifestations

A wide range of skin manifestations may be seen in up to 40% of patients with typical psoriasis, mucous membrane lesions such as circinate balanitis (Figure 16.4), or pustular psoriasis on the soles of the feet known as keratoderma blennorrhagica (Figure 16.5). Less commonly oral ulceration or nail dystrophy is seen.

Other manifestations

Constitutional symptoms of malaise, fatigue, and fever occur in 10% of individuals. Cardiac and renal pathology is usually asymptomatic and results in electrocardiograph abnormalities and proteinuria.

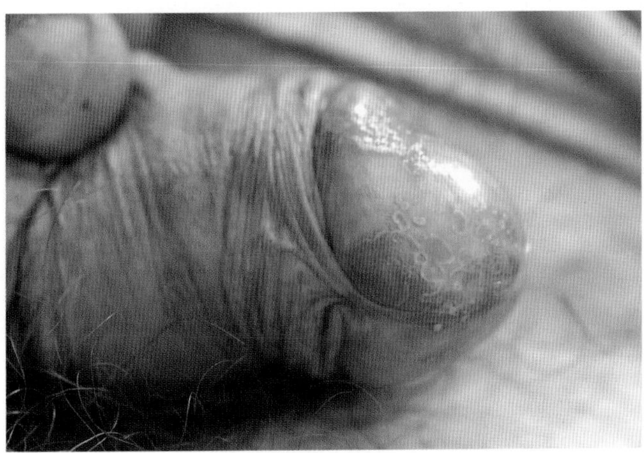

Figure 16.4 Circinate balanitis. Courtesy of Nottingham University Hospitals NHS Trust/Dr Sheelagh Littlewood.

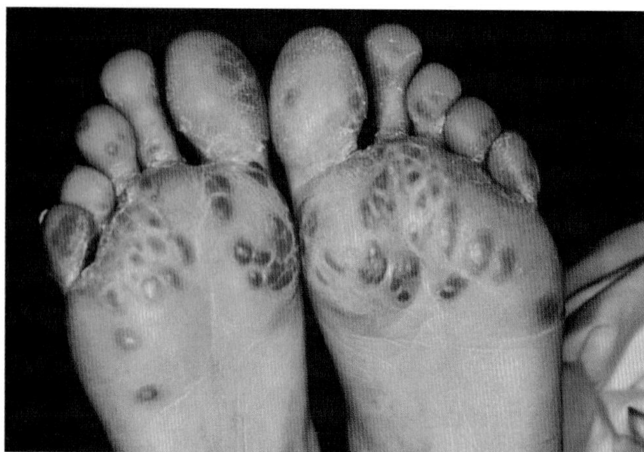

Figure 16.5 Keratoderma blennorrhagica. Courtesy of CDC/Dr MF Rein.

Progress of the condition

SARA is usually a self-limiting condition with the average first episode lasting 4–6 months and being followed by a full recovery. About 50% of cases will have recurrent episodes at varying frequency. Chronic symptoms for over 1 year occur in 17%, are more likely in HLA-B57-positive individuals, and are usually due to aggressive arthritis. Long-term disability may occur due to erosive joint damage or sacro-iliitis. Ankylosing spondylitis is seen in individuals with SARA but it is unclear whether this is a component of SARA or as a result of both conditions being more likely in certain genetic groups.

Acute anterior uveitis may lead rapidly to cataract formation and blindness if it is inadequately treated or recurrent, so although this is rare it is essential to detect it early.

Management

An STI screen and investigations for arthritis are required (Box 16.2). HLA typing to look for HLA-B27, X-rays of affected joints and sacro-iliac joints, and stool culture to detect a gastrointestinal infection (e.g. *Salmonella, Shigella* or *Campylobacter*) may be useful. Other investigations may be needed if other conditions with rheumatological features are being considered. Seek specialist rheumatology advice if tests such as ultrasonography, magnetic resonance imaging, or synovial fluid analysis are proposed.

Box 16.2 **Investigations for sexually acquired reactive arthritis (SARA)**

- Screen for STIs, including HIV
- Erythrocyte sedimentation rate (ESR), C-reactive protein (CRP), or plasma viscosity
- Full blood count
- Urinalysis

In most cases SARA is a self-limiting condition. Referral to specialist services may be required for those with significant systemic involvement and where second line therapy is being considered.

All patients with SARA should be referred to an ophthalmologist, where possible, for slit lamp assessment

The first line treatment for constitutional symptoms, arthritis, and enthesitis is rest, physical therapy such as cold pads or orthototics, and non-steroidal anti-inflammatory drugs (NSAIDs) (Figure 16.6). The NSAIDs should be taken regularly to obtain maximum anti-inflammatory effect but for the shortest time period possible. A cyclo-oxygenase 2 (COX-2) selective drug should be used in those with a high risk of gastrointestinal complications. Adding gastroprotective agents to non-selective NSAIDs can also reduce the gastrointestinal risks. Intra-articular corticosteroid injections may be useful for single joints and enthesitis if they are failing to settle with more conservative therapy.

Second line therapy options include systemic corticosteroids, or, where disabling symptoms have been present for 3 months or more, sulfasalazine, methotrexate, or azathioprine. Gold salts and D-penicillamine are occasionally used. Biological agents, tumour necrosis factor (TNF) α blockers, are not routinely used in SARA because of concerns that they may reactivate the infective trigger.

Any STI that is identified requires treatment and partner notification. Short course antibiotic therapy does not alter the course of the arthritis, although it may reduce the risk of arthritis developing in those with previous reactive arthritis. There is conflicting evidence about the effect of longer duration antibiotic therapy on the arthritis and they are not generally used.

Mild mucous membrane and skin lesions do not require treatment. If they are more severe topical salicylic acid ointments, corticosteroid preparations, or vitamin D3 analogues may be used. In severe cases methotrexate or retinoids may be required. It is essential to manage eye lesions with ophthalmological advice and slit lamp assessment to diagnose uveitis, which requires treatment with topical or oral corticosteroid and mydriatics.

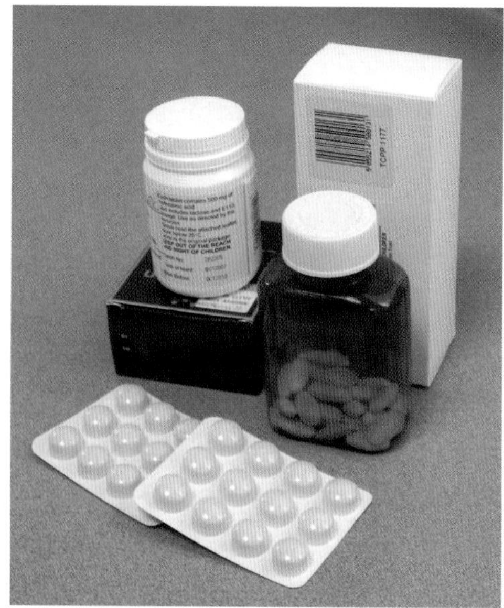

Figure 16.6 Non-steroidal anti-inflammatory drugs (NSAIDs) are the main first line treatment for arthritis.

Patients should be advised to avoid potentially 'triggering infections' in the future so safer sexual practice and food hygiene should be discussed.

Disseminated gonococcal infection

A small minority of patients with gonorrhoea develop gonococcal bacteraemia resulting in disseminated gonococcal infection (DGI). It usually develops within 1 month of acquiring gonorrhoea and is more common in women than men, often occurring within 1 week of menstruation.

Clinical presentation

A fever is often, but not invariably, present and it may be low-grade. Most patients have tenosynovitis and arthralgia with many having an acute asymmetric arthritis, usually of several joints, commonly the wrist, ankle, knee, or small joints. About two-thirds of patients have skin lesions, which typically are tender necrotic pustules on an erythematous base distributed towards the extremities but variations on this pattern can occur (Figure 16.7). Occasionally, endocarditis, usually involving the aortic valve, may occur and this can be rapidly progressive. Gonococcal meningitis is exceeding rare.

Many patients with DGI have no genital symptoms. This may contribute to under-recognition and a delayed diagnosis

Progress of the condition

Untreated gonococcal arthritis may result in joint damage, residual arthritis, and long-term disability in some cases.

Management

Screen for *N. gonorrhoeae* from oral and genital sites, skin lesions, synovial fluid from affected joints and blood. Cerebrospinal fluid should be cultured if meningeal symptoms are present. The bacteraemia with disseminated gonorrhoea is not continuous and repeat blood cultures are required. The detection of gonorrhoea is highest in genital samples but is at best only 30% from synovial fluid and blood.

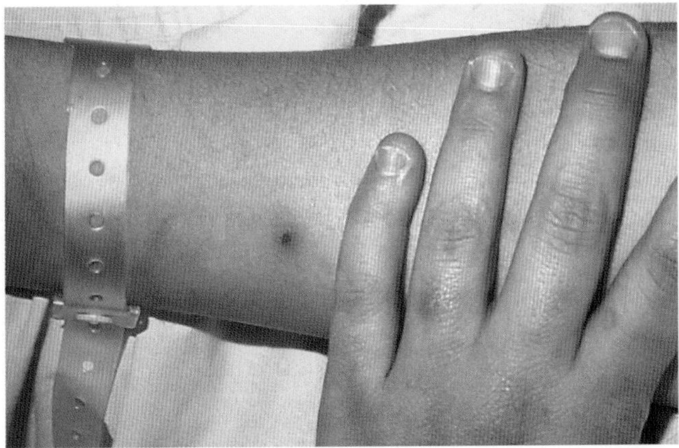

Figure 16.7 Typical skin lesions of disseminated gonococcal infection (DGI). Courtesy of CDC/Dr SE Thompson, VDCD/J Pledger.

Intravenous antibiotic therapy is required and a clinical response to treatment is usually seen within 48 hours. If DGI is suspected empirical antibiotic therapy should be started, according to local sensitivity patterns, while awaiting culture and sensitivity results.

Fitz-Hugh–Curtis syndrome

Fitz-Hugh–Curtis syndrome is a rare condition consisting of peri-hepatitis and salpingitis mostly due to *C. trachomatis*, although *N. gonorrhoeae* can also cause the condition. The infection initially extends locally to cause endometritis and salpingitis and then spreads to the liver by intraperitoneal, haematogenous, or lymphatic dissemination. In the liver it causes inflammation and fibrinous adhesions between the liver capsule and the abdominal cavity.

Clinical presentation

It is most commonly seen in women, occurring in 5% of those with salpingitis. The usual presentation is with acute onset, right upper quadrant, abdominal pleuritic pain, fever, nausea, or vomiting and a tender liver. Features of pelvic inflammatory disease may be present. If salpingitis is not present clinically it is usually identified at laparoscopy.

Progress of the condition

The liver capsule inflammation and the development of adhesions continues until antibiotic therapy is given, after which the acute pain, resulting from liver capsule inflammation, settles rapidly. The adhesions usually remain indefinitely and are mostly asymptomatic but in some chronic upper quadrant abdominal pain persists.

Management

Perform STI screening, full blood count, liver function tests, erythrocyte sedimentation rate (ESR), C-reactive protein (CRP) or plasma viscosity, and a chest X-ray. An abdominal ultrasound is useful in differentiating between peri-hepatitis and acute cholecystitis. Peri-hepatitis can be confirmed by computed tomography or by visualising the liver capsule and adhesions at laparotomy or laparoscopy.

Antibiotic therapy is required with adequate cover for *C. trachomatis* and *N. gonorrhoeae* and should continue for at least 2–3 weeks.

Other conditions with systemic manifestations

Syphilis

Syphilis has so many multiple systemic manifestations it has been called 'the great imitator'. It is described fully in Chapter 13. Systemic features include fever, malaise, anorexia, weight loss, headache, sore throat, arthralgia, and skin rashes including the palms and soles (Figure 16.8). Other features include lymphadenopathy, mucous patches in the mouth, condylomata lata, hepatomegaly and abnormal liver function tests, meningitis,

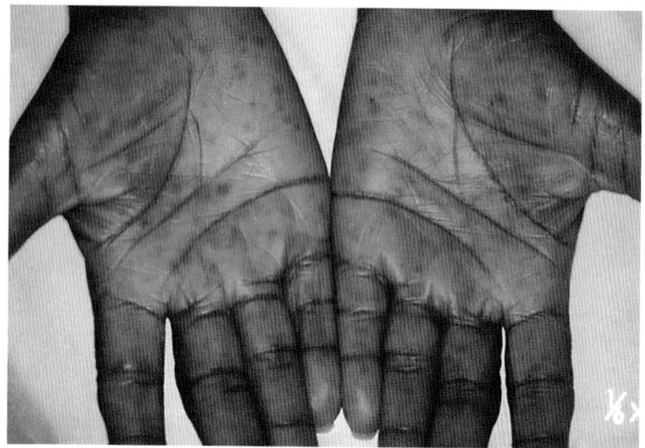

Figure 16.8 Syphilitic rash on the palms. Courtesy of CDC/Dr MF Rein.

transverse myelitis, cranial nerve palsies, and alopecia. Late complications include aortic valve disease or aneurysm, coronary ostia stenosis; meningovascular syphilis with meningitis, cerebrovascular accident (CVA), general paresis, tabes dorsalis, optic neuritis and neural deafness; and with chronic skin and bone lesions.

Genital herpes

In the primary episode constitutional symptoms, including fever, malaise, headache, and myalgia, are very common. In a minority, benign viral meningitis can occur presenting with neck stiffness, headache, and photophobia. Transverse myelitis and autonomic nervous dysfunction is extremely rare.

Donavanosis (Granuloma inguinale)

Donavanosis is caused by *Klebsiella granulomatis*. In rare cases haematogenous distribution to liver and bone occurs, usually associated with pregnancy or cervical lesions.

Further reading

Csonka GW. The course of Reiter's syndrome. *Br Med J* 1958;**1**:1088–90.

Holmes KK, Sparling PF, Stamm WE, Piot P, Wasserheit JN, Corey L, *et al.* *Sexually Transmitted Diseases*, 4th edn. McGraw Hill, New York, 2008.

Rihl M, Klos A, Köhler L, Kuipers JG. Reactive arthritis. *Best Pract Res Clin Rheumatol* 2006;**20**:1119–37.

Sexually Transmitted Infections: UK National Screening and Testing Guidelines. Available at http://www.bashh.org/guidelines.

UK National guideline for the management of genital tract infection with *Chlamydia trachomatis*. Available at http://www.bashh.org/guidelines.

UK National guideline on the management of sexually acquired reactive arthritis. Available at http://www.bashh.org/guidelines.

CHAPTER 17

HIV

Ian Williams[1], *David Daniels*[2], *Keerti Gedela*[2], *Aparna Briggs*[3] *and Anna Pryce*[3]

[1]UCL Research Department of Infection and Population Health, London, UK
[2]West Middlesex University Hospital NHS Foundation Trust, Isleworth, UK
[3]Sheffield Teaching Hospitals NHS Foundation Trust, Sheffield, UK

OVERVIEW

- HIV is predominantly sexually transmitted and heterosexual intercourse is the main route of transmission worldwide
- Decreasing the prevalence of undiagnosed cases of HIV infection, earlier diagnosis, and improved access to care are essential to reduce the incidence of AIDS and AIDS-related death
- Acute primary HIV infection is the time of highest infectivity. Untreated HIV infection results in primary immune dysfunction
- In the United Kingdom, AIDS is defined as an illness characterized by one or more indicator diseases predominantly associated with severe immunosuppression. In the developed world, pneumocystis pneumonia (PCP) remains the most common AIDS-defining opportunistic infection
- Combined antiretroviral therapies have led to dramatic falls in the incidence of new AIDS and AIDS-associated deaths
- Providing effective antiretroviral treatment to the developing world remains an immense challenge. Global initiatives have improved access to treatment; however, despite progress the HIV pandemic remains the most serious infectious disease challenge to global public health

HIV infection results in progressive damage to the immune system, which leads to severe immunodeficiency, opportunistic infections, cancers, and death. In recent years marked improvements have been made in treatments, resulting in dramatic decreases in the incidence of AIDS and death in the developed world. Life expectancy in the developed world for an HIV-infected person aged 35 years starting antiretroviral therapy (ART) is estimated to be a further 37 years, approximately 80% of that expected for someone of the same age in the UK general population. However, HIV remains a major cause of mortality and morbidity and is also making a substantial contribution to the increase in the incidence of tuberculosis (TB), including drug-resistant TB, globally.

The classification and staging of HIV disease have been defined by the Centres for Disease Control (CDC) in the United States and the World Health Organization (WHO) (Table 17.1). The CDC system was used widely in the developed world, and the WHO system is used in the developing world. However, in resource rich settings measurement of peripheral CD4 cell counts reduce the importance of clinical staging systems, although presence of HIV-related clinical disease is an important factor in determining when to start ART.

ABC of Sexually Transmitted Infections, Sixth Edition.
Edited by Karen E. Rogstad.

Epidemiology

HIV is transmitted sexually, in blood or blood products, and perinatally. Worldwide, heterosexual transmission is the main route of transmission although in resource poor settings mother-to-child transmissions (MTCT) make a substantial contribution and, in some parts of the world, intravenous drug use causes a significant proportion of infections (e.g. Eastern Europe and Asia) (Figures 17.1 and 17.2).

In 2008, the WHO estimated globally:

- There are 33.4 million people living with HIV
- 71% of all new HIV infections are in sub-Saharan Africa
- There are 2 million deaths worldwide (1.4 million in sub-Saharan Africa)
- The ratio of men to women infected with HIV is virtually 1:1

In 2008, the Health Protection Agency reported in the United Kingdom:

- There are 77 400 people living with HIV
- 28% are unaware of infection
- 31% are diagnosed late (with a low CD4 count of <200 cells/mm^3)
- Of 7495 new HIV diagnoses: 40% in men who have sex with men (MSM), 40% heterosexual acquisition abroad, 13% heterosexual acquisition in the United Kingdom

Sexual transmission

The risk of transmission per exposure is relatively low. For receptive anal intercourse it is estimated to be 0.1–3.0% per sexual exposure. Transmission risk when performing fellatio may be as high as 0.04%. Oral sex is often inaccurately considered 'safe' and there is a resulting absence of condom use (Table 17.2). The risk of sexual transmission may be increased by a number of factors:

- HIV viral load in plasma and in genital secretions
- Co-existing sexually transmitted infections (STIs)

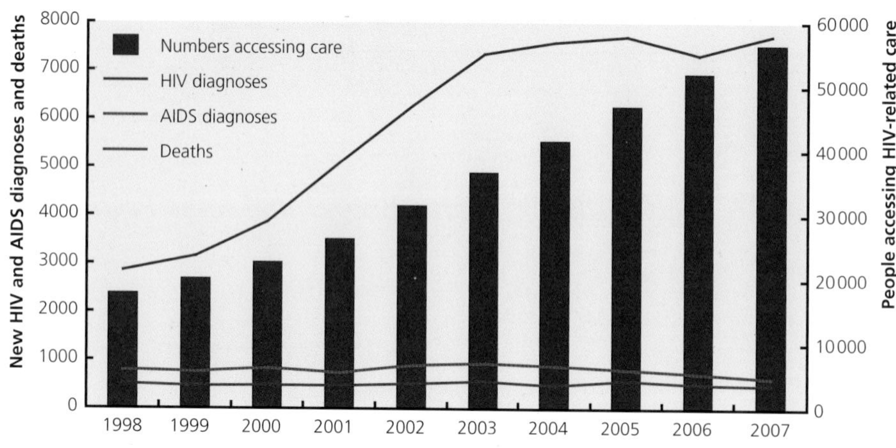

Figure 17.1 New HIV and AIDS diagnoses, HIV infected patients accessing care and deaths among HIV infected persons, UK. HIV diagnoses, AIDS case reports, and deaths in HIV-infected individuals in the United Kingdom, by year of diagnosis or occurrence. From the Health Protection Agency website (www.hpa.org.uk).

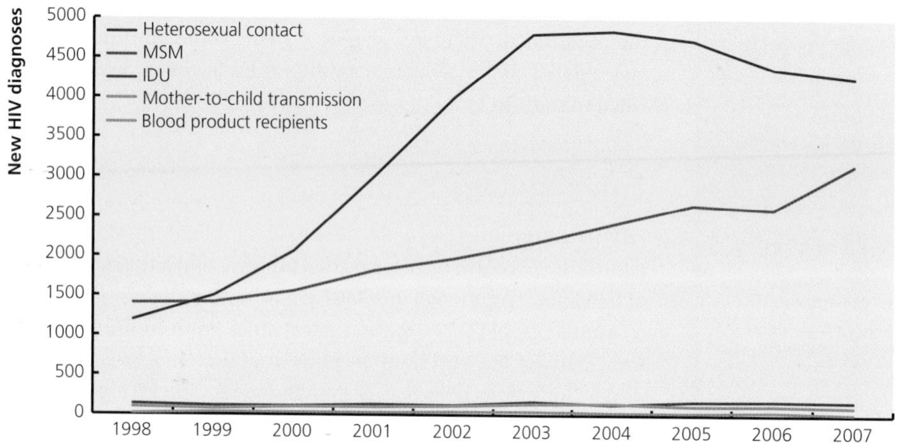

Figure 17.2 New HIV infections by prevention group. Reports to Communicable Disease Surveillance Centre of all HIV-infected individuals by year of diagnosis. From the Health Protection Agency website (www.hpa.org. uk).

- Type of sexual activity and frequency
- Breach in mucosal barrier (e.g. trauma, possibly menstruation)
- Genital herpes simplex virus (HSV) infection. The high prevalence of genital HSV is of global importance in facilitating HIV-1 transmission. It increases genital HIV shedding and also increases susceptibility to HIV acquisition

Male circumcision and condom use are protective for HIV acquisition.

Perinatal transmission

MTCT is about 1 in 3 if no intervention occurs. About 10% of transmission occurs *in utero*, late in pregnancy. Significantly, around 40% occurs postnatally, primarily through breastfeeding. The remaining majority of MTCT occurs at delivery. These data come from middle and low income countries where breastfeeding may be recommended because of lack of clean water. In this setting exclusive breastfeeding poses a lower risk of transmission than mixed infant feeding.

Prevention and control

Since 1996 in resource rich settings, the incidence of AIDS and HIV-related mortality have fallen dramatically as a result of the use of highly active antiretroviral therapy (HAART). No cure or vaccine is currently available to prevent HIV acquisition (Box 17.1).

Box 17.1 **Prevention and control**

- Surveillance and provision of HIV testing
- Counselling and health education
- Screening of people and donated blood
- Heat treatment of blood products
- Strategies to reduce high risk behaviour in targeted populations (e.g. safer sex and risk reduction counselling, condom promotion and provision)
- Antiretroviral therapy to reduce mother-to-child transmission
- Infant feeding counselling and support
- Provision and exchange sterile injecting equipment for injecting drug users
- Protection of health care staff
- Detection, treatment, and control of STIs
- Male circumcision
- Family planning, counselling, and contraception
- Reduction in number with undiagnosed HIV infection
- Earlier diagnosis and access to antiretroviral therapy

Reducing the prevalence of undiagnosed HIV infection, earlier diagnosis, and improved access to care are essential for further

Table 17.1 WHO clinical staging of HIV/AIDS for adults and adolescents with confirmed HIV infection.

Clinical Stage 1

Asymptomatic
Persistent generalised lymphadenopathy

Clinical Stage 2

Moderate unexplained weight loss (<10% of presumed or measured body weight)
Recurrent respiratory tract infections – sinusitis, tonsillitis, otitis media, and pharyngitis)
Herpes zoster
Angular cheilitis
Recurrent oral ulceration
Papular pruritic eruptions
Seborrhoeic dermatitis
Fungal nail infections

Clinical Stage 3

Unexplained severe weight loss (>10% of presumed or measured body weight)
Unexplained chronic diarrhoea for longer than 1 month
Unexplained persistent fever (>37.6°C intermittent or constant, longer than 1 month)
Persistent oral candidiasis
Oral hairy leukoplakia
Pulmonary tuberculosis (current)
Severe bacterial infections (pneumonia, empyema, pyomyositis, bone/joint infection, meningitis or bacteraemia)
Acute necrotizing ulcerative stomatitis, gingivitis or periodontitis
Unexplained anaemia (<8 g/dL), neutropaenia (<0.5 × 10^9/L) or chronic thrombocytopaenia (<50 × 10^9/L)

Clinical Stage 4

HIV wasting syndrome
Pneumocystis pneumonia
Recurrent severe bacterial pneumonia
Chronic herpes simplex infection (orolabial, genital, or anorectal for more than 1 month or visceral at any site)
Oesophageal candidiasis (or candidiasis of trachea, bronchi, or lungs)
Extrapulmonary tuberculosis
Kaposi's sarcoma
Cytomegalovirus infection (retinitis or infection of other organs)
Central nervous system toxoplasmosis
HIV encephalopathy
Extrapulmonary cryptococcosis including meningitis
Disseminated non-tuberculous mycobacterial infection
Progressive multifocal leukoencephalopathy
Chronic cryptosporidiosis (with diarrhoea)
Chronic isosporiasis
Disseminated mycosis (coccidiomycosis or histoplasmosis)
Recurrent non-typhoidal *Salmonella* bacteraemia
Lymphoma (cerebral or B-cell non-Hodgkin) or other solid HIV-associated tumours
Invasive cervical carcinoma
Atypical disseminated leishmaniasis
Symptomatic HIV-associated nephropathy or symptomatic HIV-associated cardiomyopathy

reducing the incidence of AIDS and AIDS-related death. People who are unaware they have HIV cannot take steps to reduce the risk of ongoing transmission. Those who are diagnosed late tend to have higher viral loads and are more likely to transmit HIV; they also more commonly have advanced disease or an AIDS-defining illness and therefore their prognosis is worse. In 2008 in the United

Table 17.2 The risk of HIV following an exposure from a known HIV-positive individual.

Type of exposure	Estimated risk of HIV transmission per exposure (%)
Blood transfusion (one unit)	90–100
Receptive anal intercourse	0.1–3.0
Receptive vaginal intercourse	0.1–0.2
Insertive vaginal intercourse	0.03–0.09
Insertive anal intercourse	0.06
Receptive oral sex (fellatio)	0–0.04
Needle-stick injury	0.3 (95 CI 0.2–0.5)
Sharing injecting equipment	0.67
Mucous membrane exposure	0.09 (95 CI 0.006–0.5)

Source: Adapted from BASSH Guidelines.

Kingdom, 32% of newly diagnosed patients had a CD4 count of less than 200 cells/mm^3 and 55% a CD4 count of less than 350 cells/mm^3, the CD4 count at which ART should be started. A disproportionate number of these are black African men and women. Increased access to and wider HIV testing are key strategies to reduce the number with undiagnosed infection and increase earlier diagnosis.

The screening of blood donors for HIV antibodies and heat treatment of blood products have virtually eliminated the risk to recipients. People who are known to be infected with or may have been exposed to HIV are advised not to donate blood, organs, or semen, and to practice safe sex. At diagnosis people with HIV infection should notify their current sexual partners and, if at risk, previous partners where possible. They should also be encouraged to discuss their status with future sexual partners to ensure negotiated safer sex practices. In some countries there is the potential for criminal prosecution for transmission of HIV but it is controversial if such criminalisation is in the public health interest with regard to control of the epidemic.

The treatment and control of STIs are important, as they are significant cofactors in transmission; however, results of STI intervention strategies have been disappointing. There is evidence that male circumcision is protective for HIV acquisition. However, male circumcision provides only partial protection, and therefore should be only one element of comprehensive HIV prevention including the provision of HIV testing and counselling services; treatment for sexually transmitted infections; the promotion of safer sex practices and the provision of male and female condoms and education in their correct and consistent use. The role of microbiocides is being investigated but trials to date have been disappointing.

Individuals on effective ART are much less likely to transmit the virus and there is ongoing debate about the role of ART treatment programmes in the prevention of HIV transmission at a population level.

Use of pre-exposure and postexposure ART strategies to prevent transmission of HIV are being investigated. Postexposure prophylaxis for HIV following sexual exposure (PEPSE) to HIV is recommended in the United Kingdom for people exposed to HIV in certain situations and patients with HIV and their partners should be made aware of its availability.

The evidence for the efficacy of postexposure prophylaxis after either occupational or sexual exposure to HIV is limited. However, in clinical practice it is common to consider postexposure prophylaxis after considerable exposure to HIV, usually by a needlestick injury. It is recommended that combination antiretroviral therapy be started as soon after the exposure incident as possible, preferably within 24 hours, for 4 weeks' duration

Opt-out antenatal screening and the careful management of pregnant HIV positive mothers in the United Kingdom has substantially reduced MTCT to less than 1%. ART plus the option of non-instrumental vaginal delivery (for mothers with undetectable HIV viral loads at term) or the option of caesarean section (for mothers with detectable HIV viral loads at term) and avoidance of breastfeeding for all is recommended.

In resource poor settings where the benefits of breastfeeding may outweigh the risks ART strategies to protect the infant during breastfeeding are being studied.

Immunology

The primary immune dysfunction is depletion and impaired function of the T-helper lymphocyte subset (lymphocytes bearing the CD4 cluster differentiation antigen). However, the CD4 molecule is also displayed at lower density on other cells, such as monocytes, macrophages, and some B lymphocytes. HIV gains access to these cells via the CD4 receptor. The CD4 lymphocyte has a pivotal role in the immune response (interacting with macrophages, other T cells, B cells, and natural killer cells, either by direct contact or by the influence of lymphokines such as interferon and interleukin 2).

The mechanism for CD4 lymphocyte loss remains uncertain, but probably includes enhanced apoptosis (programmed cell death) and inhibition of CD4 lymphocyte growth. CD4 T cells are preferentially lost from the gastrointestinal tract within weeks of HIV infection. The gastrointestinal tract is the single largest immunological organ and harbours most of the body's lymphocytes. Preferential and profound depletion of mucosal CD4 T cells occurs in gut associated lymphoid tissue during early infection but is targeted during all stages of HIV-1 infection. Chronic immune activation has a key role in the loss of CD4 cells and the pathogenesis of AIDS.

The peripheral CD4 count is a surrogate marker of immune function and is usually greater than 500 cells/mm^3 in HIV-negative individuals. When this count falls over time individuals are at greater risk of opportunistic infections and therefore it is used to guide when to start HAART.

The virus

HIV has a cylindrical core and its nucleic acid has been cloned and sequenced (Figures 17.3 and 17.4). It has a basic gene structure common to all retroviruses, but it is very different from the other human retroviruses (human T-lymphotropic viruses I and II). The CD4 antigen is a major receptor required for cell entry. Only cells bearing this antigen are susceptible to infection. The chemokine receptors (CCR5 and CXCR4) also act as coreceptors for HIV entry and their expression on the cell surface determine the susceptibility of CD4 bearing cell lines to different HIV strains.

On entry to the infected cell, the viral reverse transcriptase enzyme makes a DNA copy of the RNA genome (proviral DNA), hence the term retrovirus. The proviral DNA is able to integrate into the host cell DNA, facilitated by the viral integrase enzyme. During productive replication, RNA transcripts are made from the proviral DNA, and complete virus particles are assembled and released from infected cells by characteristic budding. The viral encoded protease enzyme is important for the maturation of the virus particle.

There are two distinct HIV viruses: HIV-1 and HIV-2. HIV-1 is more prevalent in Europe, the United States, South America, Australia, New Zealand, Asia, and Africa, whereas HIV-2 is found predominantly in West Africa (Figure 17.5). HIV-2 is structurally more similar to the simian immunodeficiency virus (SIV), than HIV-1. HIV-1 is a more rapidly mutating virus eventually producing divergent quasi-species and is essentially more virulent than HIV-2. Patients with HIV-1 have a poorer prognosis and progress to AIDS faster than those with HIV-2.

Natural course

Primary HIV infection

Acute infection with HIV may be accompanied by a transient non-specific illness similar to glandular fever. Common symptoms include:

- Fever
- Malaise
- Myalgia
- Lymphadenopathy
- Pharyngitis
- Rash

A transient aseptic meningoencephalitis may also occur. Most acute infections, however, are subclinical.

Antibodies to the core (p24) and surface (GP 41, 120, 160) proteins develop in 2–6 weeks, and are usually detected by enzyme-linked immunoassays, and confirmed by immunofluorescence or Western blotting. Delayed seroconversion has been observed so repeat testing after 3 months should be considered. If primary infection is suspected then a viral detection assay such as p24 antigen (as found in fourth generation HIV tests) or cell-associated proviral DNA should be requested. A positive viral detection test in the presence of a negative or evolving antibody test is indicative of primary HIV infection.

Initial concentrations of plasma viraemia (the HIV 'viral load') detected by polymerase chain reaction (PCR) are very high but then decline rapidly within a few days to weeks as the immune response to HIV develops. It is not clear which immune mechanisms are primarily responsible for this initial fall in viraemia, but the breadth and strength of HIV-specific CD4 and CD8 T-cell responses that

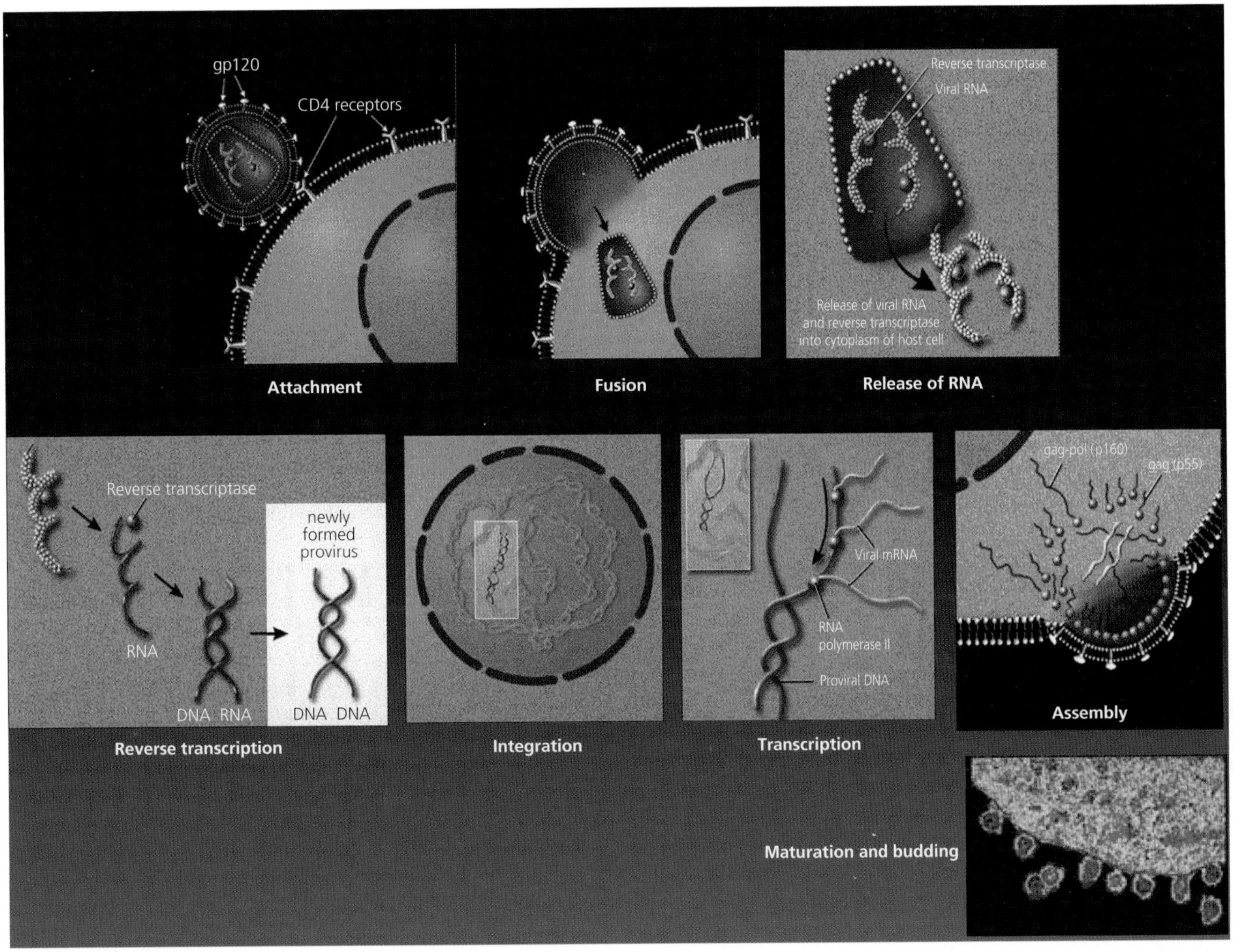

Figure 17.3 HIV lifecycle. Courtesy of Janssen.

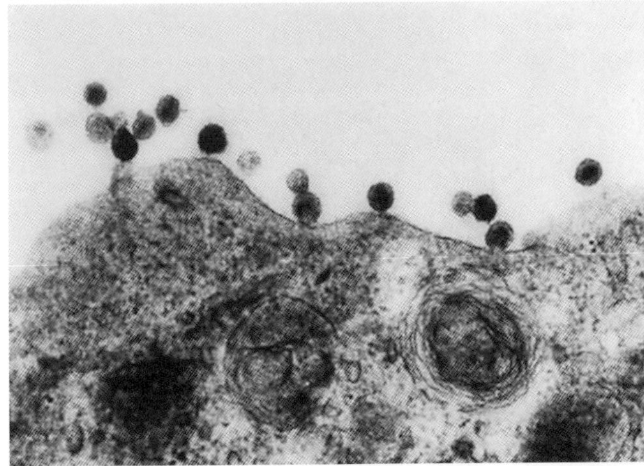

Figure 17.4 Electron micrograph of virus.

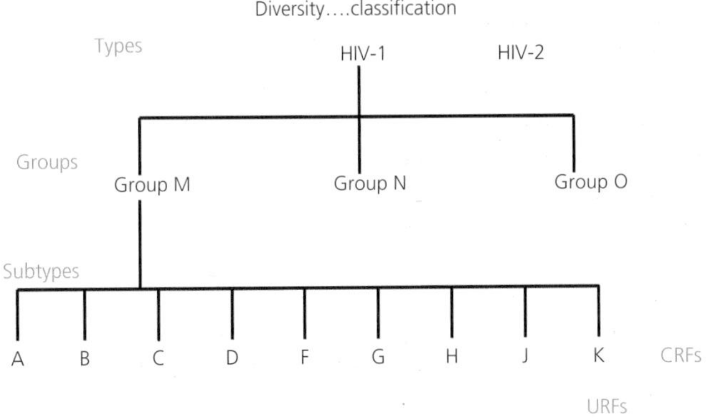

Figure 17.5 HIV diversity and classification. Courtesy of Janssen.

develop during primary infection are important for long-term virological control. They seem to determine a 'set point' around which viral replication is controlled over time, resulting in a plateau in the viral load.

A high viral load is associated with a more rapid decline in CD4 count over time and a quicker progression to symptomatic disease, whereas a very low viral load is predictive of slow or non-progression.

Primary HIV infection is the time of highest infectivity due to the high rate of viral replication and high levels of HIV RNA in the serum and other body compartments (e.g. genital tract). Diagnosing primary HIV infection is potentially important in preventing onward transmission. Whether ART given in primary infection for a defined period is of clinical long-term benefit to the individual is not known. Some patients may present with an AIDS-defining illness, neurological involvement, or a persistently low CD4 count (<200 cells/mm^3) at the time of primary HIV infection. Immediate initiation of ART would then be considered.

Chronic infection

Following seroconversion, HIV infection is initially asymptomatic for a variable period of time. Physical examination may show no abnormality, but about one-third of patients have persistent generalised lymphadenopathy. The most common sites of lymphadenopathy are the cervical and axillary lymph nodes; it is unusual in hilar lymph nodes. Biopsy usually shows a benign profuse follicular hyperplasia.

From cohort studies, it is estimated that without therapy about 75% of HIV-infected people can be expected to develop symptomatic (CDC stage B and C) disease within 9–10 years of primary infection

As the CD4 count declines, non-specific constitutional symptoms develop, which may be intermittent or persistent and include:

- Fevers
- Night sweats
- Diarrhoea
- Weight loss

Skin conditions not specifically associated with immunosuppression may develop or worsen including:

- Seborrhoeic dermatitis
- Folliculitis
- Impetigo
- Tinea infections

Patients may also have other conditions associated with immunosuppression which tend to affect the mucous membranes and skin:

- Oral candidiasis
- Oral hairy leucoplakia
- Herpes zoster
- Recurrent oral or anogenital herpes simplex

A high plasma viral load, low CD4 count (<200/mm^3) and symptoms and signs that include the above are associated with an increased risk of progression to an AIDS-defining illness (Figure 17.6).

During both the asymptomatic and symptomatic phases of chronic infection patients may present to a variety of health professionals with indicator conditions that should prompt HIV testing. The list of conditions associated with HIV is broad and covers a range of specialities (Table 17.3).

AIDS

AIDS is an illness characterised by one or more indicator diseases in the absence of another cause of immunodeficiency. Indicator diseases include opportunistic infections, malignancies, and HIV-associated dementia. The definition was initially developed when the cause of the syndrome was unknown and the HIV virus had not been identified but now the definition includes laboratory evidence of HIV infection. If the patient has not been tested or the results are inconclusive certain diseases strongly indicate AIDS.

Regardless of the presence of other causes of immunodeficiency, if there is laboratory evidence of HIV infection, other conditions may also constitute a diagnosis of AIDS. In 1993, the CDC extended the definition of AIDS to include all people who are severely immunosuppressed (CD4 count <200 cells/mm^3) irrespective of the presence or absence of an indicator disease. For surveillance purposes this definition has not been accepted within the United Kingdom and Europe. In these countries, AIDS continues to be a clinical diagnosis.

The WHO introduced a clinical case definition that could be used for epidemiological surveillance in settings where laboratory facilities are inaccessible. In 1994, this was expanded to incorporate HIV serology. If serological testing is unavailable, the clinical case definition should be used; if serological testing is available, the expanded case definition should be used.

The frequency of specific AIDS-defining illnesses differs between resource poor and resource rich settings (Box 17.2). In resource rich settings, pneumocystis pneumonia remains the most common AIDS-defining opportunistic infection and non-Hodgkin's lymphoma (Figure 17.7) is accounting for an increased proportion of AIDS diagnoses. In resource poor settings, tuberculosis is by far the most common opportunistic infection, together with diarrhoeal disease and wasting syndrome.

Box 17.2 **Common AIDS-defining diseases**

Resource rich countries

- Pneumocystis pneumonia
- Oesophageal candida
- Non-Hodgkin's lymphoma
- Tuberculosis (pulmonary and extra pulmonary)

Resource poor countries

- Tuberculosis (pulmonary and extrapulmonary)
- HIV wasting syndrome
- Cerebral toxoplasmosis
- *Cryptococcus* meningitis

Opportunistic infections

Opportunistic infections are caused by unusual pathogens. They are often caused by:

- Reactivation of latent organisms (e.g. tuberculosis)
- Usually non-pathogenic environmental organisms (e.g. *Pneumocystis jiroveci* pneumonia)

Table 17.3 Testing for HIV infection is recommended in adults presenting with the following clinical indicator diseases.

	AIDS-defining conditions	Other conditions where HIV testing should be offered
Respiratory	Tuberculosis Pneumocystis	Bacterial pneumonia Aspergillosis
Neurology	Cerebral toxoplasmosis Primary cerebral lymphoma Cryptococcal meningitis Progressive multifocal leucoencephalopathy	Aseptic meningitis/encephalitis Cerebral abscess Space occupying lesion of unknown cause Guillain-Barré syndrome Transverse myelitis Peripheral neuropathy Dementia Leucoencephalopathy
Dermatology	Kaposi's sarcoma	Severe or recalcitrant seborrhoeic dematitis Severe or recalcitrant psoriasis Multidermatomal or recurrent herpes zoster
Gastroenterology	Persistent cryptosporidiosis	Oral candidiasis Oral hairy leukoplakia Chronic diarrhoea of unknown cause Weight loss of unknown cause Salmonella, shigella or campylobacter Hepatitis B infection Hepatitis C infection
Oncology	Non-Hodgkin's lymphoma	Anal cancer or anal intraepithelial dysplasia Lung cancer Seminoma Head and neck cancer Hodgkin's lymphoma Castleman's disease
Gynaecology	Cervical cancer	Vaginal intraepithelial neoplasia Cervical intraepithelial neoplasia Grade 2 or above
Haematology		Any unexplained blood dyscrasia including: • thrombocytopenia • neutropenia • lymphopenia
Ophthamology	Cytomegalovirus retinitis	Infective retinal diseases including herpesviruses and taxoplasma Any unexplained retinopathy
ENT		Lymphadenopathy of unknown cause Chronic parotitis Lymphoepithelial paroticl cysts
Other		Mononucleosis-like syndrome (primary HIV infection) Pyrexia of unknown origin Any lymphadenopathy of unknown cause Any sexually transmitted infection

Source: UK HIV testing guidelines 2008, © British HIV Association 2008.

Treatment usually suppresses rather than eradicates the organisms and without effective antiretroviral therapy, and subsequent immune reconstitution, relapses are common.

The main organ systems affected by opportunistic infections are the respiratory system, the gastrointestinal tract, and the central nervous system.

Pulmonary complications

Pneumocystis jiroveci (previously *carinii*) pneumonia is one of the most common life-threatening opportunistic infections. The presentation is often subacute, with symptoms developing over several weeks. These include, malaise, fatigue, weight loss, a dry cough, shortness of breath, fever, and retrosternal chest pain. Chest examination and the chest radiograph (CXR) may be normal at presentation, or the CXR may show bilateral fine infiltrates, which are typically perihilar (Figure 17.8). The resting arterial oxygen tension may be normal or low, but desaturation usually occurs on exertion. Measurement of oxygen saturation following exercise is an important bedside test. The diagnosis is confirmed by cytological examination of induced sputum or by fibre optic bronchoscopy and bronchoalveolar lavage. Bronchoscopy can exclude other causes of pneumonia or coexistent infection or disease. First line treatment is with high dose co-trimoxazole. Concomitant treatment with steroids is indicated in severe disease. Pneumothorax is a common

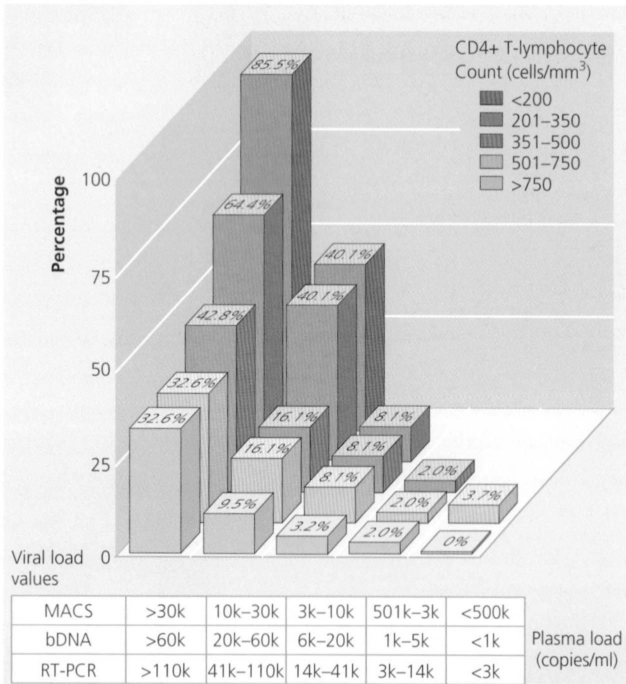

Viral load values						
MACS	>30k	10k–30k	3k–10k	501k–3k	<500k	Plasma load (copies/ml)
bDNA	>60k	20k–60k	6k–20k	1k–5k	<1k	
RT-PCR	>110k	41k–110k	14k–41k	3k–14k	<3k	

Figure 17.6 Likelihood of developing AIDS within 3 years. Adapted from Mellors *et al. Ann Intern Med* 1997;**126**(12):946–54.

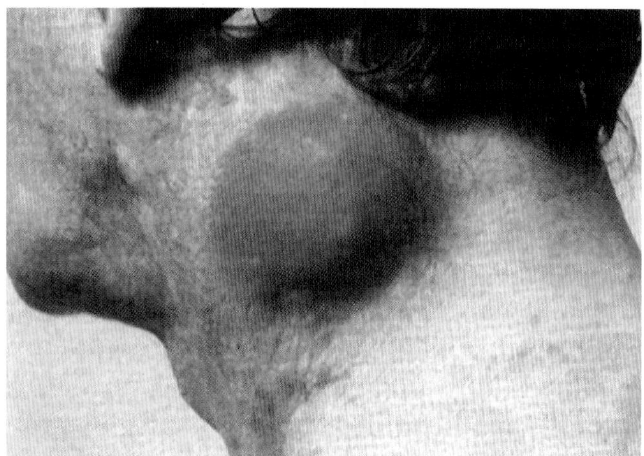

Figure 17.7 Extranodal lymphoma in the neck.

complication and should be excluded in patients with clinical deterioration. Antiretroviral therapy is indicated and secondary prophylaxis with co-trimoxazole is given until patients consistently maintain a CD4 count above 200 cells/mm^3.

Bacterial pneumonia is not an opportunistic infection but is more frequent in HIV-positive patients with any CD4 count. It should always be considered particularly as its presentation may be atypical and the radiological appearances may include diffuse infiltrates as well as the more typical focal or lobar patterns.

Mycobacterium tuberculosis is an AIDS defining infection and is the most common opportunistic infection and the leading cause of death in people living with HIV (PLWHIV) in Africa. It may present as pulmonary or extrapulmonary disease. The presentation of pulmonary tuberculosis may be atypical and should be considered

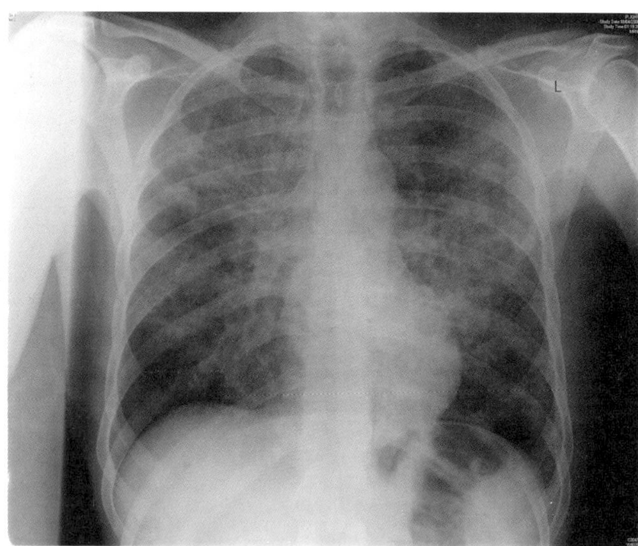

Figure 17.8 Chest radiograph of pneumocystis. Courtesy of Dr Vincent Lee.

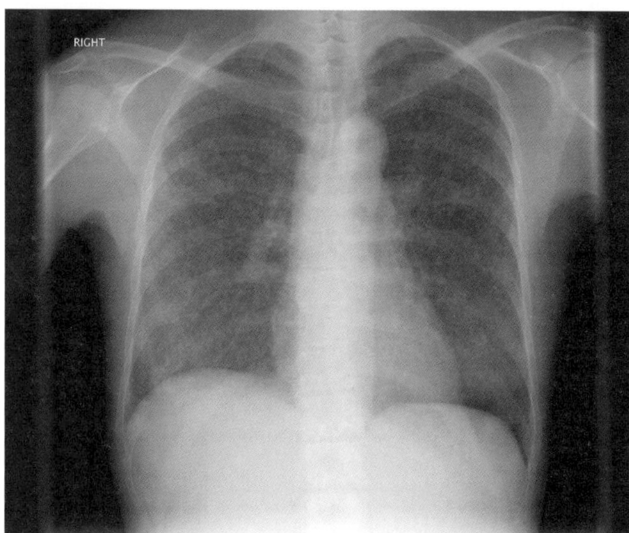

Figure 17.9 Chest X-ray of miliary TB. Courtesy of Ann Chapman.

in all patients with respiratory symptoms (Figure 17.9). Likewise, the diagnosis of extrapulmonary tuberculosis should be considered in all patients with lymphadenopathy, night sweats, fevers, or weight loss. Multidrug resistant (MDR) and extensively drug-resistant (XDR) TB in PLWHIV present a significant global challenge. Patients should be treated with antituberculous chemotherapy and HAART.

Atypical mycobacterial infection may occur but usually complicates severe immune depression (CD4 <50 cells/mm^3) in patients with advanced AIDS.

Gastrointestinal and hepatic complications

Oro-pharyngeal and oesophageal candidiasis commonly cause dysphagia or retrosternal discomfort. Oral candidiasis alone does not fulfil the criteria for AIDS (Figure 17.10). Oesophageal infection is best confirmed by culture or biopsy at endoscopy but

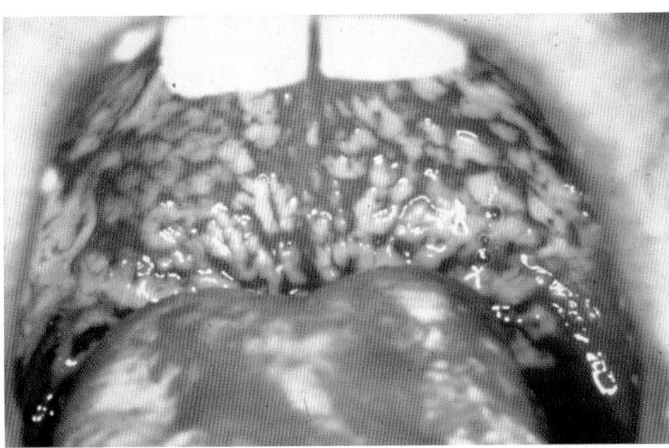

Figure 17.10 Oral candidiasis.

empirical treatment with an azole is common practice when access to endoscopic examination is limited.

Oral hairy leukoplakia is caused by EBV and is a sign of immune deficiency. It is a corrugated white lesion on the lateral borders of the tongue and occurs in about 20% of persons with asymptomatic HIV infection and occurs more frequently as the CD4 count falls.

Diarrhoea is a common symptom of patients with chronic HIV infection. In the majority of cases a pathogen is found, although an HIV enteropathy with malabsorption has been described.

Important gut pathogens are cryptosporidium (Figure 17.11), microsporidium, isospora, salmonella, and campylobacter. In resource poor settings, parasite infections are endemic and include giardia, strongyloides, and hookworm. When investigating diarrhoea, a variety of different pathogens should be considered depending on CD4 count. These include other bacteria, tuberculosis, *Mycobacterium avium* complex (MAC) and cytomegalovirus (CMV). Small bowel overgrowth, lymphoma, and Kaposi's sarcoma can also cause diarrhoea.

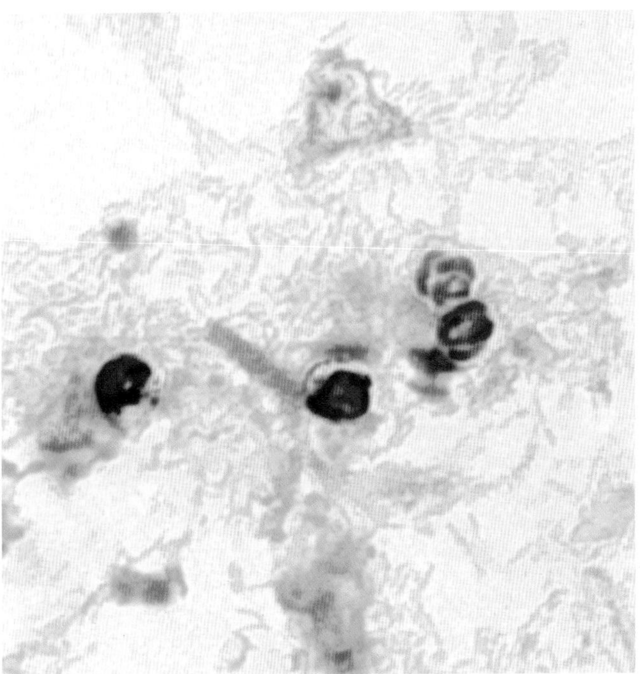

Figure 17.11 Cysts of cryptosporidium. *Source*: CDC/DPDx.

Investigation should comprise stool specimen for:

- Microscopy and culture
- Ova, cysts, and parasites (three separate specimens increase diagnostic yield)
- Requests for specific stains (e.g. cryptosporidium)

Fresh samples are more likely to yield positive results.

If the diarrhoea is persistent and no cause is identified, endoscopy with duodenal aspirate or biopsy and colonoscopy with mucosal biopsy may be indicated.

Cryptosporidium is the most common protozoal cause of diarrhoea and one of the most common pathogens isolated from AIDS patients. In immunocompetent human hosts, cryptosporidium produces a transient diarrhoeal illness. In people infected with HIV, it can cause transient, intermittent, or persistent diarrhoea ranging from loose stools to watery diarrhoea, colic, and severe fluid and electrolyte loss. The diagnosis should not be discounted without examining multiple specimens.

CMV and herpes simplex virus (HSV) can cause focal or diffuse ulceration of the gut, from the mouth to the anus. Herpes simplex virus most commonly causes mucocutaneous lesions at the upper and the lower ends of the gastrointestinal tract, whereas CMV may mimic inflammatory bowel disease or cause oral and oesophageal ulceration in patients with severe immunosuppression.

Hepatitis in patients with HIV may present as fever, abdominal pain, and hepatomegaly. Alternatively elevated liver function test (LFT) results may be the only indicator of liver disease. The most common infectious causes of hepatitis are coinfection with hepatitis B or C viruses. This occurs most often among homosexual and bisexual men, injecting drug users, and in patients originating from countries with high rates of endemic infection. Drugs, including antiretrovirals and antituberculous chemotherapy, are also a common cause of abnormal LFTs. Patients with lymphoma may present with fever, night sweats, and weight loss accompanied by abnormal LFTs. A granulomatous hepatitis, usually caused by atypical mycobacteria rather than *M. tuberculosis*, may occur. The herpes viruses and syphilis also occasionally may cause hepatitis as part of a disseminated infection.

Acalculous cholecystis and cholangitis show an endoscopic retrograde cholangiographic picture similar to that of primary sclerosing cholangitis, with strictures and dilatation of the biliary tree. *Cryptosporidium* and CMV are implicated as a cause of this syndrome.

Neurological complications

The nervous system is often affected by opportunistic infection and tumours. *Cryptococcus neoformans* is the most common fungal pathogen within the CNS, predominantly causing meningitis. This usually presents subacutely as headache, fever, vomiting, and confusion but may present acutely with seizures. The differential diagnosis includes tuberculous, bacterial and viral meningitis. Examination findings may include pyrexia, papilloedema, and meningism. Serum cryptococcccal antigen testing is useful in supporting the diagnosis but lumbar puncture, following computed tomography (CT)

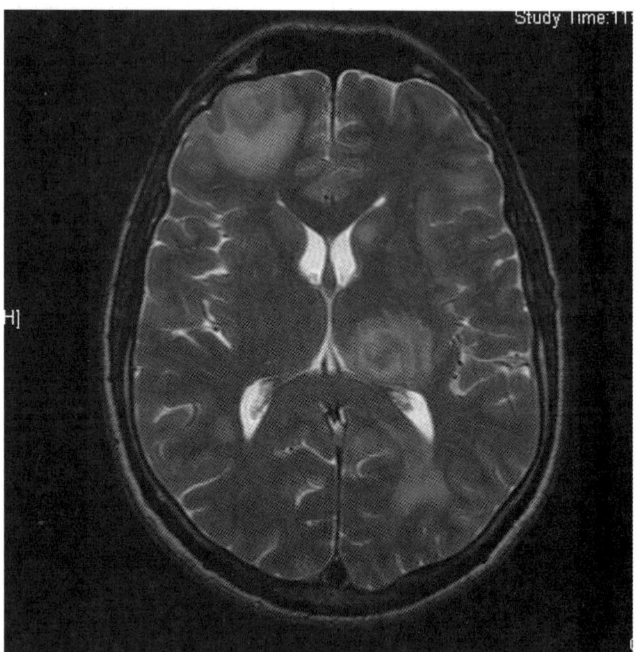

Figure 17.12 Cerebral toxoplasmosis: CT brain scan.

to exclude a space-occupying lesion, is the definitive diagnostic test. Cerebrospinal fluid (CSF) opening pressure may be extremely high and the diagnosis is confirmed with india ink staining and cryptococcal antigen testing of CSF samples. Treatment is with amphotericin and flucytosine and an important aspect of management is reduction of CSF pressure to reduce long-term neurological sequelae including loss of vision.

Cerebral toxoplasmosis is the most common cause of intracranial mass lesions and usually presents with focal symptoms and signs (Figure 17.12). Patients usually have a CD4 count of <100 cells/mm^3. The differential diagnosis includes primary cerebral lymphoma and cerebral abscess. Treatment is with sulfadiazine and pyrimethamine. If biopsy of an intracranial lesion is inadvisable then treatment may be initiated empirically with follow-up imaging at 2 weeks to assess response. A lack of radiological response indicates an alternative diagnosis such as lymphoma.

Many viruses may cause symptomatic CNS infection in immunosuppressed patients including HSV, varicella zoster virus (VZV), meningoencephalitis, and Creutzfeldt–Jakob virus-associated progressive multifocal leucoencephalopathy (PML).

Acute HIV infection may be associated with transient meningoencephalitis, myelopathy, and peripheral neuropathy. Chronic infection can cause many neurological complications.

AIDS-related dementia, also referred to as 'HIV associated motor cognitive complex', was estimated to occur in 10–40% of patients with symptomatic disease before the era of HAART. The clinical features are cognitive and behavioural changes that include memory loss, apathy, and impaired concentration. Neurological examination may show hypereflexia, hypertonia, and frontal signs. Computed tomography or magnetic resonance imaging often show cerebral atrophy and non-specific changes in the white matter. Opportunistic infections, intracranial mass lesions, metabolic encephalopathy, and neurosyphilis should be excluded.

HIV also causes vacuolar myelopathy (affecting primarily the posterior and lateral spinal cord), meningitis, and the following neuropathies: axonal sensory, chronic inflammatory demyelinating, and mononeuropathies.

Eye complications

HIV retinopathy is an essentially benign, often intermittent condition that can commonly occur in patients with HIV. Retinal changes are predominantly cotton wool spots without haemorrhages.

CMV may cause eye disease, usually in patients with a CD4 count less than 50 cells/mm^3 as a consequence of reactivation of previously acquired CMV (Figure 17.13). The most common manifestation is a destructive, potentially blinding retinitis. It usually presents with multiple floaters, blurring, loss of central vision, flashing lights, and scotomas. It is mostly unilateral but may be bilateral. Optic nerve involvement occurs in around 5%. Patients with CD4 counts less than 50 cells/mm^3 should have regular direct fundoscopy as a proportion will be found to have asymptomatic CMV retinitis involving the peripheral retina.

Fundoscopy reveals areas of retinal pallor and multiple granular white dots with haemorrhages, usually in a peri-vascular distribution. Atrophic changes and retinal thinning can occur. Changes normally start in the periphery and rapidly progress to involve the macula, leading to blindness. Complications include retinal detachment, branch retinal artery occlusion, cataract, and persistent iritis. CMV blood viraemia may be detectable by PCR testing and a high CMV viral load is associated with increased risk of developing CMV disease. First line treatment is with intravenous ganciclovir, but haematological toxicity needs to be monitored. Initiation of HAART is important in the prevention of recurrence.

Acute retinal necrosis is a rare condition caused by reactivation of varicella zoster. In patients with advanced HIV infection (CD4 counts <50 cells/mm^3) rapidly progressive herpetic retinal necrosis can occur. It is usually preceded by dermatomal herpes zoster and often presents with blurring of vision and pain in the affected eye, although it is frequently bilateral. Visual deterioration may be associated with a uveitis. Suggested therapy is a combination of intravenous foscarnet and ganciclovir (or aciclovir).

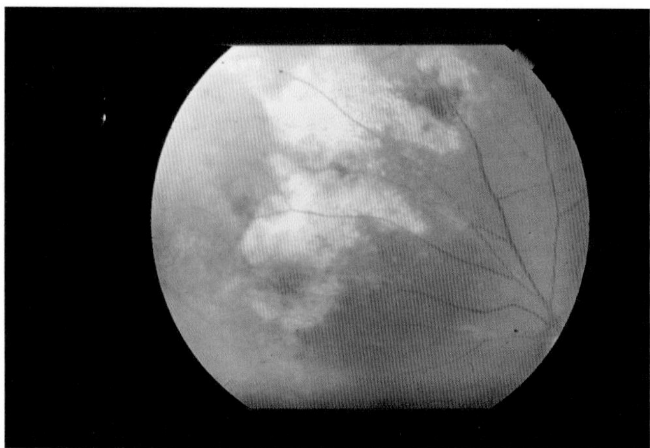

Figure 17.13 Cytomegalovirus retinitis. Courtesy of KE Rogstad.

Acute toxoplasma choroidoretinitis may resemble CMV retinitis; however, it tends to result in distinctive retinal scarring after treatment. It is more common in countries that have a higher background prevalence of toxoplasmosis such as Brazil and France. Choroidoretinitis is also a complication of cryptococcosis and histoplasmosis.

Renal complications

Kidney disease arises as a direct and indirect complication of HIV at all stages of infection, and includes HIV associated nephropathy (HIVAN), immune complex nephropathies, drug-related toxicities, and thrombotic microangiopathies.

HIVAN is thought to be caused by direct action of HIV and is diagnosed on renal biopsy. It is associated with characteristic glomerular and tubulointerstitial lesions, the most consistent finding being a collapsing focal segmental glomerular sclerosis.

HIVAN occurs in individuals of black African ethnicity and typically presents with nephrotic range proteinuria and rapidly progressive renal dysfunction in the setting of untreated advanced HIV disease. Ultrasound usually reveals large echogenic (bright) kidneys. Untreated HIVAN will progress to end-stage renal disease (ESRD) requiring dialysis. Early treatment with HAART is recommended and can produce significant renal recovery and preservation of renal function.

Tumours

The incidence of almost all tumours is increased by HIV infection. However, there does appear to be a decreased incidence of prostate and breast cancer. There are three AIDS defining malignancies:

- Kaposi's sarcoma
- High grade B-cell non-Hodgkin's lymphoma
- Invasive cervical cancer

Kaposi's sarcoma

Kaposi's sarcoma (KS) is the most common neoplasm that occurs in patients with AIDS, although the incidence has fallen over recent years. The risk is increased in all HIV-positive individual but most markedly in MSM.

KS-associated herpes virus (KSHV or human herpes virus 8) has been identified in nearly all KS lesions, and when detected in blood predicts the subsequent development of KS. Epidemiological evidence is supportive of sexual transmission and a causal role for KSHV in the pathogenesis of KS. Other malignancies associated with KSHV in HIV-positive patients include Castleman's disease (a multicentric lymphoproliferative condition) and primary effusion lymphoma.

The presentation of KS varies from indolent to aggressive. Cutaneous lesions are often characteristic violaceous plaques, macules, papules, or nodules but non-pigmented lesions may occur (Figure 17.14). Diagnosis is confimed histologically: KS lesions consist of spindle-shaped cells arranged in nodules and broad bands that contain vascular slits filled with extravasated erythrocytes (Figure 17.15).

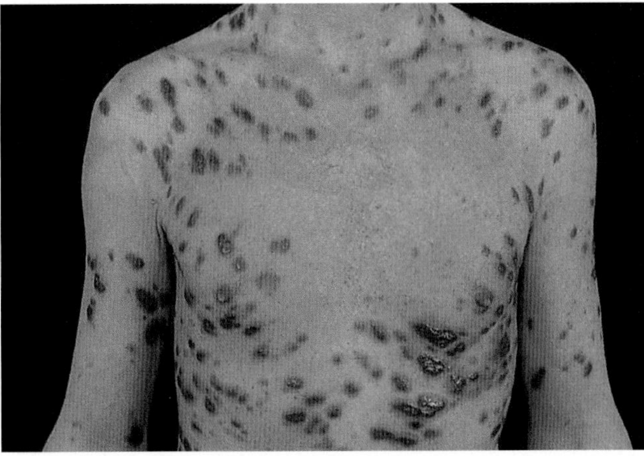

Figure 17.14 Patient with Kaposi's sarcoma.

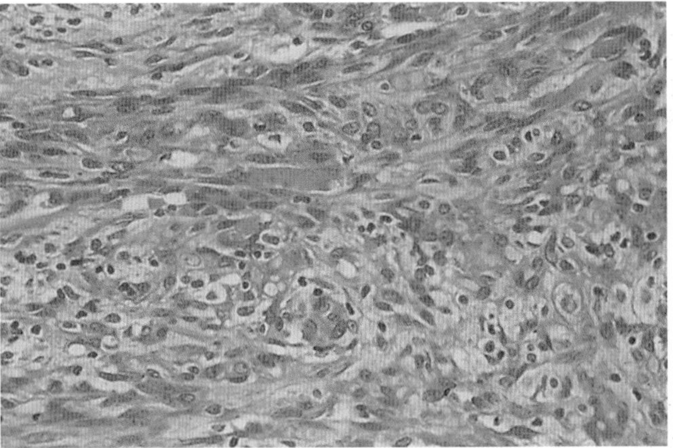

Figure 17.15 Kaposi's sarcoma histology: spindle cell proliferation of nodular Kaposi's sarcoma.

Visceral KS commonly affects the gastrointestinal tract and lymph nodes. KS of the hard palate is strongly suggestive of visceral involvement. Asymptomatic gastrointestinal tract involvement and lymph node involvement may be of no clinical consequence and only requires investigation if symptoms develop: these include pain, oesophageal or intestinal obstruction, and bleeding. Pulmonary involvement is usually symptomatic with dyspnoea, haemoptysis, and cough. Chest radiograph appearances vary from confluent irregular masses to interstitial nodularity. Computed tomography of the thorax may be useful in differential diagnosis. At bronchoscopy, endobronchial lesions may be seen.

Prior to HAART, median survival with KS was about 2 years; death was usually caused by a supervening opportunistic infection. Current good prognostic factors include CD4 count >150 cells/mm^3 and KS as the first AIDS defining illness. Poor prognostic indicators are age >50 and systemic 'B' type symptoms of fever, weight loss, or night sweats.

Non-Hodgkin's lymphoma

The incidence of AIDS-related lymphoma has fallen as a result of HAART but it accounts for an increased proportion of AIDS-related deaths. Compared with HIV-negative populations, non-Hodgkin's lymphoma (NHL) in HIV-positive patients tends to be more advanced at diagnosis and is less responsive to cytotoxic chemotherapy. Extranodal disease is common and affects the central nervous system, bone marrow, and gastrointestinal tract. More than 50% of AIDS-related lymphomas have been associated with Epstein–Barr virus (EBV) or KSHV infection, or both.

A diagnosis of NHL should be considered in patients with weight loss, constitutional symptoms, and anaemia.

The prognosis is beginning to approach that of the HIV-negative population, when adjusted for grade of disease, and median survival is around 24 months. Recent improvement is due to HAART – administration allowing the use of more potent chemotherapy.

Invasive cervical carcinoma

The definition of AIDS has included invasive cervical carcinoma since 1993. HIV-positive patients have an increased risk of cervical intra-epithelial neoplasia (CIN), anal intra-epithelial neoplasia (AIN), and vulval intra-epithelial neoplasia (VIN) related to co-infection with human papilloma virus (HPV).

Currently, there appears to be only a modest increase in the incidence of ICC in the HIV population that is independent of CD4 count. The clinical presentation of cervical cancer in HIV-positive women tends to be more aggressive with many patients presenting with advanced-stage disease; thus, HIV-positive women should have annual cervical cytology.

Non-HIV-related comorbidity

In resource rich settings, the leading causes of death in HIV patients on HAART are non-HIV-related. In resource poor settings, the leading causes of death are still AIDS defining illnesses.

HIV infected individuals have an increased risk of non-AIDS comorbidites such as cardiovascular, renal and liver disease, neurocognitive impairment as well as non-AIDS cancers. All of these diseases are traditionally associated with ageing. Pathogenesis is uncertain but may be due to additional effects of immunodeficiency and immune activation state as a consequence of HIV.

As life expectancy of patients with HIV increases as a consequence of effective ART, the proportion living into older age will also increase. It is expected that by 2015, 50% of people living with HIV in the United Kingdom will be above 50 years of age. Thus, the incidence and management of non-AIDS comorbidities is likely to become an increasing challenge. This highlights the need for HIV physicians and primary care physicians to work together to manage patients' comorbidities.

Treatment

Antiretroviral therapy

Sustained inhibition of viral replication with highly active antiretroviral therapy (HAART) results in reconstitution of the immune system in most patients, even those with advanced disease and very

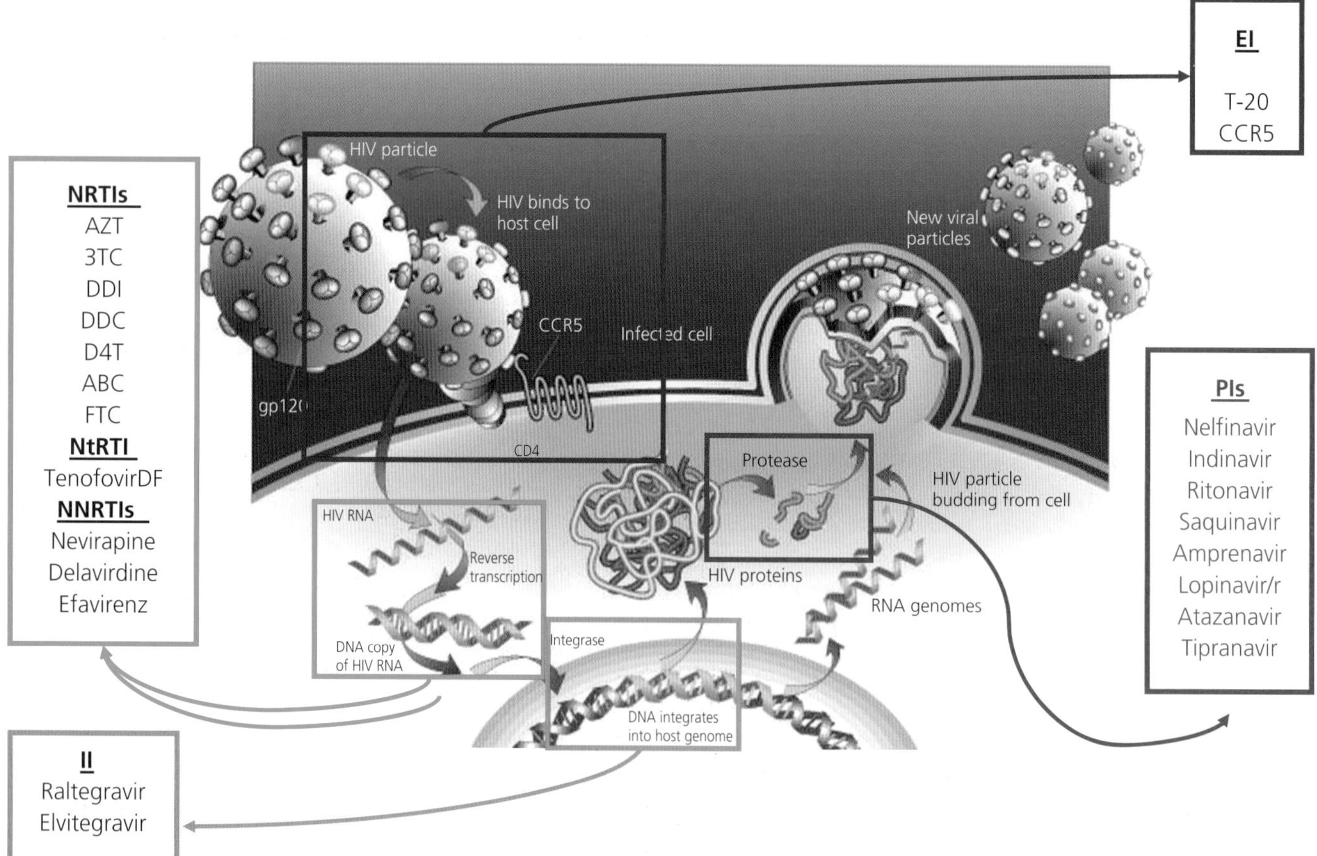

Figure 17.16 Targets for therapy. Courtesy of Janssen.

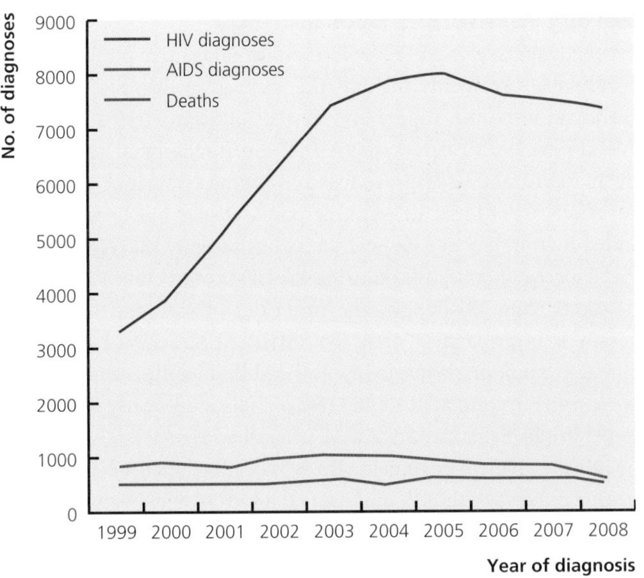

Figure 17.17 UK HIV diagnoses, AIDS case reports, and deaths in HIV-infected individuals by year of diagnosis/occurrence (see HPA HIV report 2009).

low CD4 counts, substantially reducing the risk of clinical disease progression and death (Figures17.16 and 17.17). The incidence of new AIDS illnesses or death in patients with CD4 counts below 50 cells/mm^3 is 55–70 events per 100 person years, whereas in patients whose CD4 count is above 200 cells/mm^3, this event rate falls to 3–6 (Figure 17.6).

Five main classes of antiretroviral drugs are currently licensed. The nucleoside/nucleotide analogues (NRTIs) and non-nucleoside agents (NNRTIs) inhibit the viral reverse transcriptase enzyme that produces a DNA copy from the single strand of viral RNA. The protease inhibitors (PIs) inhibit post-translational processing of viral proteins (Figure 17.16).

New drug classes include entry inhibitors, fusion inhibitors, CCR5 antagonists, and integrase inhibitors. These are often used in patients who have failed previous ARV treatments or who have developed ARV drug resistance.

Current standard regimens combine two NRTIs with either one NNRTI or a PI. The choice of therapy for an individual depends on the drug toxicity profile, pill burden, dosing schedule, likelihood of adherence to a particular regimen, comorbidities, and drug interactions. HAART is usually prescribed life-long.

The objective of antiretroviral therapy is to reduce and sustain plasma viral load concentrations to below what can be detected by sensitive viral load assays (e.g. <50 copies/mL). Failure to suppress to this level is associated with increased risk of viral load rebound and the emergence of viral genotypic mutations associated with reduced drug susceptibility. More than 80% of patients maintain undetectable viral loads at 1 year following the initiation of HAART. Patients who are able to tolerate and adhere to their treatment regimen successfully are more likely to achieve and sustain suppression of plasma viral load. Addressing adherence is an important aspect of clinical care.

Recommendations on when to initiate therapy are based on the knowledge of the risk of clinical disease progression (as determined by clinical status, CD4 count, and plasma viral load) and the likelihood of clinical benefit of therapy versus the likelihood of drug toxicity. Clinical practice across Europe and North America varies, but current guidelines recommend initiating therapy when the CD4 count falls to 350 cells/mm^3 or below, and in all patients who have symptomatic disease (Table 17.4). Similar CD4 guidance has recently been recommended by the WHO including in resource poor settings (Box 17.3). Following the initiation of HAART, at 4 weeks a viral load fall of greater than 1 log, and by 3–6 months an undetectable viral load should be expected. Patients who are stable

Table 17.4 Recommendations for starting antiretroviral therapy in adults.

Presentation/ clinical condition	BHIVA guidelines, Oct 2008	USDHHS, Dec 2009
Primary HIV infection	Treatment in clinical trial or neurological involvement or CD4 <200 cells/mm^3 >3/12 or AIDS-defining illness	Treat
Established HIV infection:		
CD4 <200 cells/mm^3	Treat	Treat
CD4 201–350 cells/mm^3	Treat as soon as possible when patient ready	Treat
CD4 351–500 cells/mm^3	Treat in specific situations when high risk of clinical events, e.g. HIVAN, hepatitis B co-infection when HBV treatment indicated	Treatment optional
CD4 >500 cells/mm^3	Consider enrolment into 'when to start trial'	Treat if HIVAN or HBV co-infection when HBV treatment indicated
AIDS diagnosis	Treat (except for TB when CD4 >350 cells/mm^3)	Treat

BHIVA - British HIV Association Guidelines, USDHHS - United States Department of Health and Human Services

Box 17.3 **WHO recommendations for antiretroviral therapy in adults and adolescents, November 2009**

When to start:

- Start antiretroviral treatment in all patients with HIV who have a CD4 count <350 cells/mm^3 irrespective of clinical symptoms
- CD4 testing is required to identify if patients with HIV and WHO clinical stage 1 or 2 disease need to start antiretroviral treatment
- Start antiretroviral treatment in all patients with WHO clinical stage 3 or 4 irrespective of CD4 count

Recommended first line regimens

Zidovudine + lamivudine + nevirapine or efavirenz
Tenofovir* + lamivudine or emtricitabine + nevirapine or efavirenz

*First line regimens for people with active hepatitis B should contain tenofovir plus lamivudine or emtrictabine and avoid nevirapine whenever possible
Boosted protease inhibitor reserved for treatment failure to first line regimen

on therapy and those who are not yet requiring treatment should have clinical and blood parameters monitored at regular intervals (e.g. 4–6 monthly).

Problems with current therapies include drug resistance and long-term drug toxicity (Table 17.5). For some drugs, the emergence of a single point mutation confers a large decrease in susceptibility, whereas for others the decrease in susceptibility is less and multiple mutations may be required to confer high-level resistance. Genotypic resistance testing should be performed prior to starting therapy and to repeat testing to guide second and third line treatment regimens is recommended. Patients may be infected with drug-resistant virus and recent studies in the developed world have shown that 10–15% of patients who present with primary HIV infection have genotypic mutations.

Table 17.5 Drug toxicities.

Drug	Toxicity
NRTIs	
Class associated	Lactic acidosis Hepatic steatosis Lipodystrophy (peripheral fat wasting)
Drug specific	
Zidovudine	Bone marrow suppression, nausea, vomiting, peripheral neuropathy
Stavudine	Peripheral neuropathy, hepatitis
Didanosine	Pancreatitis, dry mouth, peripheral neuropathy
Abacavir	Hypersensitivity reaction, nausea
Tenofovir	Renal impairment, renal Fanconi's syndrome, osteomalcia
NNRTIs	
Nevirapine	Rash, hepatitis, Stevens–Johnson syndrome
Efavirenz	Rash, dysphoria, mood change, vivid dreams, hypercholesterolaemia, hepatitis
Etravirine	Rash
Protease inhibitors	
Class associated	Lipodystrophy (fat wasting or accumulation), hyperlipidaemia, diabetes mellitus
Drug specific	
Indinavir	Hyperbilirubinaemia, nephrolithiasis, nail changes, dry skin
Ritonavir	Perioral dysathesia, flushing, hepatitis, diarrhoea, nausea, vomiting
Saquinavir	Few side effects, diarrhoea
Fos-amprenavir	Rash, diarrhoea
Lopinavir	Diarrhoea, nausea
Darunavir	Few side effects, rash, diarrhoea
Atazanavir	unconjugated hyperbilirubinaemia, nephrolithiasis
Tipranavir	Nausea, diarrhoea, abdominal pain
Integrase inhibitors	
Raltegravir	Nausea, diarrhoea, headache, rhabdomyolysis (very rare)
Entry inhibitors	
Enfuvirtide (fusion inhibitor)	Injection site reaction, respiratory tract infections
Maraviroc (CCR5 antagonist)	Nausea, diarrhoea, headache

NNRTI, non-nucleoside agents; NRTI, nucleoside/nucleotide analogues.

Therapy in resource poor settings

The challenge to provide effective therapy in resource poor settings is immense. Problems include the lack of availability of HIV diagnostic tests, the supply and cost of antiretroviral drugs, the pressure on health care systems that are ill-equipped to deliver effective care, and widespread fear and stigma associated with HIV and AIDS. Treatment in resource poor settings has largely been guided by the patient's clinical status but recently the WHO have placed a greater emphasis on using the CD4 count (Box 17.3).

Despite these challenges, the provision of care and access to therapy is improving in many countries. At the end of 2008, an estimated 4 million people in low and middle-income countries had access to ART compared to 400 000 in 2003, and nearly 3 million people in sub-Saharan Africa were prescribed HAART.

Multiple challenges remain. Every day more than 6800 people become infected with HIV and more than 5700 die, mostly because they have no access to HIV prevention, treatment, and care services. Despite progress made in scaling up the response over the last decade, the HIV pandemic remains the most serious infectious disease challenge to global public health (Box 17.4).

Box 17.4 **United Nations Declaration of commitment on HIV/AIDS (2001): features of comprehensive care for people living with HIV and AIDS**

- Available, accessible voluntary counselling and testing services
- Prevention and treatment of HIV-related illnesses
- Provision of antiretrovirals
- Prevention and treatment of tuberculosis and other infections
- Prevention and treatment of STIs
- Prevention of further HIV transmission
- Palliative care
- Family planning
- Good nutrition
- Social, spiritual, psychological, and peer support
- Respect for human rights
- Reduction of the stigma associated with HIV and AIDS

The Millennium Development Goals include a target to combat HIV/AIDS: to halt and reverse the spread of HIV/AIDS by 2015, and to achieve universal access to treatment for all those who need it by 2010. However, in 2008 only 42% of those requiring treatment had access and only 45% of HIV-positive women received treatment to prevent MTCT of HIV.

Immune reconstitution syndrome

Immune reconstitution syndrome (IRS) describes a phenomenon associated with restoration of immune function with subsequent worsening of diagnosed opportunistic infections (OIs) of unmasking of previously undiagnosed OIs. It occurs after the initiation of HAART in patients with low CD4 counts. IRS most commonly involves mycobacterial infections (TB and disseminated MAC) but is also seen with cryptococcal disease, toxoplasmosis, PCP, hepatitis B and C viruses, CMV infection, histoplasmosis, and PML. Manifestations may be non-specific but patients usually present with fever and worsening of the clinical manifestations of the underlying OI. It usually occurs within the first 4–8 weeks after starting ARVs. Management is to continue treatment of the underlying OI, continue HAART and provide supportive care. Symptoms may take weeks or months to subside. Adjunctive use of immunosuppressive or immunomodulatory therapy has been used but there is no definitive evidence of clinical benefit.

Preventing opportunistic infections and tumours

Primary and secondary prophylaxis of opportunistic infections remains important in patients with severe immunodeficiency (Tables 17.6 and 17.7). Both can be discontinued once the CD4 count rises (consistently >200 cells/mm^3) without risk of recurrence. However, the most effective strategy to prevent OIs is treatment with antiretroviral therapy. Challenges occur when deciding whether to start HAART in patients recently diagnosed with an OI. Clearly, one advantage is that HAART initiation will usually improve immune function and contribute to faster resolution of the infection. Certain OIs are effectively treated only with HAART such as PML, Kaposi's sarcoma and microsporidiosis. However, starting HAART in patients with acute OIs can be associated with an increased risk of drug toxicity and the development of IRS. Recent data suggest that there is potential clinical and survival benefit if ART is started early, at 10–14 days after initiation of treatment for an acute OI excluding mycobacterial disease. The risk of IRS and overlapping drug toxicity should be weighed against clinical benefit.

Table 17.6 Opportunistic infections: recommendations for initiation of primary prophylaxis.

Opportunistic infection	CD4 count	Standard drug	Comments
Pneumocystis jiroveci pneumonia	<200 cells/mm^3	Co-trimoxazole	
Cerebral toxoplasmosis	<100 cells/mm^3	Co-trimoxazole	if + serology
Mycobacterium avium complex	<50 cells/mm^3	Azithromycin	
Cytomegalovirus disease	Consider if CD4 <50 cells/mm^3	Valganciclovir	if CMV viraemia

Tuberculosis prophylaxis if recent close contact of smear positive index patient and no evidence of active clinical disease. National guidelines for use of tuberculin skin testing for screening varies.

Table 17.7 WHO Recommendations for Initiation of co-trimoxazole prophylaxis among adults and adolescents living with HIV in resource limited settings.

Based on who clinical staging criteria alone (when CD4 count is not available)	Based on who clinical staging and CD4 cell count criteria*
WHO clinical stage 2, 3, or 4	Any WHO clinical stage and CD4 <350 cells per mm^3† OR WHO clinical stage 3 or 4 irrespective of CD4 level

Universal option: Countries may choose to adopt universal co-trimoxazole for everyone living with HIV and any CD4 count or clinical stage. This strategy may be considered in settings with high prevalence of HIV and limited health infrastructure

*Expanded access to CD4 testing is encouraged to guide the initiation of antiretroviral therapy and to monitor the progress of antiretroviral therapy.
†Countries may choose to adopt a CD4 threshold of <200 cells per mm^3.

Primary care

GPs will increasingly be involved in testing patients and they should be knowledgeable of who should be offered a test. Including patients from high prevalent populations, those with a history of risk behaviour, and those presenting with indicator diseases. Additionally, although the care of HIV-infected patients has primarily been the responsibility of specialist centres, the GP's role is likely to increase as patients survive longer, require management of metabolic and cardiovascular complications of therapy, and develop other non-HIV-related conditions. Primary care physicians should be aware of potential severe drug interactions with antiretroviral therapy. A good source of information is www.hiv_druginteractions.org.

Patients with good CD4 counts, particularly those on ART with undetectable viral loads, are unlikely to present with opportunistic infections and in the primary care setting should be investigated in the same manner as those patients without HIV infection.

Primary care involvement in the management of social, mental health, and palliative care issues is important. In addition, doctors can have an important role in HIV prevention by promoting safer sex behaviour and by improving diagnosis and treatment of STIs in primary care. GPs are in a unique position to support HIV-positive patients during pregnancy and facilitate the testing of children of HIV-positive patients as well as providing contraception and managing non-HIV-related medical problems. A knowledge of HIV and its management, common complications related to low CD4 counts and drug interactions will assist GPs in providing the most appropriate care for their patients.

Further reading

Adler MW. *ABC of AIDS*. BMJ Books, Oxford, 2001.

British Association of Sexual Health and HIV Guidelines. Available at www.bashh.org.uk.

British HIV Association Clinical Guidelines. Available at http://www.bhiva.org/ClinicalGuidelines.aspx.

Holmes KK, Sparling PF, Stamm WE, Piot P, Wasserheit JN, Corey L, *et al*. *Sexually Transmistted Diseases*, 4th edn. McGraw Hill, New York, 2008.

Palfreeman A, *et al*. UK National Guidelines for HIV Testing 2008. British HIV Association, British Association for Sexual Health and HIV, British Infection Society. Available at www.bhiva.org.

CHAPTER 18

Diagnosis of Sexually Transmitted Infections

Sarah Alexander [1] *and Monique Andersson* [2]

[1]Sexually Transmitted Bacteria Reference Laboratory, Health Protection Agency, London, UK
[2]Health Protection Agency Regional Laboratory South West, Bristol, UK

OVERVIEW

- To describe the range of laboratory methods available for detecting individual STIs and detail their advantages and limitations
- To describe STI point of care tests
- To define both 'sensitivity and specificity' with regards to laboratory testing

The accurate and timely laboratory identification of sexually transmitted infections (STIs) is pivotal to supporting a presumptive clinical diagnosis and for detecting cases of asymptomatic infection. This chapter provides a brief overview of the range of different testing methods that are used to detect STIs in the laboratory and also introduces some of the newer point of care or rapid tests, which are becoming more widely available.

Gonorrhoea

Gonorrhoea is caused by the obligate human pathogen *Neisseria gonorrhoeae*, and the accurate detection of this bacterium is paramount for successful control. Methods of detection vary considerably in cost, technical complexity, and performance. Historically, presumptive diagnosis was by microscopy, where a patient's genital smear was stained and examined directly for intracellular gram-negative diplococci. This technique is still used in many parts of the world, and can be performed even where resources and laboratory facilities are limited.

Bacteriological culture followed by full identification of gonococcal colonies is regarded as the gold standard diagnostic method (Figure 18.1). This is because where transport links between clinic and laboratory are good or where direct plating takes place in the clinic, culture has a high specificity and sensitivity. Culture also provides an isolate upon which susceptibility testing can be performed. This is important as the prevalence of *Neisseria gonorrhoeae* resistance is increasing and therapeutic options are becoming limited.

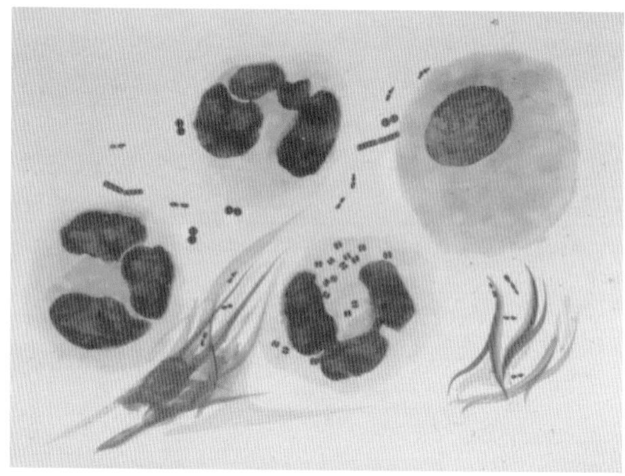

Figure 18.1 Urethral exudate containing *Neisseria gonorrhoeae* showing typical intracellular gram negative diplococci.

However, culture can be labour intensive and slow. Consequently, molecular techniques, which do not require viable bacteria can be used on non-invasive specimens, are becoming more widely available (Table 18.1).

Chlamydia

The laboratory confirmation of *Chlamydia trachomatis* has been historically difficult because this bacterium has a unique growth cycle and can only be propagated in tissue cultured cell lines (Figure 18.2). Methods for detecting *C. trachomatis* include cell culture, direct fluorescence microscopy, and enzyme-linked immunosorbent assays (ELISA). Molecular tests are now the mainstay of diagnosis in the developed world and are regarded as the gold standard because of high sensitivity and specificity. With the exception of some newly available rapid tests, all *C. trachomatis* testing is confined to the laboratory environment (Table 18.2).

Lymphogranuloma venereum

All *C. trachomatis* tests will detect lymphogranuloma venereum (LGV) strains, but there is currently no commercial test available for the specific detection of LGV-associated serovars. However, LGV-specific real-time polymerase chain reaction (PCR)

ABC of Sexually Transmitted Infections, Sixth Edition.
Edited by Karen E. Rogstad.

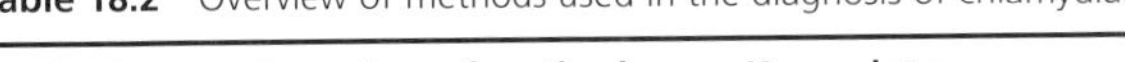

Table 18.1 Overview of methods used in the diagnosis of gonorrhoea.

Overview of method and specimen collection	Key points
Direct microscopy (Presumptive diagnosis)	
Production of a clinical smear followed by gram staining. Slide is examined for the presence of intracellular gram-negative diplococci	• Rapid: performed while patient waits in clinic • Sensitive in symptomatic males (95%) • Lacks sensitivity in: women, asympomatic males and extragenital samples
Bacteriological culture – Definitive diagnosis	
Inoculated swab or loop is either: (i) streaked onto culture plate directly in clinic, or (ii) placed into a transport media (Amies or Stuarts). Commonly both a selective and non-selective culture media is used Subsequent colonies can be identified using a range of different testing methods including: gram stain, oxidases test, biochemical tests (carbohydrate fermentation or chromogenic enzyme substrates tests) and immunological tests (latex agglutination test, immunfluoresence test)	• High specificity (~100%) in all sites • Medium sensitivity (80–90%) in genital sites • Isolate available for antimicrobial susceptiblity testing • Transport/storage critical • Labour intensive • Requires invasive specimens (urethral/cervical swabs)
Molecular Methods	
The nucleic acid amplification tests (NAATs) amplify sequence specific regions of *N. gonorrhoeae* RNA or DNA	• Automated and rapid • High sensitivity (90–100%) • Suitable for non-invasive specimens (self-taken vaginal swabs and urines) • Some commercial platforms lack specificity and therefore false positive results can occur • Implementing confirmatory testing (employing a second molecular test with a different target site), reduces the chance of false positive results

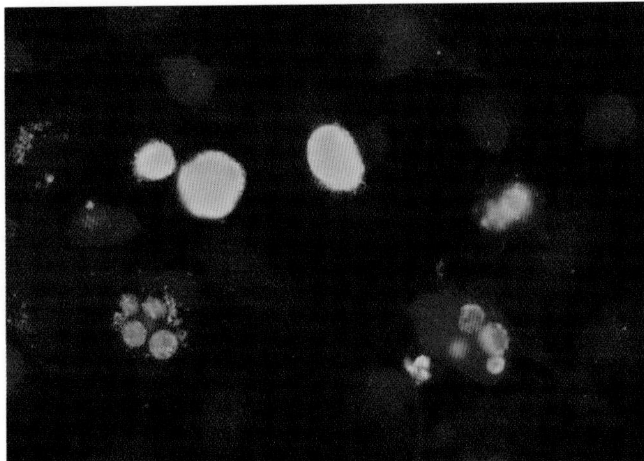

Figure 18.2 Green and yellow fluorescent stained inclusions of *Chlamydia trachomatis* in tissue culture cells.

Table 18.2 Overview of methods used in the diagnosis of chlamydia.

Method	Overview of method and specimen collection	Key points
Tissue culture	The direct growth of CT in tissue cultured cell lines (e.g. McCoy cells) followed by microscopic examination for inclusion bodies	• High specificity (~100%) • Low sensitivity (~65–75%) • Requires invasive specimens (urethral/cervical swabs) • Transport/storage critical • Technically complex
Direct Immunoflu-orescence	Direct staining of clinical smear with fluorescence labelled antibody and microscopic examination for the presence of inclusion bodies	• High specificity (~99%) with experienced personnel • Rapid: ~2 hour turnaround time • Low sensitivity (70–80%) • Labour intensive and non-automatable
ELISA	ELISA based tests which utilise labelled antibodies to detect the presence of CT lipopolysaccharide (LPS) in clinical samples	• Intermediate sensitivity (~60–70%) • High specificity in genital specimens (~80–90%) • Semi-automated: suitable for large-scale screening • Low specificity in extragenital specimens
Molecular methods	Nucleic acid amplification tests (NAATs) amplify sequence specific regions of *C. trachomatis* RNA or DNA	• High sensitivity and specificity (>90% and >90%) • Automated and rapid • Suitable for non-invasive specimens (vaginal swabs and urines) • Specificity can be compromised by contamination

methods are available in some national reference laboratories and research settings. High risk samples should undergo confirmatory testing.

Mycoplasma genitalium

Mycoplasma genitalium is extremely difficult to grow. Molecular tests are used in detection, but no commercial test is currently available. Testing is confined to specialist centres using in-house PCR tests.

Chancroid

Culture of *Haemophilus ducreyi* is the method available to most laboratories. However, the fastidious nature of *H. ducreyi* means that direct bedside inoculation on specialist media is required for optimal sensitivity. This can be difficult to provide in many clinical settings. No commercial molecular assay is currently available, but several specialist laboratories have in-house real-time PCR assays. These are commonly multiplexed, allowing the simultaneous detection of multiple agents responsible for genital ulcer disease (e.g. herpes simplx virus (HSV), *Treponema pallidum* and *H. ducreyi*).

Syphilis

Treponemal serology

In the United Kingdom it is common practice to screen serum specimens using an ELISA test and any reactive specimens are then confirmed using either a *Treponema pallidum* haemagglutination assay (TPHA) or the more sensitive *Treponema pallidum* particle agglutination assay (TPPA). A reactive TPPA and ELISA test is indicative of either past or current treponemal infection. In most instances a patient with only one reactive treponemal serology test is regarded as a false positive (Table 18.3).

The differentiation between past and active treponemal infection can be problematic as the TPPA and ELISA usually remain positive for life. To confirm an active infection either a rapid plasma reagin (RPR) or a venereal disease reference laboratory (VDRL) test can be used, where a high titre (>1:16) is indicative of active infection. T pallidum IgM assays are available and can play a role in differentiating active from past infection.

Direct detection of *Treponema pallidum*

In addition to serological testing, it is possible to detect *T. pallidum* directly from genital lesions by either the use of dark ground microscopy or molecular assays (see Chapter 13).

Herpes simplex

There are two distinct genital herpes simplex types (HSV-1 and HSV-2). Detection methods include culture and molecular tests (Table 18.4). The screening of asymptomatic patients by serological methods is not routinely performed because of the implications of both false positive results and/or the unknown clinical significance of HSV-1 positive result in causing genital disease. However, there are specific scenarios in which serological testing for HSV may be initiated, for example:

1 In symptomatic pregnant women, to determine whether they have primary HSV infection
2 In undiagnosed vaginal soreness, and
3 In serodiscordant couples who wish to have unprotected sex.

Table 18.3 Summary of serological assays for detecting treponemal infection.

Method and setting	Key points
Screening and confirmatory tests *EIA:* detection of treponemal antibody (IgG and IgM) in a sandwich assay *TPPA:* gelatine particles sensitised with *T. pallidum* antigens are mixed with patient serum. Visual agglutination occurs in the presence of treponemal antibodies	• High sensitivity and specificity (>95%) • Cheap to perform • EIA tests can be automated and electronically reported • Reactive tests do not discriminate between past/recent infections • Tests can be insensitive if used in early infection • In low prevalence populations the absence of confirmatory testing will result in a high number of false positive results
Assays for detecting active infection *RPR and VDRL tests:* agglutination tests that detect host antibody to lipoidal (present on treponemal and host cells)	• Active infection is assumed when serum is reactive at high titer (>1:16) • Biological false positives can occur (<1:4) • Cheap, reproducible, easy to perform • In some countries RPR/VDRL are used as screening tests

Table 18.4 Methods used in the diagnosis of herpes simplex.

Method and setting	Key points
Direct detection of HSV material from lesions • *Virological culture:* Propagation and identification of HSV virus in cultured cell lines. • *Molecular detection:* The PCR amplification of HSV: directly from lesions	• Culture has high specificity (~100%) • Culture detects replicating virus • Culture has intermediate sensitivity (50–90% from vesicles, 40–70% from ulcers) • Culture requires viable specimen: transport and storage critical • Culture is non-automatable, untimely, and expensive • Molecular testing is highly sensitive • Molecular testing is automatable, rapid, and labour efficient
Serological tests • The examination of clotted blood for the presence of HSV type-specific antibodies: ◦ *HSV2 antibodies:* usually indicative of genital herpes ◦ *HSV1 antibodies:* either oral pharyngeal or genital infection A range of different serology tests are available including Western blot, ELISA IgG tests, and immunoblot (IgG)	• Relatively high sensitivity (90–97%: depending on test) • Specificity (61%–98%: depending on test) • Serology can be insensitive if used in early infection

Trichomonas vaginalis

Trichomonas vaginalis is a motile flagellated protozoa, and is the causative agent of trichomoniasis. Detection is by microscopic examination of a wet mount smear. This is insensitive when compared with culture, which is considered to be the gold standard, although it is rarely available. Some in-house PCR assays have shown high sensitivity, but availability is limited to research laboratories.

Bacterial vaginosis

Two criteria exist for the diagnosis of bacterial vaginosis:

1 Clinical criteria (Amsel criteria), or
2 By the microscopic examination of a gram-stained vaginal smear using the Hay–Ison criteria (Table 18.5)

Point of care testing for STIs

Point of care tests (POCT), near patient tests, and rapid tests are synonymous terms used to describe analytical procedures performed

Table 18.5 Methods for the diagnosis of bacterial vaginosis (BV).

Clinical diagnosis (Amsel criteria)	Microscopic diagnosis (Ison & Hay criteria, 2002)
At least 3 out of the following 4 criteria should be present:	Gram-stained vaginal smear examined by microscopy and graded as follows:
• Homogeneous discharge (thin, white) • Clue cells in wet mount (20%) • Vaginal fluid pH >4.5 • Whiff test (fishy odour on adding alkali)	1 *Normal:* dominance of Lactobacillus 2 *Intermediate:* mixed flora (some Lactobacilli, but also some Gardnerella/or Mobiluncus present) 3 *BV:* Dominance of Gardnerella and/or Mobiluncus morphotypes. Few or absent Lactobacilli

Table 18.6 Potential advantages and disadvantages of point of care testing (POCT).

Advantages	Disadvantages
• Useful in specific clinical scenarios (e.g. HIV POCT for late presentation labour and PEPSE) • Useful for community outreach • Ease of use • May have a role in destigmatising testing • Uses small volume of blood • May be perceived as more confidential • Knock on public health benefits with more infections being diagnosed • Improves patient acceptability, therefore increasing testing • Reduce pressure on STI clinics	• Requires rigorous control of quality assurance • High burden of training • Second sample required for confirmation of positives • May reduce testing for other STIs • Loss of epidemiological data

*PEPSE, postexposure prophylaxis for HIV following sexual exposure.

for patients within a limited time period outside of the conventional laboratory. In the UK, POCT for the diagnosis of STIs has expanded rapidly (Table 18.6), although inappropriate use and inaccurate results lead to poor patient outcomes. Quality assurance procedures in conjunction with support from microbiology and virology is essential.

How do they work?

Most POCT tests for STIs are immunochromatographic tests that detect either antibody (e.g. syphilis); antigen (e.g. HbsAg) or both antigen and antibody (e.g. fourth generation HIV test). The presence of the specific antigen or antibody is demonstrated by a colour change on the test strip (Figure 18.3). To ensure the individual test is valid a control bar is incorporated into the device. If this bar is absent the test is invalid and should be repeated.

Tests

Blood-borne viruses

POCT using whole blood from a finger prick are available for diagnosing HIV and hepatitis B virus (HBV) infection.

Third generation HIV tests (HIV-1 and HIV-2 antibody only) are used routinely in many genitourinary clinics and in some

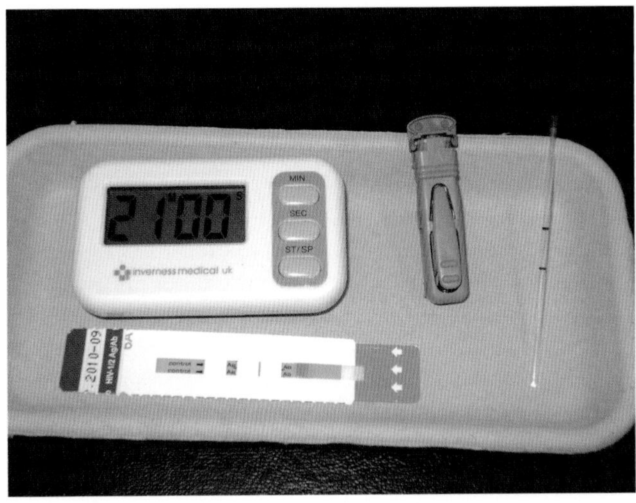

Figure 18.3 Point of care HIV test showing HIV test strip, chase buffer, capillary tube and timer.

specialist wards (e.g. labour ward). Oral fluid tests have the benefit of being non-invasive, thus increasing their utility and patient acceptance, although there have been concerns about the specificity of these tests. Their use is limited predominantly to epidemiological studies. A fourth generation HIV rapid test is available. This test detects antibodies against HIV-1 and HIV-2, and p24 antigen. It can therefore detect HIV during the seroconversion phase. Patients whose last risky exposure was three months previously, who are negative, can be reassured that they are truly negative. All positive HIV POCT tests should be confirmed by laboratory-based tests.

The sensitivity and specificity of the newer HBV POCTs, which detect HBV surface antigen (HBsAg) are acceptable in circumstances where laboratory testing is difficult. Some of these assays measure HBsAg to less than 1 IU/mL HBsAg. Laboratory-based tests measure HBsAg to 0.05 IU/mL. All positive results should be confirmed with laboratory testing, including anti-HBc immunoglobulin M (IgM), anti-HBe and HBe antigen.

Syphilis serological test

A syphilis POCT test is available for use in the UK. This test only detects total antibody and therefore does not discriminate between past infection and active infection. Its use in a developed world setting, other than in outreach situations to high-risk individuals, is not currently recommended. A positive test should be confirmed with a full syphilis screen including RPR, TPPA/TPHA, Treponemal pallidum total IgG, and Treponemal pallidum IgM.

Gonorrhoea and chlamydia testing

While the identification of an acceptable POCT for gonorrhoea is lagging, there has been much progress in developing such a test for chlamydia. Data are emerging of an acceptable POCT for professional use using vaginal swabs in women and first pass urine in men with the provision of results within one hour. It has been proposed that this test has a role in the management of symptomatic patients and may also have a role in high prevalence areas where return rates are low or where access to nucleic acid testing is limited. In addition to some high quality POCT tests for chlamydia there are also some poorly performing home use tests, which are not recommended.

Dried blood spot testing

Over the past few years dried blood spot testing for HIV, HBsAg, and hepatitis C (HCV) antibody, and HCV PCR testing has become more widely available in the UK. Following finger prick testing, blood spots are collected on a card similar to a Guthrie card and submitted for laboratory testing. Its use should be reserved for the testing of those who are at high risk of infection such as injecting drug users, in whom venepuncture is difficult.

Test performance

Ultimately, no laboratory diagnostic test is perfect and clinicians who request STI tests or issue the results should be aware of the potential for both false positive and negative results. The performance of any diagnostic test is judged by two key measurements.

1 **Sensitivity:** The percentage of positive patients who are correctly identified with the condition
2 **Specificity:** The percentage of negative patients who are correctly excluded

However, in order to determine how a test actually performs in any given patient group having sensitivity and specificity data alone is not enough, the prevalence of the infection in that current population must also be taken into consideration. Ultimately, the lower the prevalence of an infection in any given population, the greater the proportion of reactive test results that will be false positives (even if using a highly specific test) (Box 18.1).

Box 18.1 **Defining positive and negative predictive values**

Positive predictive value (PPV): The proportion of patients with positive test who actually have the infection

Negative predictive value (NPV): The proportion of patients with a negative test result, who do not have the infection.

Both the NPV and PPV will vary according to the prevalence of an infection in any given population.

		Test A	Test B
Test sensitivity		99%	99.9%
Test specificity		99%	99.9%
PPV	1% prevalence	50%	91%
	10% prevalence	92%	99%

Above is an example of the PPVs of two different hypothetical tests (Test A and B) with very high sensitivities and specificities, when used in a high (10%) and low (1%) prevalence population.

It can be seen that when used in a low prevalence population even the very specific 'Test A' only achieves a 50% PPV. This means that half the test results issued in this population will be false positives.

Quality control

The reliability of any STI test result is not only influenced by the performance of the test itself, but also the quality of the specimen, storage and transportation, training and experience of the operator, and quality of the testing procedures. Great care must be taken in the laboratory to implement best practice by the use of standard operating procedures, strict adherence to training programmes, and the competency checking of laboratory staff. The implementation of both internal quality control (where clinical specimens are blinded and retested) and external quality control (where a panel of specimens of known identity from a second laboratory are sent for testing) will ensure that specimen results are both reproducible and accurate.

Further reading

Amsel R, Totten PA, Spiegel CA, Chen KC, Eschenbach D, Holmes KK. Nonspecific vaginitis: diagnostic criteria and microbial and epidemiologic associations. *Am J Med* 1983;**74**(1):14–22.

Health Protection Agency. Serological Diagnosis of Syphilis. National Standard Method. VSOP44. Issue 1. 2007. Available at www.hpa-standardmethods.org.uk/pdf_s_ops.asp.

Ison CA, Hay PE. Validation of a simplified grading of Gram stained vaginal smears for use in genitourinary medicine clinics. *Sex Transm Infect* 2002;**78**(6):413–5.

Kingston M, French P, Goh B, Goold P, Higgins S, Sukthankar A, *et al.*; Syphilis Guidelines Revision Group, Clinical Effectiveness Group. UK National Guidelines on the Management of Syphilis 2008. *Int J STD AIDS* 2008;**19**(11):729–40.

Lin YH, Wang Y, Loua A, Day GJ, Qiu Y, Nadala EC Jr, *et al.* Evaluation of a new hepatitis B virus surface antigen rapid test with improved sensitivity. *J Clin Microbiol* 2008;**46**(10):3319–24.

Mahilum-Tapay L, Laitila V, Wawrzyniak JJ, Lee HH, Alexander S, Ison C, *et al.* New point of care chlamydia Rapid Test: bridging the gap between diagnosis and treatment – performance evaluation study. *Br Med J* 2007;**335**(7631):1190–4.

Michel CE, Saison FG, Joshi H, Mahilum-Tapay LM, Lee HH. Pitfalls of internet-accessible diagnostic tests: inadequate performance of a CE-marked chlamydia test for home use. *Sex Transm Infect* 2009;**85**(3):158.

Sexually Transmitted Infections: UK National Screening and Testing Guidelines 2006. *Sex Transm Infect* 2006;**82**:Supplement 4.

Walensky RP, Arbelaez C, Reichmann WM, Walls RM, Katz JN, Block BL, *et al.* Revising expectations from rapid HIV tests in the emergency department. *Ann Intern Med* 2008;**149**(3):153–60.

CHAPTER 19

Contraception

Rak Nandwani and Alison Bigrigg

The Sandyford Initiative, Glasgow, UK

OVERVIEW

- Heterosexual individuals attending services for the diagnosis and treatment of sexually transmitted infections (STIs) are often at risk of unwanted pregnancy
- STI clinicians should have sufficient knowledge to discuss the range of contraceptive options that are available and to administer emergency contraception
- Long-acting reversible contraception (LARC) is now the preferred first line method of preventing pregnancy, combined with barrier methods to protect against HIV and STIs

Why is contraception important for those requesting STI services?

Heterosexual individuals at risk of sexually transmitted infections (STIs) are also at risk of either becoming pregnant themselves or of getting their partner(s) pregnant. A sexual history provides opportunities to review contraception as well as to offer testing for HIV and other STIs. Contraception is focused on the prevention of unplanned or unwanted pregnancy in women and this chapter discusses contraception choices for women who present for STI care. Specialised advice should be sought for those with particular needs (e.g. HIV).

Discussion of contraceptive needs

The full range of available contraceptive methods should be presented to all women, using a leaflet, video, or discussion. A woman's willingness to use back-up strategies, such as emergency contraception or abortion, and perceived risk of STIs will affect choice (Figure 19.1).

The most suitable method will vary over the course of life, so contraception should be reviewed at every visit.

Effectiveness of contraceptive methods

The effectiveness of a particular contraceptive method is a crucial element of any woman's decision about her contraceptive strategy (Box 19.1). Popular beliefs regarding risk of pregnancy with unprotected sex or various contraceptive methods are often incorrect.

Box 19.1 **Factors affecting a woman's choice of contraceptive method**

Method related

- Effectiveness
- Common side effects
- Serious adverse medical complications
- Access/availability
- Need to interact with health professional
- Non-contraceptive benefits

User related

- Sexual lifestyle
- Frequency of intercourse
- Plans around future fertility
- Experiences and view of friends/close relatives
- Attitudes to emergency contraception and abortion
- Personal medical history

It is more appropriate to quote 'typical effectiveness' than 'perfect use effectiveness' to inform discussion (Table 19.1). A typical effectiveness rate of 92% means that if 100 women use this method of contraception for 1 year, 8 women would become pregnant. Therefore, over a 4-year university course, a student using the combined oral contraceptive pill in a typical manner would have approximately a 1 in 3 chance of becoming pregnant (4 years with 8 pregnancies each year = 32 pregnancies per 100 women during the university course).

Long-acting reversible contraception

Long-acting reversible contraception (LARC) is a contraceptive method that requires administration less than once per cycle or month. Advice from the National Institute of Health and Clinical Excellence (NICE) led to wide acceptance that LARC methods should be a first line contraceptive choice in the UK (Box 19.2).

Copper intrauterine device

Copper intrauterine devices (IUDs) work by preventing fertilisation and inhibiting implantation. A device with greater than 380 mm^2

ABC of Sexually Transmitted Infections, Sixth Edition.
Edited by Karen E. Rogstad.

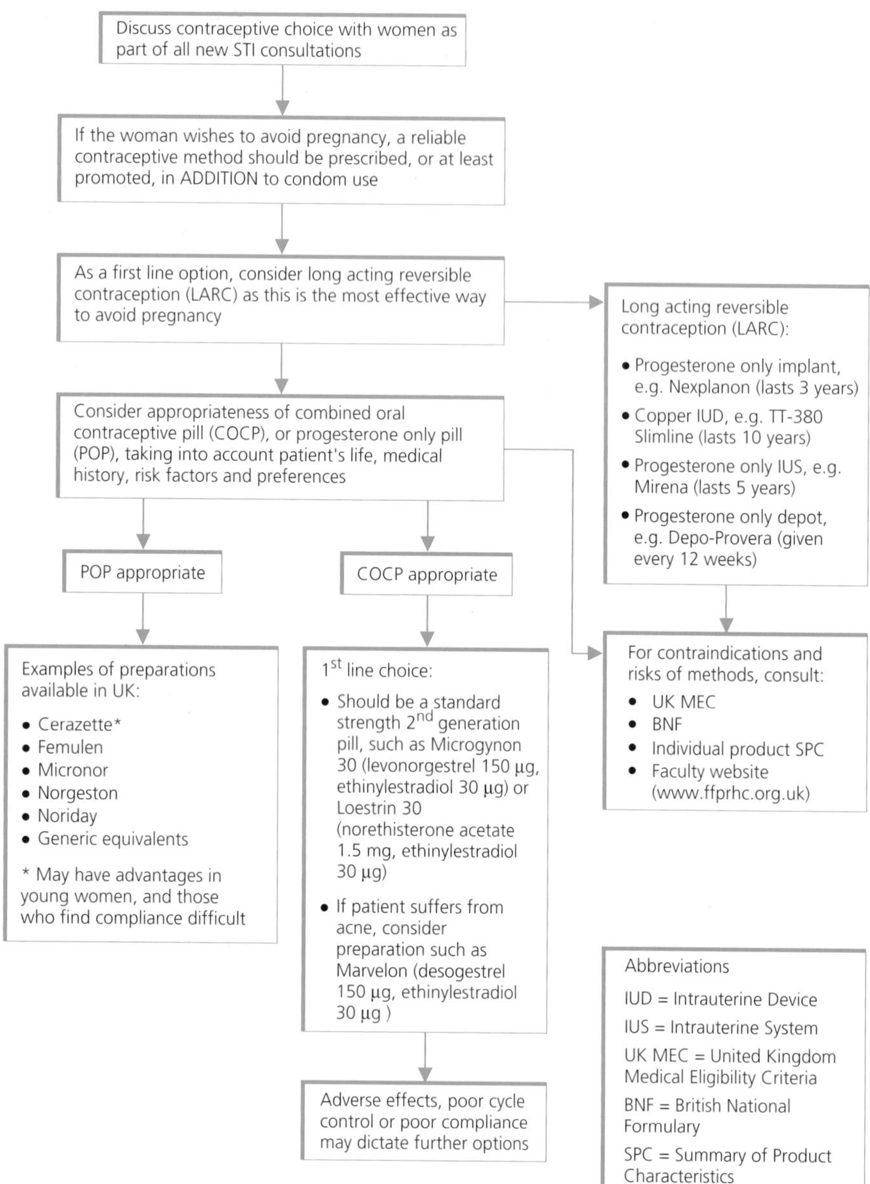

Figure 19.1 Contraception options flowchart.

copper will provide contraceptive cover for 5–10 years. If inserted in a woman aged over 40 years, it will be effective until contraception is no longer needed. IUDs generally cause heavier and more painful periods. There is no delay in the return of fertility following removal (Figures 19.2 and 19.3).

> Box 19.2 **Types of long-acting reversible contraception (LARC)**
>
> - Copper intrauterine device (IUD)
> - Progesterone-only intrauterine system (IUS)
> - Progesterone-only injectable contraceptive
> - Progesterone-only subdermal implant

Risks from using an IUD include pelvic inflammatory disease (PID) following insertion, uterine perforation, and iron deficiency anaemia. Although PID affects less than 1% of women who are at low risk of an STI, screening should be performed prior to insertion

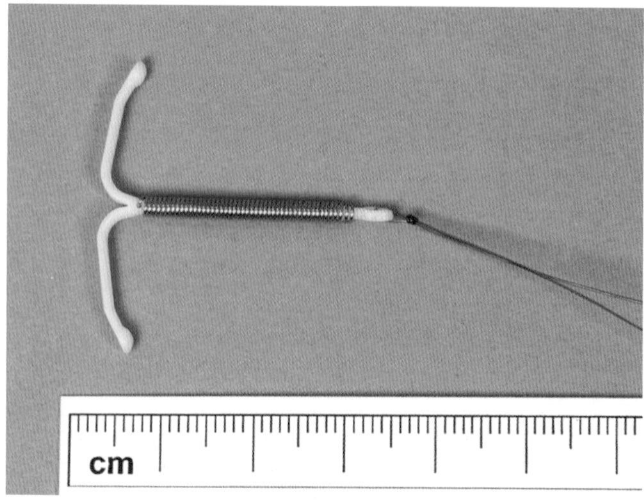

Figure 19.2 Nova T 380 copper intrauterine device (IUD) showing threads.

Table 19.1 Effectiveness of contraceptive methods: percentage of US women experiencing an unintended pregnancy during the first year of use (failure rates).

Method	Pregnant (%)	
	Typical use	Perfect use
No method	85	85
Spermicides	29	18
Withdrawal	27	4
Periodic abstinence	25	
Calendar	9	
Ovulation method	3	
Sympto-thermal	2	
Cap		
Parous women	32	26
Nulliparous women	16	9
Diaphragm	16	6
Condom		
Female	21	5
Male	15	2
Combined pill and mini-pill	8	0.3
Combined hormonal patch (Evra)	8	0.3
Combined hormonal ring (NuvaRing)	8	0.3
DMPA (Depo-Provera)	3	0.3
IUD		
Copper T	0.8	0.6
LNG-IUS (Mirena)	0.1	0.1
Implant	0.05	0.05
Female sterilisation	0.5	0.5
Male sterilisation	0.15	0.10

Adapted from: Trussell J, Kost K. Contraceptive failure in the United States: A Critical review of the literature. *Studies in Family Planning* 1987;**18**(5): 237–83.

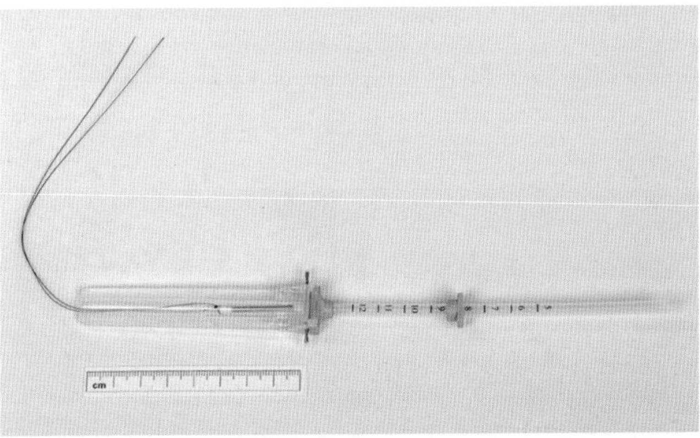

Figure 19.3 TT380 Slimline intrauterine device (IUD) with applicator prior to insertion.

or antibiotic cover administered. Uterine perforation affects less than 1 in 1000 women. Ectopic pregnancy rates are lower than without use of contraception, but if a woman becomes pregnant with an IUD in place the risk rises to 1 in 20.

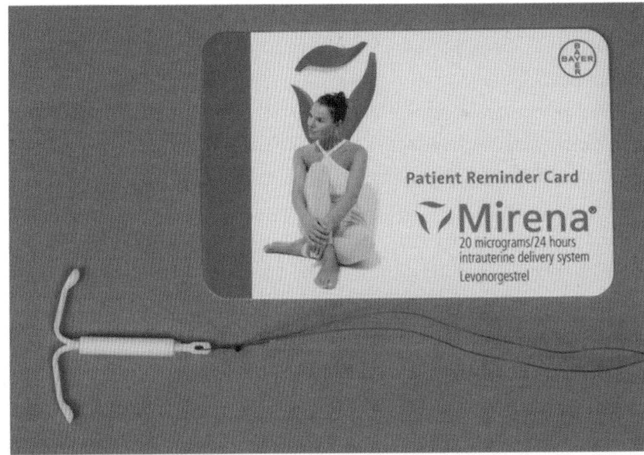

Figure 19.4 Mirena intrauterine system (IUS) and credit-card sized patient reminder.

Progesterone-only intrauterine system

The most popular intrauterine system, the progesterone-only intrauterine system (IUS) releases 20 μg/day levonorgestrel (Mirena; Figure 19.4). It prevents implantation, and sometimes fertilisation. It is recommended for 5 years, or until contraception is no longer needed if the woman is over 45 at the time of insertion and does not have periods with the IUS in place.

Irregular bleeding and spotting are common during the first 6 months, but oligomenorrhoea or amenorrhoea are likely by 12 months. The most common reason for stopping an IUS is unacceptable vaginal bleeding. There is no evidence of weight gain but there may be a small increased risk of acne and mood change. The risk of PID, ectopic pregnancy, or uterine perforation is comparable with the copper IUD.

Progesterone-only injectable contraceptive

The most commonly used progesterone-only injectable contraceptive method is depo medroxyprogesterone acetate (DMPA Depo-Provera; Figure 19.5). It works primarily by preventing ovulation. Repeat injections are needed every 12 weeks. A subcutaneous self-administered form is currently in development.

The most common reason for stopping Depo-Provera is altered bleeding. Thirty per cent of women may complain of prolonged

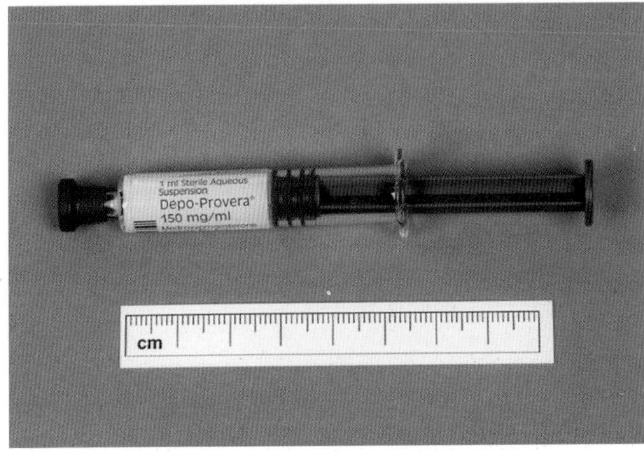

Figure 19.5 Progesterone-only injectable contraceptive: Depo-Provera.

bleeding episodes (greater than 10 days) but this decreases to 10% at 12 months. Amenorrhoea is common in 55% of users at 1 year and 70% at 2 years.

There is no evidence of adverse effects of Depo-Provera on depression, acne, or headaches. It may cause weight gain of 2–3 kg over 1 year. Its use is associated with a small loss of bone mineral density which appears to largely recover on discontinuation. There is no evidence that fracture risk is increased, but this small risk has led to a recommendation of caution in use for adolescents and women over 40.

Pregnancies have been reported as early as 14 weeks after the last injection, with the mean time to ovulation being 5.3 months and to conception 9 months. Therefore, on discontinuation, even if amenorrhoea persists, another method of contraception should always be used immediately to avoid an unplanned pregnancy.

Progesterone-only subdermal implant

Implanon is a non-biodegradable single semi-rigid rod (40 × 2 mm) containing 68 mg etonogestrel (Figure 19.6 and Box 19.3). From 2010 onwards, it is being replaced by a newer version, Nexplanon, which is radio-opaque and has a different application device/insertion technique. The duration of action remains 3 years. After removal, etonogestrel serum levels become undetectable within 1 week.

Box 19.3 **Example of UK Medical Eligibility Criteria (UKMEC) for use of contraceptive implants**

UK Category 4 (conditions that represent unacceptable health risks)

- Known or suspected pregnancy
- Breast cancer diagnosed within the last 5 years
- Hypersensitivity to any of the components of the implant

(N.B. If these develop during use, the implant should be removed)

UK Category 3 (condition where the risks usually outweigh the advantages)

- Current venous thrombo-embolism
- Continued use after myocardial infarction or stroke
- Continued use after new onset of migraine with aura
- Gestational trophoblastic neoplasia if human chorionic gonadotrophin (hCG) is abnormal
- Past history of breast cancer with no active disease for 5 years
- Unexplained vaginal bleeding (if underlying pathological condition such as pelvic malignancy is suspected it must be evaluated)
- Active viral hepatitis (not including carriers)
- Hepatic tumours (benign or malignant), primary sclerosing cholangitis, decompensated cirrhosis
- Concurrent use with hepatic enzyme-inducing drugs

Category 3 for continuation of method if migraine with aura, stroke, ischaemic heart disease.

UK Category 2 (condition where the advantages usually outweigh the risks)

- Multiple risk factors for arterial cardiovascular disease
- Current or past history of myocardial infarction or stroke (initiation)
- Hypertension with vascular disease
- Blood pressure (>160 mmHg systolic or >100 mmHg diastolic) unless other conditions which may predispose to arterial cardiovascular disease
- Diabetes mellitus
- Hyperlipidaemia
- Past history of venous thromboembolism or pulmonary embolism
- Known thrombogenic mutation
- Surgery with immobilisation
- Undiagnosed breast mass (should be evaluated as soon as possible)
- Migraine without aura (any new headaches or changes should be fully evaluated)
- Cervical intra-epithelial neoplasia
- Gallbladder disease
- Compensated cirrhosis, combined oral contraceptive-related cholestasis
- Irregular, heavy, or prolonged vaginal bleeding
- Carriers of known gene mutation associated with breast cancer
- Secondary Raynaud's disease with lupus anticoagulant
- Antiretroviral therapy for HIV

Full UKMEC available at http://www.ffprhc.org.uk/

Implanon works by preventing ovulation and altering the quality of the cervical mucus. Changes in bleeding patterns are common and tend to remain irregular, with 20% of women having no periods and almost 50% having infrequent, frequent, or prolonged bleeding. Dysmenorrhoea is likely to improve. There is no evidence of effect on weight, mood, libido, headaches, or bone mineral density, although a small increased risk of acne is possible. There is no evidence of a delay in return to fertility.

Choice of appropriate LARC method

Intrauterine device/system (IUD/IUS), progesterone-only injections, and implants are suitable for women with contraindications to oestrogen (Box 19.4). Good counselling prior to initiation of the method is likely to make the woman more tolerant of her menstrual pattern. IUD/IUS and implants are suitable, without restriction, for

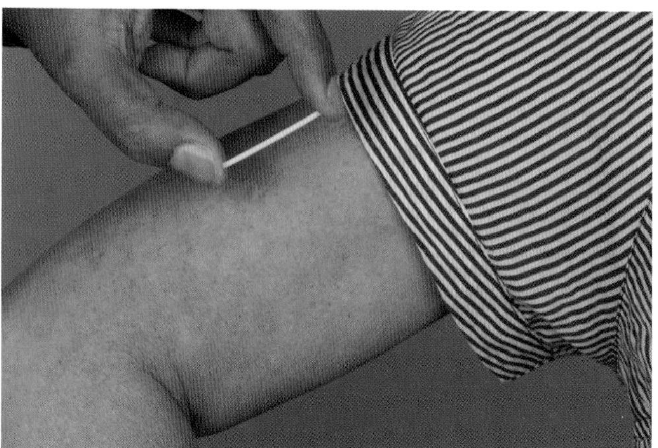

Figure 19.6 Progesterone-only subdermal implant: Implanon.

adolescents and women over 40, but because of concerns regarding possible effect on bone mineral density of Depo-Provera discussion is needed before women in these groups choose this method.

> Box 19.4 **Groups for whom IUD/IUS, progesterone-only implants, and injections are suitable**
>
> - Nulliparous women
> - Women who are breastfeeding
> - Women who have had an abortion – at time of abortion or later
> - Women with body mass index (BMI) greater than 30
> - Women with HIV – encourage condom use
> - Women with diabetes
> - Women with migraine, with or without aura

Short-acting reversible contraception

Male condoms

Emphasis should be placed on consistent and correct use and use of lubricants (Box 19.5). There is a high failure rate in typical use, and the need for a back-up or alternative contraceptive strategy should be discussed. Advanced provision of emergency contraception should be offered to women using condoms as their sole method of contraception.

> Box 19.5 **Lubricant use**
>
> - Condoms lubricated with non-spermicidal lubricant are recommended for use
> - Additional lubricant should be recommended for use with condoms for anal sex
> - Non-oil based lubricants are recommended for both latex and non-latex condoms
> - It is not recommended that lubricant be applied to the penis under a male condom

If a condom used for contraception breaks, individuals need to know that emergency contraception is required as soon as possible.

Female barrier methods

Female barrier methods include diaphragms and cervical caps (fitted by a practitioner) and the female condom (Figures 19.7 and 19.8). Female barrier methods do not confer the same degree of protection against STIs, must remain in place for at least 6 hours after the last episode of intercourse, and be regularly checked for damage. Spermicide must be used with diaphragms and caps.

Combined oral contraceptive pill

The most commonly prescribed combined oral contraceptive pill (COCP) contains 30 or 35 µg ethinyl oestradiol, combined with the progesterones: levonorgestrel or norethisterone (Figures 19.9 and 19.10). Lower strength preparations with 20 µg ethinyl oestradiol can be used, as can pills with 30 µg ethinyl oestradiol containing desogestrel, drospirenone, and gestodene, if women have side effects such as acne, headache, depression, weight gain, breast

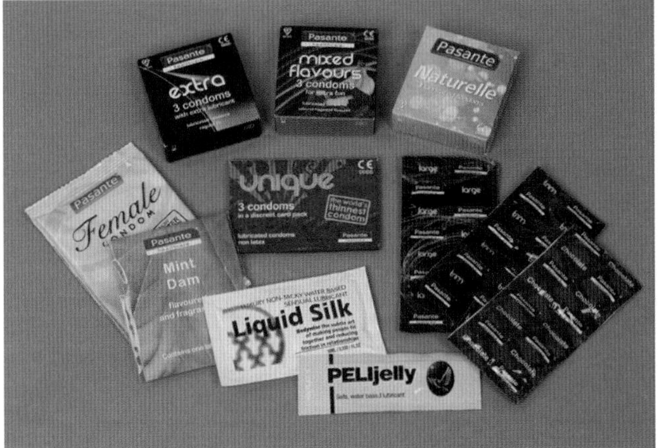

Figure 19.7 Selection of male and female condoms with lubricants.

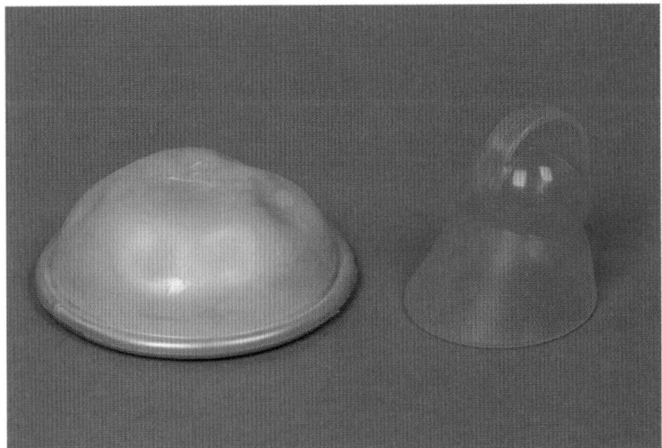

Figure 19.8 Flat spring diaphragm and FemCap.

symptoms, and breakthrough bleeding. Women should be advised that desogestrel or gestodene have been associated with increased risk of venous thrombo-embolism.

Traditionally, the COCP is taken for 21 days followed by a 7-day break, when a withdrawal bleed usually occurs. Many women, however, run two or more packs together to decrease the frequency of bleeding. Before prescribing the COCP, the woman's age, blood pressure, and body mass index should be recorded. Follow-up should be arranged at 3 months to reassess blood pressure, review, and reinstruct if required, and in the absence of problems a 12-month supply of COCP can be dispensed.

Transdermal contraceptive patch

The transdermal patch delivers combined oestrogen and progesterone into the bloodstream through the skin. It is usually applied to the buttock, abdomen, upper arm, or upper back. It works in the same way as the COCP but has the advantage that it only needs to be applied once a week for 3 weeks followed by a week off. Breast discomfort and breakthrough bleeding are common in the first 3 months. Local skin irritation can also occur.

The pharmacokinetic profile of the patch results in 60% higher steady state concentrations of oestrogen compared with COCPs containing 35 µg ethinyl oestradiol which may increase the risk of adverse events including venous thrombo-embolism. Women who use the patch are strongly advised not to smoke.

Combined contraceptive vaginal ring

The vaginal ring is an alternative method of delivering combined oestrogen and progesterone without the need for gastrointestinal absorption (and hepatic first pass metabolism), making it suitable for women with conditions such as inflammatory bowel disease. A 54-mm flexible ring (NuvaRing) is inserted into the vagina for 3 weeks before a 1-week ring-free period. Like the transdermal patch, adherence is aided by not having to remember to take take a daily pill.

It is generally well tolerated, expulsion is uncommon, and efficacy and contraindications apply as for the COCP.

Progesterone-only pill

The progesterone-only pill (POP) does not contain oestrogen. The dose of progesterone is significantly lower than that in the equivalent combined preparation. Around half of women continue to menstruate, 10–20% develop amenorrhoea, and the remainder experience irregular bleeding.

Traditional POPs (containing norethisterone, levonorgestrel, or etynodiol diacetate) work by altering cervical mucus to prevent sperm penetration and, for some women, ovulation is also inhibited. The desogestrel-only pill also alters cervical mucus; however, its main mode of action is inhibition of ovulation.

Women should be advised to take the POP at the same time every day, and without a pill-free interval. Some women may prefer the desogestrel-only pill, as its efficacy is maintained if taken within 12 hours of the usual time (Figure 19.9).

There is no evidence of a causal association with weight change, depression, headache, cardiovascular disease, or breast cancer. It is commonly used by women who are breastfeeding, when it is highly effective and does not interfere with the quantity or constituents of breast milk.

The efficacy of traditional POPs appears to be related to the age of the user, where the efficacy of the desogestrel containing POP in clinical trials is comparable to the efficacy of the COCP, which also inhibits ovulation.

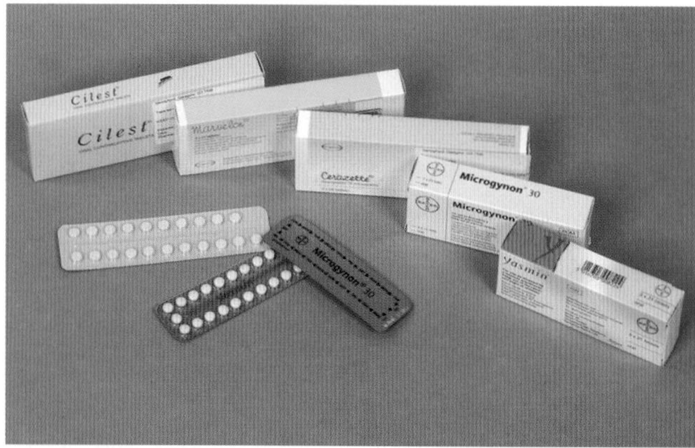

Figure 19.9 Selection of oral contraceptive pills.

Other methods of contraception

Coitus interruptus is the withdrawal of the erect penis from the vagina before ejaculation. Oral and anal sex are widespread sexual practices that avoid the need for contraception.

The lactational amenorrhoea method (LAM) is highly effective as long as the woman is fully, or nearly fully, breastfeeding, amenorrhoeic, and less than 6 months postpartum. Other methods of natural family planning are not so successful and all involve 'periodic abstinence'. The simplest is the calendar, or rhythm, method, when the woman calculates her fertile period according to events of the menstrual cycle (Figure 19.10). Other methods, such as the mucus method, use symptoms that reflect fluctuating levels of hormone during the menstrual cycle.

Emergency contraception

Hormonal methods

Hormonal emergency contraception involves taking a single dose of 1.5 mg levonorgestrel (Levonelle) as soon as possible after unprotected sex. Side effects include an early or late period, nausea, and vomiting. The woman must be warned of failure and, if she does not have a menstrual bleed or if it is abnormally light, heavy, or brief, she must return for a pregnancy test. If vomiting occurs within 2 hours of taking levonorgestrel, a repeat dose should be given. It may be given more than once within a menstrual cycle. If an antiemetic is required, domperidone is preferred.

Hormonal emergency contraception can prevent 84% of expected pregnancies if taken within 72 hours, and may prevent 63% if taken between 73 and 120 hours, although data is limited and use after 72 hours is unlicensed.

Ulipristal (EllaOne) has recently been licensed in the United Kingdom. It is a synthetic selective progesterone receptor modulator (SPRM) derived from 19-norprogesterone. It is an important development as it can be taken up to 120 hours after unprotected sex, and therefore it will decrease the need for IUD fitting (see below).

Intrauterine device

Insertion of an interutering device (IUD) is more effective than hormonal methods of emergency contraception. A copper IUD can be inserted up to 120 hours (5 days) after unprotected intercourse. Additionally, if intercourse has occurred more than 5 days previously, the device can still be inserted up to 5 days after the earliest likely calculated date of ovulation (i.e. within the minimum period before implantation). STIs should be tested for, and insertion of a device would usually be covered with antibacterial prophylaxis (e.g. azithromycin 1 g).

At least 99% of expected pregnancies can be prevented by emergency use of a copper IUD. A woman can decide whether to have the device removed, or to continue to use it as a long-term method of contraception.

Male and female sterilisation

Sterilisation involves interrupting the fallopian tubes, or the vas deferens in a man, to prevent the egg and sperm meeting. It

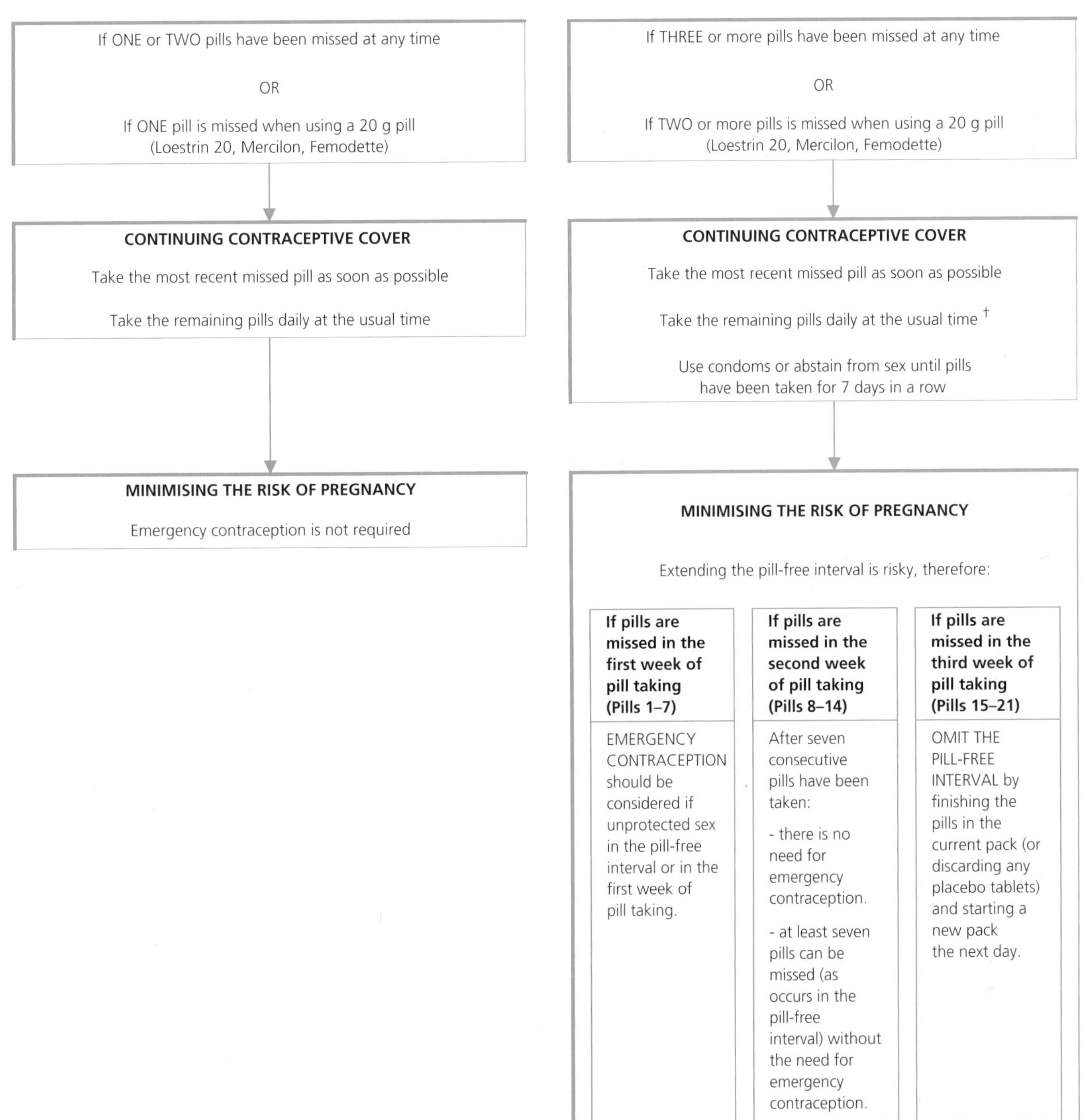

† Depending on when the missed pill is remembered, two pills can be taken on the same day (one at the moment of remembering and the other at the regular time) or even at the same time.

Any pills missed in the last week of the previous packet should be taken into account when considering emergency contraception.

Figure 19.10 Missed pill advice.

is intended to be permanent and should not be undertaken at emotional times, such as a relationship or personal crisis. If a woman does become pregnant after a tubal ligation, an ectopic pregnancy must be excluded.

Vasectomy is usually performed under local anaesthetic, in an outpatient setting, in around 20 minutes. It is only considered to be effective when two consecutive negative semen samples have been produced, normally after 3–4 months (up to 36 ejaculations). Until then an additional contraceptive method should be used.

Acknowledgements

The authors wish to thank Elle Carpy for typing the draft and Kirsty Lattka at Gartnavel General Hospital Medical Illustration Services.

Further reading

Faculty of Sexual and Reproductive Healthcare website. Available at www.ffprhc.org.uk. Includes guidance on all contraceptive methods.

NHS National Institute for Health and Clinical Excellence (NICE). Clinical guideline CG30: long-acting reversible contraception 2005. Available at http://guidance.nice.org.uk/CG30.

UK medical eligibility criteria for contraceptive use (UKMEC 2005/2006). Available at http://www.ffprhc.org.uk/admin/uploads/298_UKMEC_200506.pdf.

UK national family planning statistics. Available at http://www.statistics.gov.uk/CCI/nscl.asp?ID = 6376.

World Health Organization information, publication, and statistics on family planning. Available at http://www.who.int/topics/family_planning/en/.

CHAPTER 20

Care of Specific Risk Groups

Paul A Fox [1] *and Karen E Rogstad* [2]

[1]Ealing Hospital, London, UK
[2]Department of Sexual Health and HIV, Sheffield Teaching Hospitals NHS Foundation Trust, Sheffield, UK

OVERVIEW

- Men who have sex with men (MSM) are more at risk of STIs and these may be different to those seen in heterosexuals
- MSM require careful history-taking, full examination, and prevention in the form of vaccinations, postexposure prophylaxis for HIV (PEP), and risk-reduction advice
- Young people may be victims of sexual abuse and exploitation – risk assessments may be necessary
- Sex workers often do not disclose their work without direct questioning
- Those attending travel clinics should have sexual health advice

Men who have sex with men

Many men who identify themselves as heterosexual have engaged in homosexual activity, but because of taboos attached to this behaviour it may be denied even on direct questioning. This is an important issue to address, in order to provide adequate sexual health screening, health promotion, and STI prevention. One avenue would be to ask the patient 'Have you thought about any sexual encounters that might have put you at higher risk (e.g. of HIV); have you, for instance, ever experimented in sex with another man?' In some cultures only passive anal intercourse is regarded as a truly homosexual activity, and active anal intercourse is not. Men who identify as homosexual tend to congregate in large cities where they feel more accepted and where the opportunities for sexual relationships (and the acquisition of STIs) are greater.

Sexual behaviour of MSM and associated health risks

Men who have sex with men (MSM) have more needs and are more time consuming as regards sexual health provision (examination, STI testing, health promotion and prevention). They have a higher burden of STIs, including infections such as lymphogranuloma venereum (LGV), syphilis, HIV, and viral hepatitis and STIs may cause a proctitis (Box 20.1). The widespread availability of gay venues such as saunas, bars, and clubs means that a man might have sex anonymously with many other men in a short space of time, sometimes in a completely darkened room ('dark rooms').

Box 20.1 **Causes of proctitis in MSM**

- Gonorrhoea
- Chlamydia
- LGV
- Herpes simplex (Figure 20.1)
- Inflammatory bowel disease

It should not be assumed that a gay man who only reports insertive anal intercourse never adopts the passive role, or vice versa. The majority of gay men are 'versatile' in this regard and will adopt different roles in the context of different relationships. Nevertheless, it is not really necessary to screen the anal canal for infections in asymptomatic gay men who have not engaged in passive anal intercourse for a year a more.

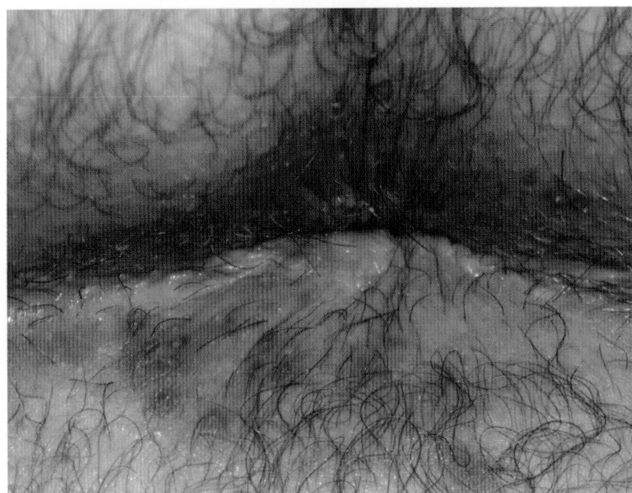

Figure 20.1 Peri-anal herpes. Courtesy of Dr Colm O'Mahoney.

ABC of Sexually Transmitted Infections, Sixth Edition.
Edited by Karen E. Rogstad.

Frequent misconceptions which may need to be corrected include a belief that insertive anal sex is a low risk activity for HIV acquisition, and the belief that oral sex carries no risk. Vaccination against hepatitis B is extremely important because of its high prevalence in MSM. Oro-anal contact, known as 'rimming', carries its own risks'; especially common is acquisition of threadworms and Giardia, but any organism transmitted by the faeco-oral route might be thus acquired. Hepatitis A may be slightly increased (see Chapter 15).

Testing for STIs in MSM

In addition to the usual male STI screen the asymptomatic MSM is recommended to have serology for hepatitis B and swabs taken from the throat and anus for gonorrhoea and chlamydia. Rectal chlamydia infection prevalence is typically 5% or more in large city clinics, and the infection is frequently asymptomatic. Pharyngeal prevalence is much lower.

Infections specific to MSM

Rectal lymphogranuloma venereum

This tropical disease emerged worldwide as a disease affecting MSM in 2003, and is strongly associated with sexual networking for unprotected group sex between men (Figure 20.2). The majority of men affected are HIV-positive. It presents with anal pain, tenesmus, pain on defaecation, and sometimes systemic symptoms. Proctoscopy typically reveals a bloodstained purulent discharge and there may be visible ulceration, linear or otherwise. Unlike in the genital form of LGV, seldom seen in MSM, the inguinal lymph nodes are not enlarged. Rectal nucleic acid amplification tests (NAATs) for *Chlamydia trachomatis* will be positive, and specific analysis for the L1, L2, and L3 serovars that cause LGV should be requested. Most cases in the developed world have been associated with the L2 serovar. Treatment is with a prolonged course of doxycyline 100 mg twice daily for 3 weeks. Chronic untreated cases are at risk of anal stenosis and fistulas.

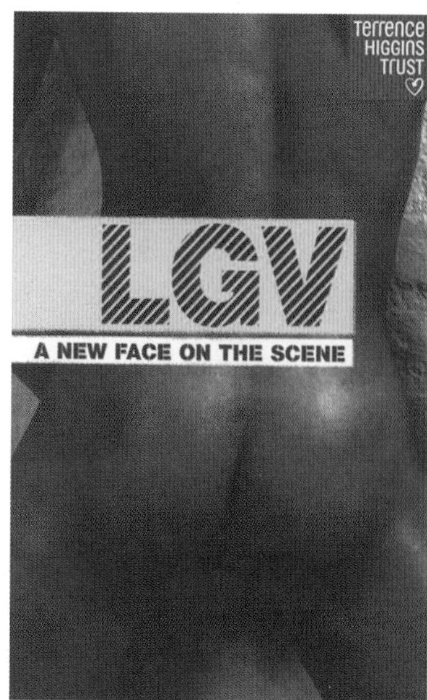

Figure 20.2 Poster highlighting risk of lymphogranuloma venereum. Courtesy of the Terrence Higgins Trust.

New variant syphilis

Syphilis frequently presents in MSM in a manner that differs from the classic primary stage of the painless genital ulcer or chancre. This is the result of the evolution of a new strain, which causes painful primary lesions which are often multiple, and can be quite similar in appearance to herpetic lesions. Medical advice is often sought at a relatively early stage, before the chancres have fully developed, and the hallmark lesion of this condition is the small erosion. If new variant syphilis presents in the secondary stage, with a skin rash, it may be pruritic, in contrast to the rash of classic syphilis. Thus far the new strain has not spread significantly into the heterosexual population. Testing and treatment are the same as for classic syphilis (see Chapter 13).

Anal canal warts and anal intra-epithelial neoplasia

While perianal warts are not a marker of receptive anal intercourse, warts within the anal canal usually are (Figure 20.3). Symptoms of anal canal warts are itching and bleeding, an anal lump, and non-specific anal discomfort. MSM with such symptoms should be examined proctoscopically. Both podophylotoxin and imiquimod creams can be inserted in the anus to treat the warts, although neither drug is licensed for this indication. Treatment should begin very cautiously, and be interrupted if soreness occurs, until it resolves. If both treatments fail then surgery can be considered, but should not be undertaken lightly as recovery can take several weeks. Low-grade anal intra-epithelial neoplasia (AIN 1) may be present on histology. This will typically be caused by the same non-oncogenic HPV virus that caused the warts. It requires follow-up, but need not cause undue concern unless the patient is HIV-positive. Higher grades of AIN require monitoring either by periodic surgical examination under anaesthetic or by high resolution anoscopy. MSM are at higher risk of developing anal cancer in later life than the general population, but in HIV-negative men

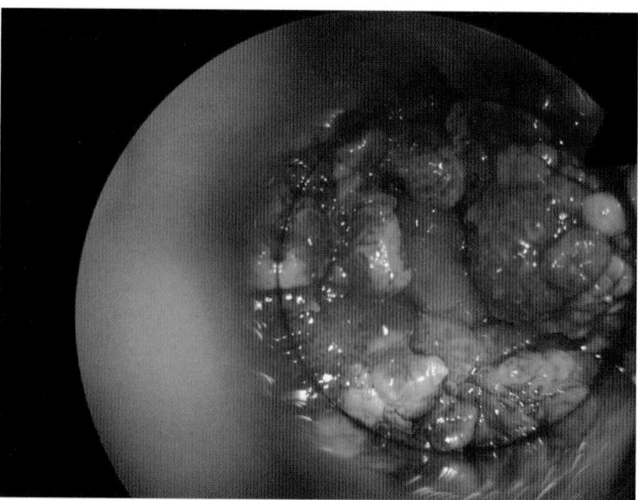

Figure 20.3 Anal canal warts.

this would be a rare occurrence before the age of 50. Screening is not advocated at the present time, but elderly MSM should be encouraged to self-examine and to report any new anal lumps.

Postexposure prophylaxis for HIV

Because of the high prevalence of HIV amongst MSM it is recommended that antiretroviral postexposure prophylaxis is taken as soon as possible following unprotected anal intercourse (see Chapter 22). In the UK it is available at GUM clinics, and out of hours from accident and emergency departments. It is ideally commenced within 4 hours of exposure but might be of benefit up to 72 hours. Individuals who have take PEP tend to adopt a more cautious approach in subsequent sexual encounters. The concept of pre-exposure prophylaxis for HIV with antiretrovirals in MSM is currently being evaluated.

Children and young people

The legal age of consent for sexual intercourse is 16 years in the United Kingdom, but varies across the world. Many young people are sexually active below the legal age, with 25% of 15-year-olds being sexually active in England. When providing sexual health services to underage boys and girls, practitioners must take into consideration the needs of that young person for a confidential service and the provision of STI screening and management and fertility services, with the need to protect them from sexual abuse and exploitation. Although most will be in consensual sexual relations with a similar-aged peer, this should not be assumed. Additionally, there may be both consensual and abusive sexual activity occurring. Assessment should be undertaken on those below the age of consent to consider issues that may either indicate current exploitation, or risk for the future. Issues such as age of their partner(s), alcohol, and drug use, can indicate a cause for concern; the younger the adolescent the lower the threshold should be for the need for intervention.

The issue of competence to accept investigation and treatment also needs to be addressed, for example use of the Fraser Guidelines in England for young people who attend sexual health services without a parent or guardian.

The use of a standardised proforma (see Appendix 3) is useful to assess risk factors and document competence. Where there is cause for concern or a young person is at risk, then practitioners should access advice or refer to Child Protection Services according to their local, national, and professional body guidance.

Sexually transmitted infections in children

STIs in a prepubertal child may be a result of vertical transmission from mother to child before, during, or after delivery or through breastfeeding. Some may be passed on horizontally (e.g. hepatitis B). The possibility of child sexual abuse should also be considered, and the likelihood of abuse is high for some STIs (e.g. genital gonorrhoea, chlamydia, trichomonas), and a somewhat lower but still significant for others (e.g. genital warts). Assessing the significance of an STI in children is a difficult area and advice and referral to specialist services is essential.

The diagnosis of ophthalmic gonorrhoea or chlamydia in a neonate requires treatment not only of the infant, but also testing and treatment of the mother and her sexual partner(s).

Sex workers

Sex work takes many different forms and some will not result in increased risk of STI (Figure 20.3). Many men and women working in the industry may be more at risk of acquiring STIs from their regular partner than from clients, as non-condom usage is used to differentiate between sex with clients and partners. Sex workers may not disclose voluntarily and routine questioning can be helpful. History should include the nature of sexual activity and condom usage, as well as enquiring whether work is voluntary, coerced, or forced. Trafficking either from another country or within the country can occur. Vaccination against hepatitis B should be offered, and regular STI screening. Support should be offered either in-house or by referral to specialised agencies.

Sexual assault, rape, and historical abuse

Both men and women can be victims of sexual assault and rape. In the United Kingdom there were more than 12 000 rapes of women in 2008–2009 reported to the police, with many more cases that were not reported. Twenty-one per cent of girls and 11% of boys under 16 in the UK are victims of child sexual abuse, but may not present until many years later, as adults. Victims of acute assault will need forensic testing (if they wish), testing for STIs, contraception, hepatitis B vaccination, and consideration of postexposure prophylaxis for HIV (PEP). Counselling and other psychological services should also be offered to both acute and historical victims. A chain of evidence needs to be in place for forensic samples, otherwise the information gained would not be accepted in a court of law. Referral to a specialist sexual assault referral centre (SARC in the UK), if available, should be offered to victims of recent rape, where a comprehensive forensic and medical service can be provided.

Travellers

The chances of acquiring an STI depend on the country of travel and the demographic features of new partners. Those who have had sex abroad in a less affluent nation are at increased risk of acquiring infections that may be resistant to antibiotics, or to more unusual infections such as LGV, chancroid, syphilis, and other tropical ulcerative conditions. A travel history is therefore an integral part of a sexual health history especially in someone presenting with genital ulcer disease, or with symptoms or signs consistent with syphilis or HIV. That having been said, there is a strong tendency for travellers to have sex with someone from their own country of origin, or from a country that shares a common heritage, and this often mitigates against risk. Those attending for pre-travel health care such as vaccinations/anti-malarials may not be planning to engage in sexual activity overseas, but should be warned about the dangers of doing so, and advised to take condoms with them. Hepatitis B vaccination should be considered for people travelling for some time to developing countries (e.g. gap year students).

Sex tourists are usually, but not necessarily, men who travel with the express purpose of having sex, with the exchange of sex for money or gifts. They rarely spontaneously admit to their reason for travel, but if suspected then hepatitis B vaccination should be offered. Advice can also be given on HIV risk.

Further reading

eHIV-STI (Module 8). An e-learning programme for health care professionals. Available at www.eHIV-STI.com.

Fisher M, Benn P, Evans B. UK Guideline for the use of post-exposure prophylaxis for HIV following sexual exposure. Available at www.bashh.org.uk.

Report from the Task Force on the health aspects of violence against women and children. Available at http://www.dh.gov.uk/en/Publicationsandstatistics/Publications/PublicationsPolicyAndGuidance/DH_113727.

Richardson D, Goldmeier D. Lymphogranuloma venereum: an emerging cause of proctitis in men who have sex with men. *Int J STD AIDS* 2007; **18**(1):11–4.

Rogstad K, Thomas A, Williams O, *et al.* United Kingdom National Guideline on the Management of Sexually Transmitted Infections and Related Conditions in Children and Young People (2010). Clinical Effectiveness Group, British Association for Sexual Health and HIV. Available at www.bashh.org.

Rogstad KE. Sex, sun, sea and STIs; sexually transmitted infections acquired on holiday. *Br Med J* 2004;**329**:214–7.

www.sigmaresearch.org.uk has a wide range of reports on sexual behaviour in MSM.

Royal College of Paediatrics and Child Health in collaboration with the Royal College of Physicians of London, and its Faculty of Forensic and Legal Medicine. *Physical signs of child sexual abuse. An evidence-based review and guidance for best practice*. London, Royal College of Paediatrics and Child Health, 2008.

CHAPTER 21

Sexual Health Care in Resource Poor Settings

David A Lewis

Sexually Transmitted Infections Reference Centre, National Institute for Communicable Diseases, National Health Laboratory Service, Johannesburg, South Africa

> **OVERVIEW**
>
> - The challenges of managing STIs in resource poor settings are reviewed
> - The syndromic management approach is described
> - Advantages and disadvantages of the syndromic management approach are discussed
> - Components of STI surveillance in resource poor settings are outlined
> - Periodic presumptive therapy may be a useful adjunct to syndromic therapy in areas of high bacterial STI prevalence

The management of sexually transmitted infections (STIs) in resource poor settings frequently requires the provision of STI clinical services at significantly reduced cost compared with those provided in more affluent areas of the world. This inherently lowers the quality of services provided to individual patients but ensures access and equitable treatment and care to all individuals within a country, regardless of whether they live in rural areas or major cities. In comparison with more affluent regions, resource poor regions of the world tend to have a higher prevalence of most STIs, as well as HIV infection, which adds to the health care burden faced by individual countries.

The World Health Organization (WHO) has advocated the adoption of the syndromic management approach for STI treatment and care in resource poor settings. Syndromic management relies on the identification by a clinician of a specific clinical syndrome, or a collection of signs and symptoms, that may be caused by a recognised group of pathogens. Examples include male urethral discharge (Figure 21.1), vaginal discharge, genital ulceration (Figure 21.2), scrotal swelling, and lower abdominal pain syndromes (Box 21.1). Other conditions included in the syndromic management approach, which are not syndromes per se, include buboes, genital warts, balanitis, ophthalmia neonatorum, pubic lice, scabies, molluscum contagiosum, positive rapid plasmin reagin (RPR) serology, and altered drug management to cover the presence of multiple STI syndromes in the same index patient (Box 21.2).

ABC of Sexually Transmitted Infections, Sixth Edition.
Edited by Karen E. Rogstad.

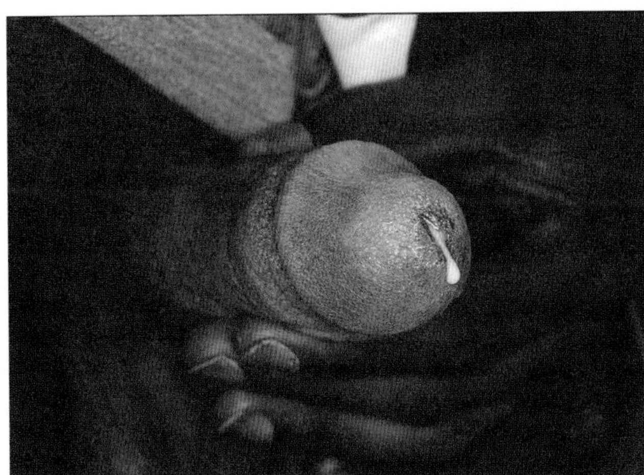

Figure 21.1 Male urethral discharge.

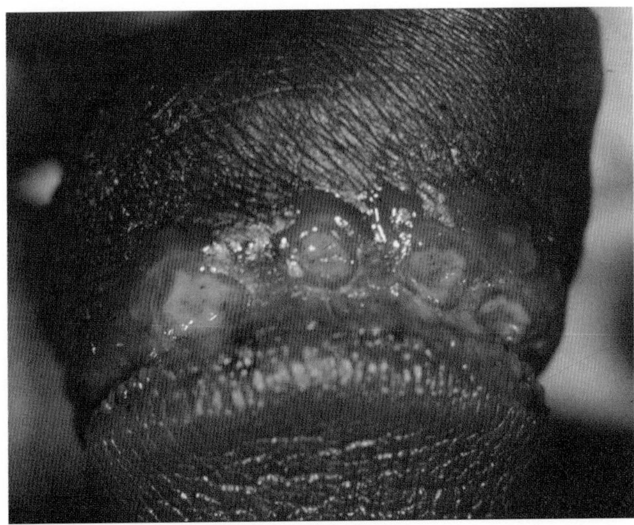

Figure 21.2 Genital ulceration in a male patient.

The syndromic management approach utilises flow charts, which allow the majority of STIs to be treated by nurses rather than doctors (Figures 21.3 and 21.4). The flow charts outline the main steps required to manage the patient correctly, along with the relevant antimicrobial agents. In resource poor settings this is of critical

Box 21.1 **Main STI syndromes**

- Male urethral discharge syndrome
- Vaginal discharge syndrome
- Scrotal swelling syndrome
- Lower abdominal pain syndrome
- Genital ulceration syndrome

Box 21.2 **Other conditions covered in syndromic management guidelines**

- Genital warts
- Buboes
- Balanitis
- Ophthalmia neonatorum
- Scabies
- Pubic lice
- Molluscum contagiosum
- RPR seropositivity
- Mixed STI syndromes

importance, as nurses' salaries are less of a burden to the state health care system and nurses are often the only health care workers accessible to patients in the primary health care sector entry point, particularly in under-resourced rural areas.

The aim of syndromic management is to ensure effective treatment of both common and serious pathogens for each syndrome through multi-antibiotic therapy (Boxes 21.3–21.5). This is an important principle as syndromes with mixed infections are not uncommon. For example, male urethral discharge syndrome may be caused by co-infection with *Neisseria gonorrhoeae* and *Chlamydia trachomatis*, and genital ulceration may be caused by co-infection

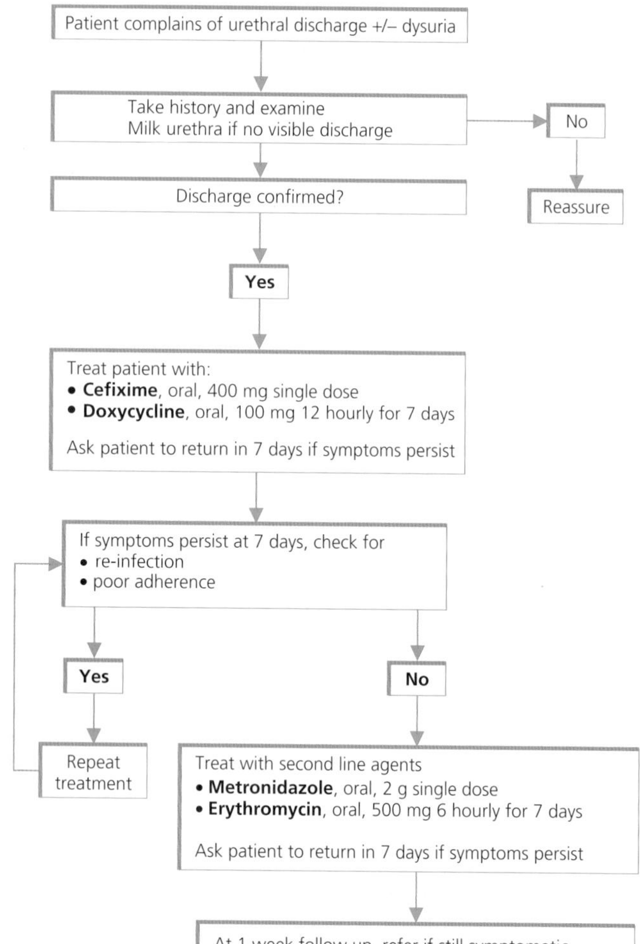

Figure 21.3 Flow chart for male urethral discharge syndrome.

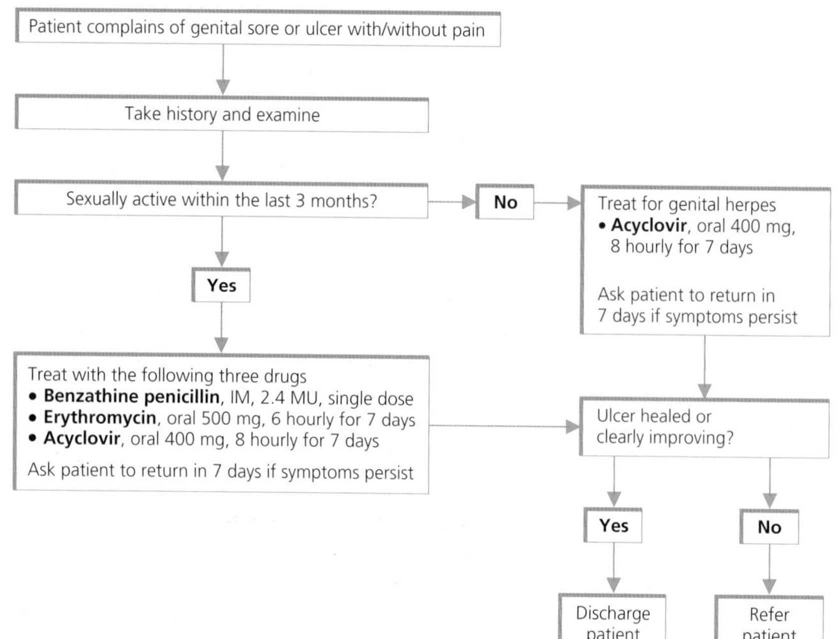

Figure 21.4 Flow chart for genital ulceration syndrome.

with herpes simplex virus and *Haemophilus ducreyi*. If patients are not better 1 week after treatment, and reinfection excluded, some flow charts encourage further treatment with the same or an alternative therapy, while others recommend referral to the next health care level, where they may be seen by either a specialised nurse or a doctor. Most countries operate with three levels of health care services, where the primary level would be the primary health care clinic, the second level would be a local hospital, and the third level would be the level of a teaching hospital or equivalent.

Box 21.3 **Main aetiological agents causing male urethral discharge and scrotal swelling syndromes**

- *Neisseria gonorrhoeae*
- *Chlamydia trachomatis* serovars D–K

Box 21.4 **Main aetiological agents and conditions causing vaginal discharge and lower abdominal pain syndromes**

- *Trichomonas vaginalis*
- *Neisseria gonorrhoeae*
- *Chlamydia trachomatis* serovars D–K
- Bacterial vaginosis
- Candidiasis

Box 21.5 **Main aetiological agents and conditions causing genital ulceration syndrome**

- Herpes simplex type 2 virus
- *Treponema palllidum*
- *Haemophilus ducreyi*
- *Chlamydia trachomatis* serovars L1–3

In addition to provision of effective medicines, the management of each patient with an STI should involve a number of non-biomedical components, including patient education, health promotion, discussion on condom use and condom provision, partner notification, and promotion of HIV counselling and testing (Box 21.6). Partner notification is essential to effective syndromic management, as it is the only way that asymptomatic infections will be treated using this approach. Effective partner management is the main weakness in STI control programmes across the world, and is generally more challenging in resource poor settings. Most resource poor settings employ patient-initiated partner notification strategies as human resource limitations make provider-initiated partner notification an impossibility.

Syndromic management saves money in terms of not requiring laboratory tests for individual patient management (Box 21.7). Another advantage of the syndromic approach is the provision of same-day treatment to patients, who often live far from the health care facility and who frequently cannot afford to return to the clinic to collect results, even if STI tests were to be performed. One key disadvantage of syndromic management is that this approach results in over-treatment of some individuals, particularly women with vaginal discharge and lower abdominal pain syndromes for whom this approach has poor specificity for detecting infection with STI pathogens. This may lead to unnecessary fears about infidelity or domestic violence for some female patients.

Box 21.6 **Non-biomedical components of syndromic management**

- Educate, ensure compliance, and counsel
- Promote abstinence during the course of treatment
- Promote and demonstrate condom use and provide condoms
- Stress the importance of partner treatment and issue notification slips
- Offer HIV counselling and testing – repeat at 3 months in case of negative test results

Box 21.7 **Advantages and disadvantages of syndromic management**

Main advantages

- No need for routine laboratory tests
- Flow charts enable nurses to manage most patients
- Patients treated at same visit
- Cost saving

Main disadvantages

- Female-only syndromes perform badly
- Most asymptomatic patients remain untreated
- Requires surveillance systems to be set up
- May induce relationship problems

The introduction of cheap and easy-to-use rapid tests for chamydial, gonococcal, and *Trichomonas vaginalis* infections in the future would certainly assist with enhancing the specificity of syndromic management as a means to treat only true STIs, and may assist with screening of asymptomatic high risk patients for STIs. Several rapid tests are currently available for HIV and treponemal antibody testing, and some rapid test kits exist for the detection of HSV-2 antibodies as well as *C. trachomatis* and *T. vaginalis* genital infections. At present, there is still a need for a sensitive and specific rapid test for gonorrhoea, given that microscopy is not practical in many busy clinics in resource poor settings.

Key to effective syndromic management, but not given priority in many resource poor settings, is the establishment of sentinel clinical and microbiological surveillance systems within countries. Most primary health care clinics collect very little information on STI presentations. At most this would be information on the total number of STI syndromes diagnosed, the number of male urethral discharge syndromes seen, and the number of STI contacts seen and treated. The number of male urethral discharge cases seen is a useful indicator of true STIs among men, given that some of the other syndromes may not be reflective of newly acquired STIs, for example non-STI related vaginal discharges or recurrent genital herpes. Sentinel clinical STI surveillance programmes collect data on each STI syndrome presenting to a defined number of sentinel sites. The syndrome data are generally collected by gender, age, and (for women) pregnancy status.

Microbiological surveillance is composed of two discrete elements: aetiological surveillance and monitoring of antimicrobial resistance. Both are critical components required to inform revision of national STI treatment guidelines. Periodic aetiological surveys using molecular diagnostic testing, which provides high diagnostic sensitivities, are required to confirm or establish rising or decreasing trends in the aetiology of particular syndromes. Such aetiological surveillance has, for example, demonstrated the rise of genital herpes and the decline in chancroid as a cause of genital ulceration in several African countries over the past decade.

In practice, given the demise of *H. ducreyi* infections worldwide, antimicrobial resistance surveillance is now only performed on *N. gonorrhoeae* isolates (Figures 21.5 and 21.6). Unless such antimicrobial resistance surveys are undertaken on a regular basis, important trends of rising resistance to first line therapies can be missed. Currently, several countries in Africa are now abandoning treatment of presumptive gonococcal infections with quinolones on the basis of recent in-country antimicrobial resistance surveys. The emergence of multidrug resistance among *N. gonorrhoeae* isolates is a cause of global concern and the WHO is currently active in trying to enhance antimicrobial resistance surveillance in several regions of the world.

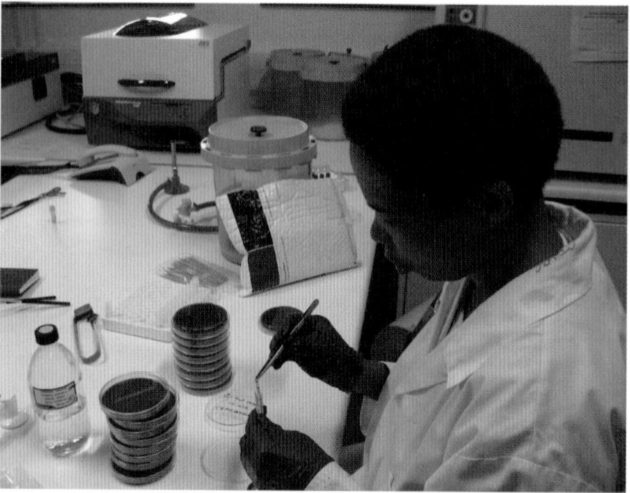

Figure 21.5 Antimicrobial resistance surveillance among *Neisseria gonorrhoeae* isolates is an essential component of the syndromic management approach. Courtesy of Professor David Lewis.

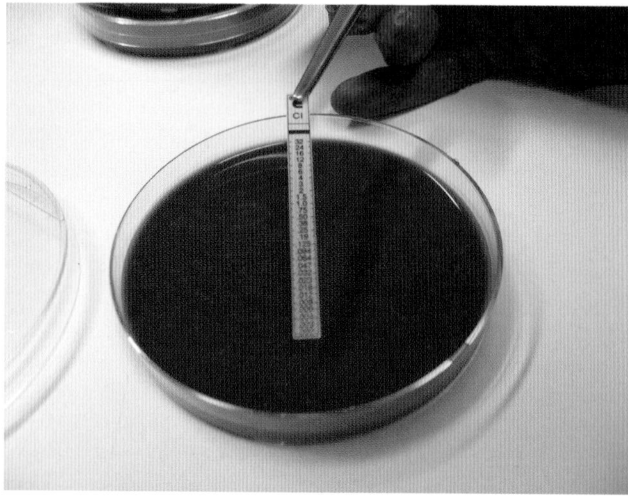

Figure 21.6 Screening for ciprofloxacin-resistant gonococci using E test technology (AB Biodisk, Sweden). Courtesy of Professor David Lewis.

In addition to weak surveillance systems and a rise in antimicrobial resistant gonorrhoea, the effectiveness of the syndromic management is hampered by the large burden of asymptomatic STIs. Although not proven, it is conceivable that syndromic management may, through selective treatment of symptomatic cases and hence natural selection, enhance the proportion of asymptomatic STIs within a population. Asymptomatic STIs, as exemplified by chlamydial and gonococcal infections, are of particular concern in women, who will only receive treatment if their partners notify them that they require STI partner therapy.

Among populations with high STI prevalence, for example commercial sex workers, introduction of short-term periodic presumptive therapy (PPT) programmes may assist by quickly reducing the prevalence of a number of bacterial STIs. Within PPT programmes, one or more antibiotics are given at intervals (typically monthly) for a defined period of time. Azithromycin is one such agent that has been used with some success in PPT programmes, because it remains at high concentrations inside polymorphonuclear leucocytes for several weeks. Azithromycin is active against chlamydial and gonococcal infections, *Mycoplasma genitalium* infections, chancroid, and syphilis. The PPT agent(s) treat both asymptomatic STIs and may provide an element of prophylaxis against acquiring bacterial STIs in the weeks following the PPT administration. Studies have shown that clinically diagnosed and laboratory detected STIs decrease not only in women at high risk of STIs who receive the PPT, but also among men residing in the locality.

In terms of STI control, resource poor countries have a number of epidemiological and structural variables that may enhance STI transmission and hamper public health efforts. Among these are economically driven migrant labour and mobility, the presence of high STI/HIV transmission areas at places such as country borders, commercial sex work, high levels of sexual assault, partner concurrency, often limited access to high quality STI/HIV health education, and inequalities in economic status, educational opportunities, and gender. Without political will and funds to deal with these variables, syndromic management on its own will always have limited success in reducing STI prevalence.

Accordingly, it is likely that STIs will remain a significant health problem in resource poor countries for some time to come. Significant reductions in STI prevalence may in the future be possible with enhanced STI services that incorporate STI screening programmes for individuals at high risk, such as commercial sex workers and their male partners, men who have sex with men, and those in professions that place them at high risk of acquiring STIs, for example long-distance lorry drivers.

Further reading

Grosskurth H, Mosha F, Todd J, Mwijarubi E, Klokke A, Senkoro K, *et al.* Impact of improved treatment of sexually transmitted diseases on HIV infection in rural Tanzania: randomised controlled trial. *Lancet* 1995;**346**:530–6.

Mayaud P, Mabey D. Approaches to the control of sexually transmitted infections in developing countries: old problems and modern challenges. *Sex Transm Infect* 2004;**80**:174–82.

Pettifor A, Walsh J, Wilkins V, Raghunathan P. How effective is syndromic management of STDs? *Sex Transm Dis* 2000;**27**:371–85.

Steen R, Vuylsteke B, DeCoito T, Ralepeli S, Fehler G, Conley J, *et al.* Evidence of declining STD prevalence in a South African mining community following a core-group intervention. *Sex Transm Dis* 2000;**27**:1–8.

CHAPTER 22

Vaccinations, Treatments, and Postexposure Prophylaxis

Ashini Jayasuriya

Nottingham University Hospitals, Nottingham, UK

> **OVERVIEW**
>
> - Vaccination is an effective tool in the prevention of hepatitis B infection and should be strongly encouraged, particularly in patients thought to be at higher risk of exposure to this virus
> - Human papillomavirus subtypes 16 and 18 are associated with more than 65% of cervical cancers in Europe and vaccination to prevent acquisition of these viruses is thought to be highly effective and safe
> - Postexposure prophylaxis following occupational, non-occupational, and sexual exposure to HIV is readily available; however, it requires prompt reporting of exposure and urgent referral to postexposure prophylaxis (PEP) providing services
> - Individuals presenting postexposure require holistic management – taking into account risks of blood-borne viruses and sexually transmitted infections (if relevant) but also the impact of exposure on the individual's social situation and psychological well-being

In order to deal with sexually transmitted infections, both preventative and therapeutic medical interventions are required. In this chapter, we summarise currently available vaccines, postexposure prophylaxis, and treatments commonly used in sexual health clinics.

Vaccinations

Hepatitis B

Hepatitis B vaccination is recommended for patients from certain risk groups seen in a sexual health clinic, including those with hepatitis C (see Chapter 15 for details of risk groups). Vaccination is also offered to individuals from countries with a high prevalence of hepatitis B if their risk of exposure is deemed to be ongoing. In other clinical settings, vaccination is recommended for newborn babies of hepatitis B infected mothers, household contacts, and renal dialysis patients.

ABC of Sexually Transmitted Infections, Sixth Edition.
Edited by Karen E. Rogstad.

Formulations and dosing schedules

Hepatitis B vaccines are inactive and unable to cause disease. The vaccine is available in several formulations, the most widely used being Engerix B™, HBVaxPro®, and Twinrix® (Figure 22.1). The latter is a combined hepatitis A and B vaccine given on the same dosing schedule as the monovalent hepatitis B vaccine. A comparison of currently marketed formulations of hepatitis B vaccine is shown in Figure 22.2.

A schematic diagram showing Engerix B dosing schedules commonly used in the United Kingdom are represented in Figure 22.3(a). Evidence suggests that if vaccine courses are not completed in immunocompetent patients, the outstanding doses can be given 4 years or more later without the need to restart a three-dose course.

Vaccine efficacy and failure

Engerix B induces specific antibodies against hepatitis B surface antigen (HBsAg). An anti-HBs antibody titre ≥10 IU/L correlates with protection against infection. Studies have demonstrated a protective efficacy of 95–100% in neonates, children, and adults at risk. Figure 22.3(b) summarizes seroprotection rates obtained in clinical studies with Engerix B, given according to the different dosing schedules.

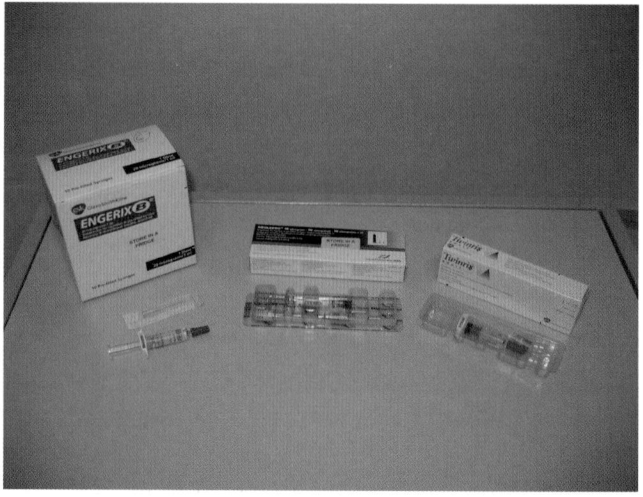

Figure 22.1 Commonly used hepatitis B vaccines.

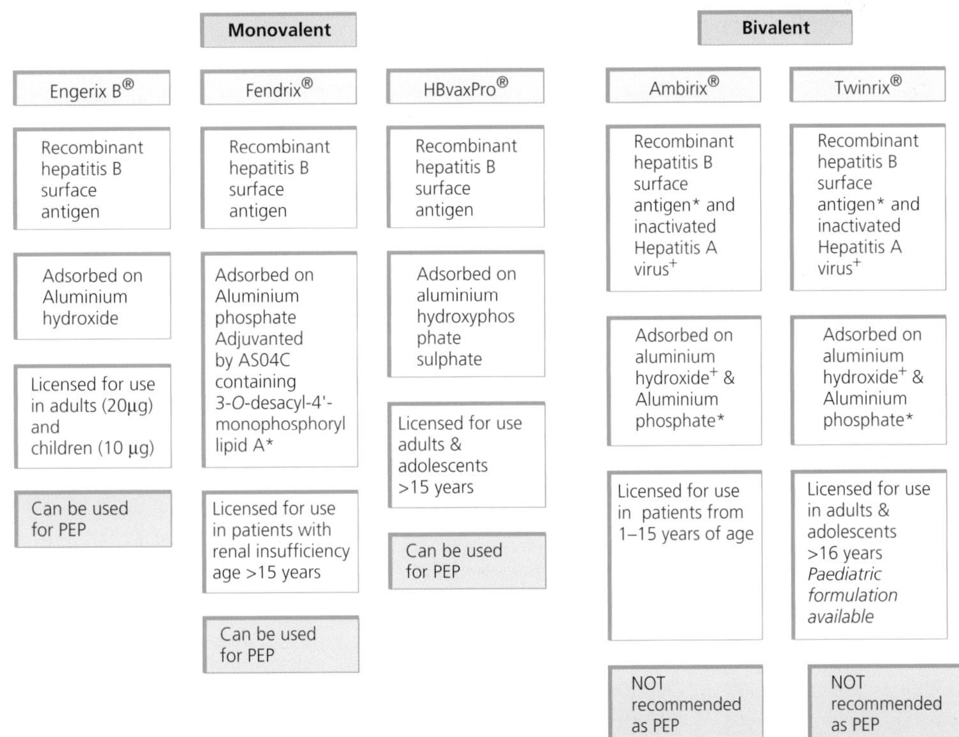

Figure 22.2 Currently available formulations of hepatitis B vaccine. *This adjuvant is thought to be responsible for increased immunogenicity of Fendrix®.

Across all vaccination schedules, 10–15% of immunocompetent individuals will fail to respond adequately. Poor responses are associated with age >40 years, obesity, smoking, and alcohol misuse. Reduced response rates are also associated with immunocompromised states. In HIV-positive patients, double-dose vaccine has been shown to increase response rates by 13%. Non-responders to a repeat (which may be double-dose) vaccination course may benefit from further vaccination once viral suppression is achieved and CD4 count maintained above >500 cells/mm^3. Third-generation vaccines, containing PreS1 and PreS2 antigens in addition to the S antigen, have demonstrated the ability to elicit seroprotective titres in previous vaccine non-responders.

Following completion of a primary course of vaccination with good immunological response, booster vaccinations may not be needed for at least 15 years (if at all). Immunocompromised patients may become anti-HBs-negative more rapidly and require more frequent monitoring and possible booster doses.

Postexposure prophylaxis

An accelerated course of hepatitis B vaccine can be offered as postexposure prophylaxis if started up to 6 weeks after exposure. In certain situations, where the donor is known to be infectious, specific hepatitis B immunoglobulin may also be administered, ideally within 48 hours but up to 7 days postexposure. Vaccination is also used in the prevention of perinatal hepatitis B transmission. Transmission to neonates can be prevented in over 90% of cases by commencement of a course of vaccination at birth.

Hepatitis A

Hepatitis A is transmitted faeco-orally and outbreaks have been reported in men who have sex with men (MSM) associated with certain risk behaviours. Most MSM are not at increased risk for hepatitis A infection and therefore universal vaccination in this group has not been firmly recommended. Nevertheless, it is the practice of several centres, particularly in larger cities where outbreaks have been reported, to offer vaccination for hepatitis A to MSM following screening for pre-existing hepatitis A exposure. A combined hepatitis A and B vaccination is often used. Intravenous drug users and hepatitis B or C positive individuals should also be vaccinated, as should travellers to developing countries, people with haemophilia or chronic liver disease, those with occupational exposure, and those at risk during an outbreak.

Monovalent hepatitis A vaccine (e.g. Havrix™) is given at 0 and 6–12 months and confers 95% protection. Currently, revaccination is advised every 10 years although accumulating evidence suggests that immunity is lifelong in immunocompetent individuals. Hepatitis A vaccine may be given as prophylaxis up to 14 days postexposure if this occurred within the infectious period of the source case (during the prodromal illness or first week of jaundice).

Human papillomavirus

Cervical cancer is the second most common cancer affecting women worldwide, with approximately 500 000 new cases and 270 000 deaths annually. Persistent infection by high risk human papillomavirus (HPV) types is detectable in more than 99% of cervical

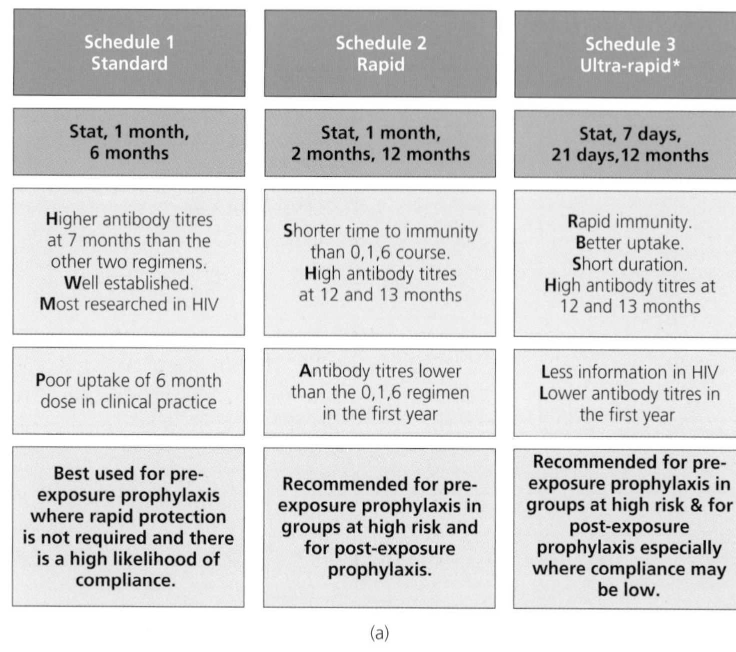

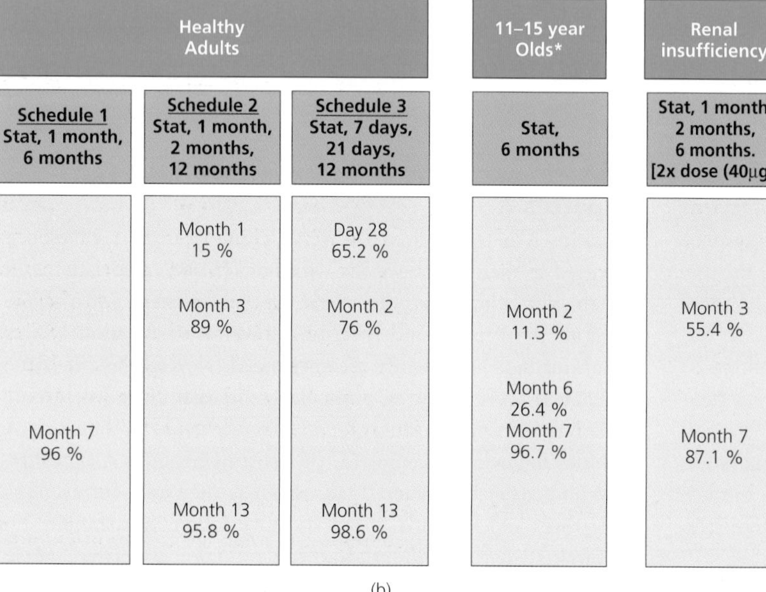

Figure 22.3 (a) Dosing schedules for Engerix B®. *As a significant proportion of patients given the 'Ultra-rapid' vaccination course will fail to demonstrate an early antibody response following the third (day 21) dose of vaccine, it is prudent to offer them booster vaccinations of up to three further doses if they are at high risk of acquiring hepatitis B. Alternatively, for those at low risk, no further action needs to be taken until the 12-month booster, by which time over 95% will be anti-HBs positive. (b) Percentage of individuals who develop seroprotection following vaccination with Engerix B®. * For teenagers between 11 and 15 years, a two-dose schedule (at 0 and 6 months) of the adult vaccine provides similar protection to three doses of the childhood vaccine (Engerix B Paed®).

cancers. Of these high risk types, HPV-16 is responsible for more than 50% and HPV-18 for more than 15% of all cervical cancers in Europe. A further 11 high risk types have been described. In addition to cervical cancer, HPV is causally associated with other less common cancers, which include cancer of the vulva, vagina, penis, and anus, and some cancers of the head and neck.

Vaccine formulations

There are currently two types of HPV vaccine available, Cervarix® and Gardasil®. The former protects against HPV types 16 and 18 and the latter protects against HPV types 6, 11, 16, and 18. The latter therefore also confers some protection against genital warts. Both are non-infectious recombinant vaccines, prepared from highly purified virus-like particles of major capsid L1 protein of HPV types 16, 18 (and 6 and 11 in the quadrivalent vaccine). A comparison of the two vaccines is shown in Figure 22.4.

Vaccine efficacy

Vaccine efficacy is mediated by the development of a humoral immune response although there is no clearly defined minimal antibody level associated with protection. The duration of immunity is expected to be at least 10 years. In studies, the vaccines produced higher antibody titres in individuals aged 10–14 years compared with those who are 15–24 years old, suggesting that vaccination is best administered in this age group. Both vaccines have a good safety record and are highly effective against the precursors of cervical cancer. Trials of Gardasil also demonstrated effective protection against genital warts. Both vaccines are preventative rather than

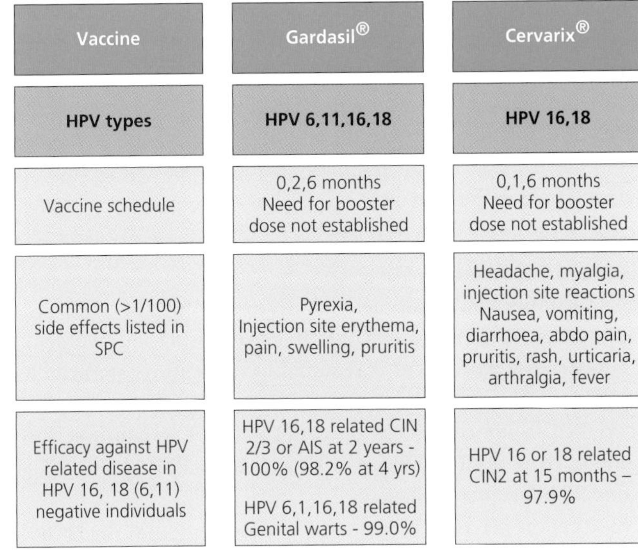

Vaccine	Gardasil®	Cervarix®
HPV types	HPV 6,11,16,18	HPV 16,18
Vaccine schedule	0,2,6 months Need for booster dose not established	0,1,6 months Need for booster dose not established
Common (>1/100) side effects listed in SPC	Pyrexia, Injection site erythema, pain, swelling, pruritis	Headache, myalgia, injection site reactions Nausea, vomiting, diarrhoea, abdo pain, pruritis, rash, urticaria, arthralgia, fever
Efficacy against HPV related disease in HPV 16, 18 (6,11) negative individuals	HPV 16,18 related CIN 2/3 or AIS at 2 years - 100% (98.2% at 4 yrs) HPV 6,1,16,18 related Genital warts - 99.0%	HPV 16 or 18 related CIN2 at 15 months – 97.9%

Figure 22.4 A comparison of currently available HPV vaccines. Data from individual SPCs.

therapeutic and are hence not currently indicated for the treatment of established HPV-associated disease. However, vaccine studies have indicated that if an individual has already been infected by one HPV type at the time of vaccination, such individuals still gain a high level of protection from the other HPV types that are included in the vaccine. Also, a degree of cross-protection is provided against infection by certain, but not all, non-vaccine HPV types. Data on use of these vaccines in immunocompromised individuals is emerging.

Vaccination programme and cervical screening

HPV vaccination is not likely to become a substitute for cytological cervical screening in the immediate future because neither vaccine is 100% effective and neither provide protection against all oncogenic HPV subtypes. However, in addition to improving health and reducing mortality, HPV vaccination programmes are predicted to be cost-effective even in countries with established cervical cancer screening programmes, especially if screening costs are subsequently reduced by increasing the age of initiation or reducing the frequency of screening. Furthermore, costs associated with the follow-up of abnormal screening tests, treating cancers and other HPV-related diseases may also be reduced.

Postexposure prophylaxis for HIV

After initial exposure, HIV replicates within dendritic cells of the skin and mucosa before spreading through lymphatic vessels and developing into a systemic infection. This delay in systemic spread (thought to be up to 48–72 hours) leaves a 'window of opportunity' for postexposure prophylaxis (PEP) using antiretroviral drugs designed to block replication of HIV. By inhibiting early viral replication, PEP may be able to prevent the establishment of systemic HIV infection. PEP is now available for use in both occupational and non-occupational settings. Following sexual exposure, it is commonly known as PEPSE (postexposure prophylaxis for sexual exposure). Clinical trials are also currently in progress to evaluate the benefit of pre-exposure prophylaxis (PreP) for HIV in sexual exposure settings.

Risk of transmission

According to currently available data, the risk of acquiring HIV infection following occupational and sexual exposure to HIV-infected blood is relatively low (Figure 22.5). The average risk of HIV transmission after percutaneous exposure to HIV-infected blood in health care settings is about 3 per 1000 injuries (0.3%). After a mucocutaneous exposure, the average risk is less than 1 in 1000 (<0.1%). It is thought that there is no risk of HIV transmission where intact skin is exposed to HIV-infected blood. In estimating risk, additional factors need to be taken into account such as the source patient's HIV viral load and, in the context of sexual exposure, the coexistence of other sexually transmitted infections (STIs), or trauma to the genital tract. In cases of sexual assault, PEPSE is considered more readily as it is believed that HIV transmission risk is increased following aggravated sexual intercourse.

Evidence for the use of PEP(SE)

Data from animal studies support the use of PEP(SE) in the prevention of HIV acquisition. Furthermore, a case-controlled study

Risk involved in type of exposure (if source HIV positive)	
Blood transfusion	90–100%
Percutaneous needle	0.3%
Receptive anal intercourse	0.1–3.0%
Receptive vaginal intercourse	0.1–0.2%
Insertive vaginal intercourse	0.03–0.09%
Insertive anal intercourse	0.06%
Receptive oral intercourse	0–0.04%
Mucous membrane exposure	0.09%

Epidemiological probability that source HIV positive		
MSM		
London	20.30%	
Scotland	3.20%	
Elsewhere UK	3.60%	
IVDU		
London	2.90%	
Elsewhere UK	0.5%	
Heterosexuals		
UK	M 0.5%	F 0.2%
Rest Europe	M 2%	F 0.2%
N America	M 2.9%	F 0.1%
Sub-S Africa:	M 6.9%	F 11.3%
Caribbean	M 1.2%	F 1.0%

Figure 22.5 Risk of transmission of HIV according to exposure type and epidemiological likelihood of HIV infection in selected populations. Adapted from the British Association for Sexual Health and HIV UK Guidelines for the use of post-exposure prophylaxis following sexual exposure (2006).

by the US Centers for Disease Control and Prevention (US CDC) demonstrated that the administration of zidovudine (AZT) prophylaxis to health care workers occupationally exposed to HIV was associated with an 81% reduction in HIV acquisition risk. In this study, factors associated with increased risk of HIV acquisition were deep injury, visible blood on the offending device, injury with a needle directly from the source patient's artery or vein, and a terminal HIV-related illness in the source patient. Several studies have also shown the protective efficacy of PEP in the prevention of mother-to-child transmission of HIV. Similarly, in non-randomised prospective studies in sexual exposure settings, PEPSE given to individuals to take immediately after sexual exposure has been shown to be protective. However, there are cases of PEP(SE) failure in both occupational and sexual settings. Failure has particularly been associated with late initiation, poor adherence, and repeated HIV exposure.

Antiretroviral therapy

There is a lack of published data comparing the efficacy of two or more antiretroviral drugs compared with monotherapy for occupational PEP. However, given that combination antiretroviral therapy is more potent than zidovudine monotherapy at suppressing viral replication, there is clear rationale to support the use of a combination of agents. Concern over the prevalence of antiretroviral drug resistance amongst HIV-infected individuals further supports the use of combination prophylaxis in PEP(SE). The UK Department of Health guidelines advocate the use of tenofovir, emtricitabine plus ritonavir-boosted lopinavir in occupational postexposure prophylaxis for a total of 28 days.

PEP(SE) in clinical practice

PEP is most likely to be efficacious if started within the first hour following exposure. Immediate reporting of exposure and an urgent preliminary risk assessment is required in order to recommend a first dose of PEP. A more thorough risk assessment can then be undertaken to inform a decision about whether to continue the regimen. There is no evidence of benefit from PEP(SE) if given beyond 72 hours postexposure.

Information needs to be gathered about the injury, the recipient, and the source (Figure 22.6). Where the source is known to be HIV-positive, information about current and previous antiretroviral therapy, known viral resistance, and viral load are important. If the source is identifiable but of unknown HIV status, it may be appropriate to ask them to be tested for HIV. Informed

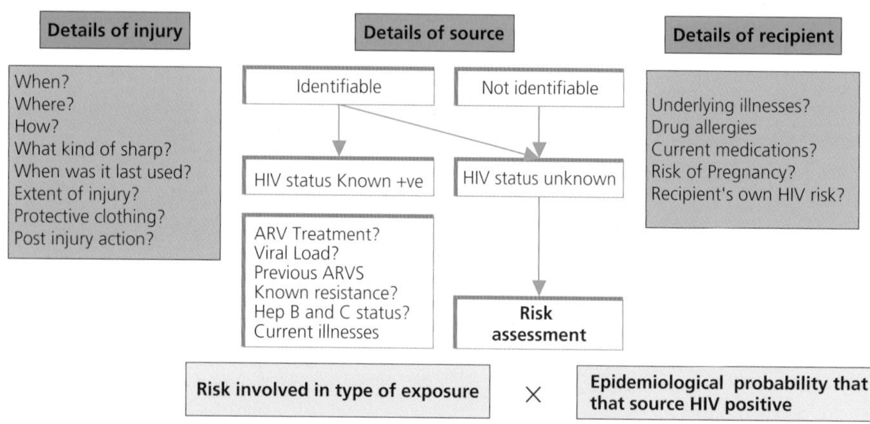

Figure 22.6 Summary of history taken in PEP(SE) scenario.

	Source known HIV positive	HIV status of source is unknown but from group or area of high HIV prevalence.	HIV status of source is unknown but from group or area of low HIV prevalence.
Receptive anal sex	PEP 'recommended'	PEP 'recommended'	PEP 'considered'
Receptive vaginal sex	PEP 'recommended'	PEP 'considered'	PEP 'not recommended'
Insertive anal sex or Insertive vaginal	PEP 'recommended'	PEP 'considered'	PEP 'not recommended'
Fellatio with ejaculation	PEP 'considered'	PEP 'considered'	PEP 'not recommended'
Fellatio without ejaculation or cunnilingus	PEP 'not recommended'	PEP 'not recommended'	Not stated
Semen in eye	PEP 'considered'	Not stated	Not stated

Figure 22.7 British Association for Sexual Health and HIV recommendations for PEPSE (2006).

consent should be taken. The use of rapid 'point of care' tests (see Chapter 18) may be useful if delays are anticipated in obtaining a laboratory test result. National or professional guidance is often available for situations in which the source patient is unable to provide consent (e.g. because they are unconscious). In the United Kingdom, this guidance is provided by the Department of Health in accordance with the Human Tissue Act 2004 and the Mental Capacity Act 2005, and the General Medical Council. Where a source patient lacks capacity to consent his/her blood/tissues can only lawfully be tested for any serious communicable disease if it is reasonably held to be in his/her best interests. In the event of a deceased patient being the source, the testing of any available tissue samples requires consent from a 'nominated representative' or a person in a 'qualifying relationship' to the deceased. The commencement of PEP(SE) should not be delayed until the availability of the source's HIV test results. In addition, the 'window period' for HIV testing must be taken into consideration before PEP(SE) is subsequently discontinued on the basis of the source patient's negative test result.

Where it is not possible to identify the source patient (e.g. the injury is caused by a discarded needle), a risk assessment is conducted on the basis of the circumstances of the exposure and the epidemiological likelihood of HIV in the source (Figure 22.7).

In practice, a case by case risk–benefit discussion is undertaken about the use of PEP(SE). The frequency, severity, duration, and reversibility of antiretroviral side effects and the potential for as yet unknown long-term complications of antiretrovirals are balanced against the risk of HIV transmission. Should PEP(SE) be prescribed, individuals are counselled on adherence, particularly as theoretically drug-resistant virus may emerge if seroconversion takes place during a period of poor adherence. They are advised on the potential for drug interactions with other medications. Baseline investigations include an HIV test to determine their own status at the time of injury. Most centres dispense a 4-day 'starter pack' (Figure 22.8) and review patients within that time period in order to assess tolerance to treatment and provide additional support.

Risk assessment should also include consideration of hepatitis B (see above) and hepatitis C. Although there is no effective postexposure prophylaxis for hepatitis C, evidence suggests that early treatment with high dose interferon can result in viral clearance in about 90% of recently infected individuals. In the case of sexual exposure, risks of transmission of other STIs should also be considered, and appropriate STI screening arranged.

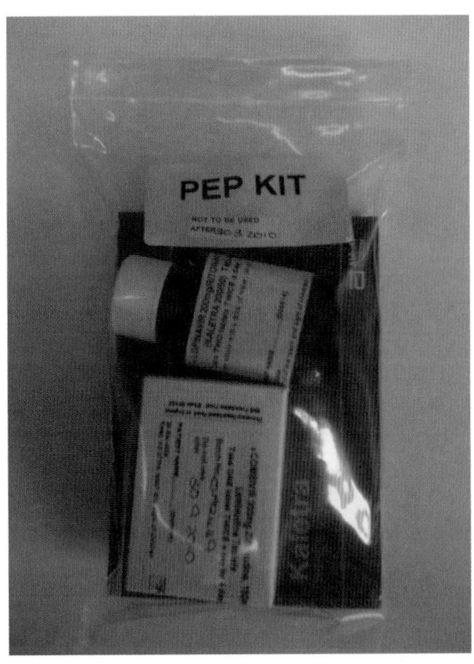

Figure 22.8 Antiretroviral 'PEP Starter Pack'.

All patients presenting for PEP(SE), whether or not taken, should be offered follow-up for testing for HIV, hepatitis B and C, and counselling as required. Patients should be advised on safer sex and the avoidance of blood donation until their follow-up period is completed. In the case of occupational exposure, the individual may also be advised to notify their occupational health service.

Treatments

First line treatments used for common conditions seen in STI clinics are summarised in Table 22.1. For alternative treatments and special circumstances (such as pregnancy and lactation) please refer to details in corresponding chapters and local and national management guidelines.

Table 22.1 Summary of first line therapies.

Condition	First line treatment
Bacterial vaginosis	Metronidazole 400 mg b.d. (5–7 days) Metronidazole 2 g (single dose)
Candidiasis	*Intravaginal* Clotrimazole 500 mg (stat), 200 mg (3 nights), 100 mg (6 nights) Clotrimazole cream 5 g (single dose) Econazole 150 mg (single dose) Econazole 150 mg (3 nights) *Oral* Fluconazole 150 mg (single dose)
Candidiasis – recurrent	*Induction* Fluconazole 150 mg every 72 hours (3 doses) *Maintenance* Fluconazole 150 mg once weekly (6 months)

(continued overleaf)

Table 22.1 *(continued)*

Condition	First line treatment	
Chancroid	Azithromycin 1 g (single dose) Ceftriaxone 250 mg IM (single dose) Ciprofloxacin 500 mg (single dose) Ciprofloxacin 500 mg b.d. (3 days) Erythromycin 500 mg q.d.s. (7 days)	
Chlamydia (uncomplicated genital, rectal, pharyngeal)	Doxycycline 100 mg b.d. (7 days) Azithromycin 1 g (single dose)	
Donovanosis	Azithromycin 1 g weekly or 500 mg o.d. Ceftriaxone 1 g IM/IV o.d. Co-trimoxazole 160/800 mg b.d.* Doxycycline 100 mg b.d.* Erythromycin 500 mg q.d.s.* Norfloxacin 400 mg b.d. Ciprofloxacin 500 mg b.d. *Duration* Until lesions healed (minimum 3 weeks)	
Epididymo-orchitis	*Most likely due to gonococcal infection* Ceftriaxone 250 mg IM (single dose) Ciprofloxacin 500 mg (single dose) Doxycycline 100 mg b.d. (10–14 days) *Most likely due to chlamydial infection/non-gonococcal/non-enteric organisms* Doxycycline 100 mg b.d. (10–14 days) *Most likely due to enteric organisms* Ofloxacin 200 mg b.d. (14 days) Ciprofloxacin 500 mg b.d. (10 days)	
Gonorrhoea (uncomplicated genital, rectal)	Ceftriaxone 250 mg IM (single dose) (inc pharyngeal infection) Cefixime 400 mg (single dose, oral) Spectinomycin 2 g IM (single dose)	
Herpes – first episode†	Aciclovir 200 mg 5x daily (5 days) Aciclovir 400 mg t.d.s. (5 days) Valaciclovir 500 mg b.d. (5 days) Famciclovir 250 mg t.d.s. (5 days)	
Herpes – recurrent	*Episodic short course* Aciclovir 800 mg t.d.s. (2 days) Valaciclovir 500 mg b.d. (3 days) Famciclovir 1 g b.d. (1 day) *Episodic therapy* Aciclovir 200 mg 5x daily (5 days) Aciclovir 400 mg t.d.s. (5 days) Valaciclovir 500 mg b.d. (5 days) Famciclovir 125 mg b.d. (5 days) *Suppressive therapy* Aciclovir 400 mg b.d. Aciclovir 400 mg q.d.s. Famciclovir 250 mg b.d. Valaciclovir 500 mg–1 g o.d.	
Genital warts	*Ablative* Cryotherapy Electrocautery/electrotherapy Laser therapy LEEP (loop electrical excision procedure) Surgical/scissor excision	*Non-ablative* Podophyllotoxin Imiquimod Trichloracetic acid
Lymphogranuloma venereum	Doxycycline 100 mg b.d. (21 days) Tetracycline 2 g daily (21 days) Minocycline 300 mg loading dose followed by 200 mg b.d. (21 days)	

Table 22.1 *(continued)*

Condition	First line treatment
Molluscum contagiosum	Cryotherapy Expression of the pearly core Podophyllotoxin cream (0.5%) Imiquimod 5% cream
Mycoplasma genitalium	Azithromycin 1 g stat Azithromycin 500 mg day 1 followed by 250 mg daily for 4 days
Non-specific urethritis	Azithromycin 1 g (single dose) Doxycycline 100 mg b.d. (7 days)
Phthirus pubis infestation	Malathion 0.5% (12 hours) Permethrin 1% cream rinse (10 min) Phenothrin 0.2% (2 hours) Carbaryl 0.5 and 1% (12 hours) *Unlicensed indication* *Infestation of eyelashes* Permethrin 1% lotion (10 min) White or yellow paraffin based ointment b.d. (8–10 days)
Pelvic inflammatory disease (outpatient management)	Ceftriaxone 250 mg IM (single dose) or cefoxitin 2 g IM (single dose) *plus* oral probenecid 1 g (single dose) *Followed by* Doxycycline 100 mg b.d. (14 days) and Metronidazole 400 mg b.d. (14 days)
Prostatitis – acute	Ciprofloxacin 500 mg b.d. (28 days) Ofloxacin 200 mg b.d. (28 days)
Prostatitis – chronic bacterial	Ciprofloxacin 500 mg b.d. (28 days) Levofloxacin 500 mg o.d. (28 days) Ofloxacin 200 mg b.d. (28 days) Norfloxacin 400 mg b.d. (28 days) *With or without* Alpha blockers
Scabies	Permethrin 5% cream (12 hours) Malathion 0.5% (12 hours)
Syphilis – incubating	Benzathine penicillin G 2.4 MU IM (single dose) Doxycycline 100 mg b.d. (14 days) Azithromycin 1 g (single dose)
Syphilis – early (primary, secondary, early latent)	Benzathine penicillin G 2.4 MU IM (single dose) Procaine penicillin G 600 000 u IM o.d. (10 days)
Syphilis – late (late latent, cardiovascular and gummatous syphilis)	Benzathine penicillin 2.4 MU IM weekly for 2 weeks (three doses) Procaine penicillin 600 000 u IM o.d. (17 days)
Syphilis – neuro/ophthalmic involvement	Procaine penicillin 1.8–2.4 MU IM o.d. plus probenecid 500 mg PO q.d.s. (17 days) Benzylpenicillin 18–24 MU daily, given as 3–4 MU IM every 4 hours (17 days)
Trichomonas vaginalis	Metronidazole 2 g (single dose) Metronidazole 400–500 mg b.d. (5–7 days)

*CDC recommended.
†Longer duration of treatment (7–10 days) advocated by CDC.
‡Avoid where gonoccocal PID likely and where high quinilone resistance rates.
Adapted from the British Association for Sexual Health and HIV STI Management guidelines (www.bashh.org/guidelines).

Further reading

British Association of Sexual Health and HIV Clinical Effectiveness Group. United Kingdom National guideline on the management of the viral hepatitides A, B and C, 2008. Available at http://www.bashh.org/guidelines.

British Association of Sexual Health and HIV Clinical Effectiveness Group. UK Guideline for the use of post-exposure prophylaxis for HIV following sexual exposure, 2006. Available at http://www.bashh.org/guidelines.

Centers for Disease Control and Prevention. Sexually Transmitted Diseases Treatment Guidelines 2010. *Morbidity and Mortality Weekly Report* **59**. Available at http://www.cdc.gov/std/treatment/2010.

UK Department of Health. Immunisation against infectious disease. 'The Green Book': Chapters on hepatitis A, B and human papilloma virus. 2006. Available at www.dh.gov.uk.

UK Department of Health. HIV post-exposure prophylaxis. Guidance from the UK Chief Medical Officers' Expert Advisory Group on AIDS. 2008. Available at www.dh.gov.uk.

US Public Health Service Guidelines for the Management of Occupational Exposures to HIV and Recommendations for Post-exposure Prophylaxis (2005). Antiretroviral postexposure prophylaxis after sexual, injection-drug use, or other non-occupational exposure to HIV in the United States. Recommendations from the US Department of Health and Human Services (2005). Available at http://www.aidsinfo.nih.gov.

Young T, Arens FJ, Kennedy GE, Laurie JW, Rutherford G. Antiretroviral post-exposure prophylaxis (PEP) for occupational HIV exposure (review). Cochrane Collaboration (2009). Available at http://www.cochrane.org/reviews.

CHAPTER 23

The Internet as a Resource for STI Education and Information

Claudia Estcourt and John Saunders

Queen Mary University of London, Barts and The London School of Medicine and Dentistry, London, UK

OVERVIEW

- The internet is a key resource for both professionals and patients
- The stigmatised nature of STIs and HIV may mean that patients access information from the internet to a greater extent than patients with other conditions
- The quality of internet information is highly variable and there is no obligation for web sites to ensure accuracy. Factually incorrect information may cause considerable anxiety
- Signposting high quality web sites to patients is good practice
- Although few educational courses are currently offered as solely online programmes, it is likely that this will change rapidly in the next few years

The internet has dramatically changed how health care professionals and patients access information about health and disease. Accessing health-related information on the internet is an extremely popular activity. Studies from Europe and the United States report that 70–80% of internet users had performed health-related searches at some time.

There are particular features of patients with sexually transmitted infections (STIs) and their infections that make the internet a key part of medical care and education. The rapid pace of change in HIV therapeutics makes the internet essential in ensuring wide access to the most relevant and up-to-date clinical and therapeutic information for clinicians. The stigma associated with STIs and HIV in many societies makes the internet a particularly appealing source of information for those who are concerned about exposure to infections, keen to self-diagnose, or those who want to find their closest clinical service quickly and discretely. Many national health organisations have worked hard to create appealing sites which can target different societal groups. These sites have often been developed creatively to include humour to underpin their messages and use features such as 'Hide this page!' buttons to enable the user to move away from sensitive material quickly if necessary (Figure 23.1).

ABC of Sexually Transmitted Infections, Sixth Edition.
Edited by Karen E. Rogstad.

The quality of health information on the internet is variable and the benefits of much greater access to information needs to be weighed against the considerable opportunities for misinformation, escalation of anxiety, and unnecessary alarm. Some believe that an objective standardized scoring system for medical information on the internet would be beneficial but this may not be feasible. In practice, it is extremely useful to guide patients to sites offering high quality accurate updated information such as sites run by national public health and professional organizations. Some of these are listed in the tables.

In this chapter, possible uses of the internet as a resource for STI and HIV information and education from both the clinician's and patient's perspective are considered. The main sites (home page) are referenced rather than specific pages of the relevant organisations to minimise problems with web site changes. Attempting to be comprehensive is impossible; instead, examples are used to guide readers in their information and education searches.

Diagnosis and management

High quality clinical images are available on a number of sites. The AIDS Images Library is an online searchable library of AIDS-related images for medical professionals. The images are downloadable and free of charge for use in assisting diagnosis or in presentations. The United States Department of Veteran Affairs web site contains sections for both patients and professionals. These contain general information about HIV diagnosis and management as well as an image bank. The web site www.dermatlas.org is a dermatology image atlas with some pictures of STIs and genital dermatoses.

Many countries offer national guidelines for management of specific conditions through either the relevant professional organisation or the relevant national public health sites. Some make reference to management in both specialist and primary care and others have a common set of guidelines (Table 23.1). These are usually updated on a regular basis but recommendations need to be assessed in context, for example those related to antimicrobial choice for *Neisseria gonorrhoeae* for which local isolate sensitivities are key, or HIV first line therapies, which will in part depend on local drug availability.

The UK National electronic Library for Infection (NeLI) contains 'on-line evidence-based, quality-tagged resources on the investigation, treatment, prevention and control of infectious disease'

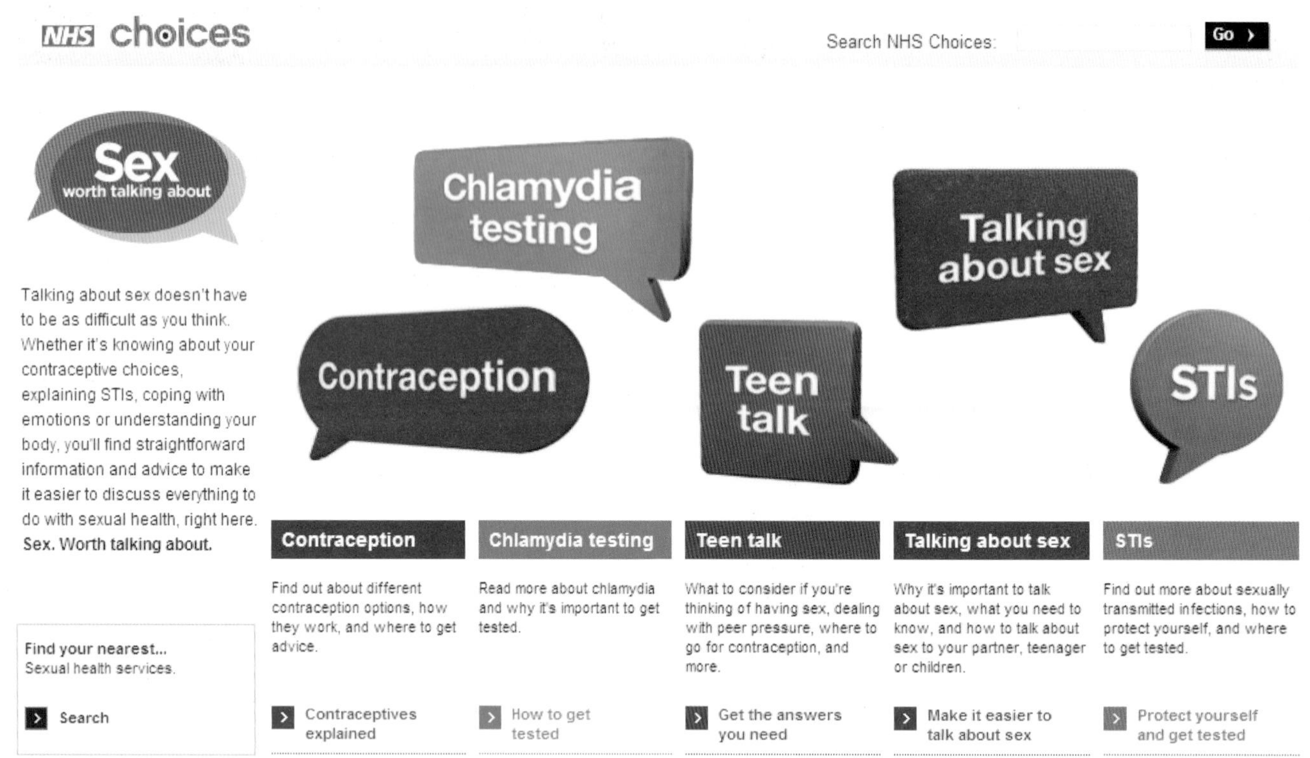

Figure 23.1 UK Department of Health patient information website. http://www.nhs.uk/worthtalkingabout/Pages/sex-worth-talking-about.aspx. © Crown copyright.

Table 23.1 Resources for STI and HIV diagnosis and management, including clinical guidelines.

STI and HIV images	AIDS Images Library	www.aids-images.ch
	Dermatology Image Atlas	www.dermatlas.org
	US Department of Veterans Affairs	www.hiv.va.gov
STI and HIV treatment guidelines, prevention and control	AIDSinfo	www.aidsinfo.nih.gov
	Australasian Chapter of Sexual Health Medicine	www.racp.edu.au
	Australasian Society for HIV Medicine (ASHM)	www.ashm.org.au
	British Association for Sexual Health and HIV (BASHH)	www.bashh.org
	British HIV Association (BHIVA)	www.bhiva.org
	Centres for Disease Control and Prevention (CDC)	www.cdc.gov
	European AIDS Clinical Society (EACS)	www.europeanaidsclinicalsociety.org
	Health Protection Agency (HPA)	www.hpa.org.uk
	International Union against STIs (IUSTI)	www.iusti.org
	National Electronic Library of Infection	www.neli.org.uk
	NHS Evidence Infection	www.library.nhs.uk/infections
	World Health Organization (WHO)	www.who.int

including STIs and HIV. Similarly, NHS Evidence – infections, formerly a specialist library of the (UK) National Library for Health, contains links to national care and service guidance.

Little is known about how patients use the internet to self-diagnose STIs. One small UK study reported that just under half of patients in an urban genitourinary clinic had looked up their symptoms on the internet prior to attendance but only around 14% of them had diagnosed their symptoms correctly.

Self-management of most STIs is limited by the need for antimicrobials, which in many countries are available on prescription only. However, a number of studies have shown that patients do try self-treatment and actively seek non-prescription remedies as an adjunct to or instead of prescribed drugs. It is probable that patients use the internet to obtain this type of information on alternative and adjunct medication.

Finding clinical services

Some countries have invested heavily in online help for people seeking health care. In the United Kingdom, the NHS Choices site

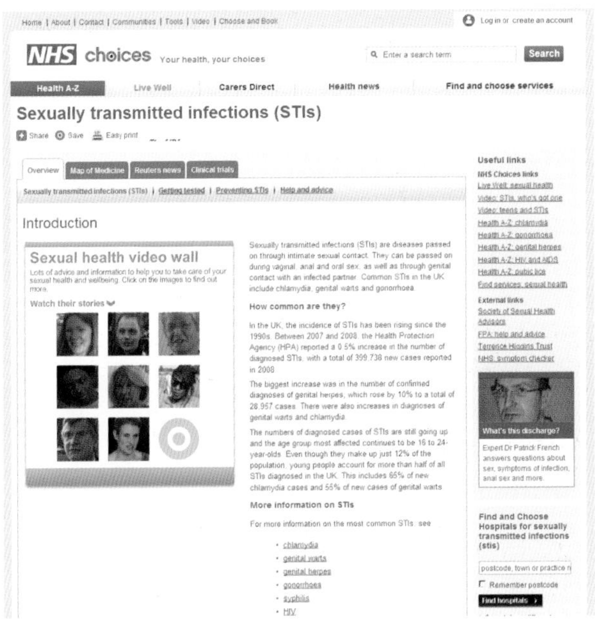

Figure 23.2 The UK NHS Choices web site, www.nhs.uk. © Crown copyright.

is designed to enable a person to quickly locate key information on local services (Figure 23.2). Information includes location, opening hours, and the range of services offered. Often these sites will have distinct sections for the public and professionals which include referral pathways and contact information.

Some sexual health clinics have developed their own sites, again designed for both public and professional visitors. These may include useful resources such as contact slips and infection specific information. A good example is the Melbourne Sexual Health Centre web site (Figure 23.3) which provides extensive partner notification information and assistance through the 'Let them

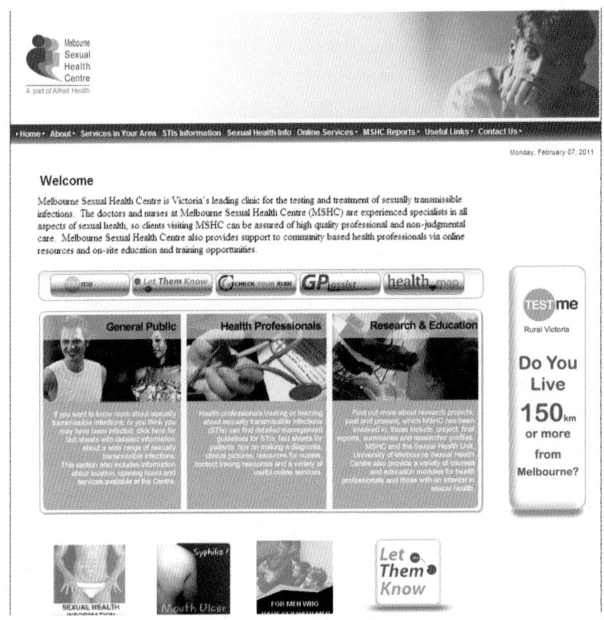

Figure 23.3 Melbourne Sexual Health Centre web site, www.mshc.org.au.

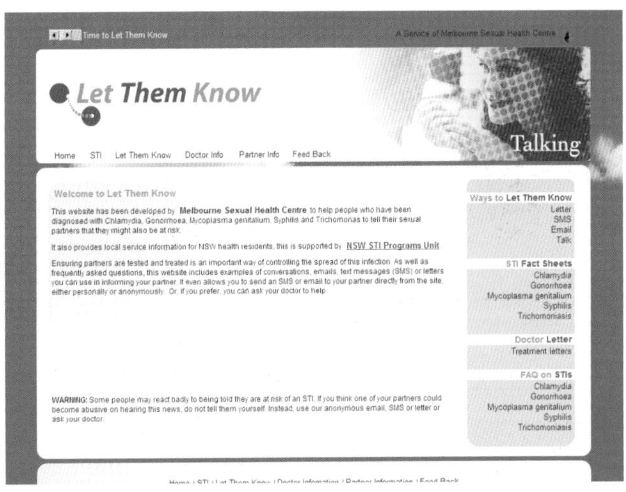

Figure 23.4 Let Them Know web site, www.letthemknow.org.au (Melbourne Sexual Health Centre).

know' site (Figure 23.4). In some centres, the web site will link to an appointment booking system which enables the person to choose a convenient time to attend. In many settings private sector providers also use the internet extensively to advertise their sexual health care services.

Information about diagnosed conditions and support groups

Many public health sites offer excellent resources in the form of downloadable printable factsheets about individual infections and conditions (Table 23.1). The availability of information electronically is also useful for those patients who do not want to take written information away with them but prefer to look at the information in privacy at a later stage. We have listed a number of reliable high quality sites in Table 23.2. These include a number of support groups that offer reliable internet resources. These sites may also be useful for non-specialists looking for brief overviews of conditions. More in-depth information about local disease epidemiology is usually published by the relevant public health services.

Education

It is likely that there will be a rapid expansion in web-based provision of STI educational resources over the next few years ranging from schools' sex education programmes to an ambitious project from the United Kingdom which will deliver all the knowledge-based curriculum components required for specialist training in GUM, called e-Learning for Healthcare (e-LfH). This is a Department of Health programme in partnership with the NHS and professional bodies which is developing an online training tool in various specialties including sexual health. Professionals providing sexual health care, either as specialists or as part of enhanced local services, will be able to access training modules specific to the level of knowledge they require.

Currently, online educational resources for a selection of sexual health competencies for pharmacists are available through the

Table 23.2 Further information and support groups.

HIV/AIDS	AIDS.gov	www.aids.gov
	AIDS Portal	www.aidsportal.org
	Avert	www.avert.org
	HIV Drug Interactions	www.hiv-druginteractions.org
	National AIDS Manual (UK)	www.aidsmap.com
	Terrence Higgins Trust (THT)	www.tht.org.uk
STIs	Australian Herpes Management Forum (AHMF)	www.ahmf.com.au
	CHAPS (gay men's sexual health)	www.chapsonline.org.uk
	Family Planning Association (UK)	www.fpa.org.uk
	GMFA (gay men's sexual health)	www.gmfa.org.uk
	National Network of STD/HIV Prevention Training Centers (USA)	www.depts.washington.edu/nnptc/
	NHS Choices (UK)	www.nhs.uk

Table 23.3 Online sexual health education programmes and conference summary web sites.

Target professional group	Organisation	Web address
Multidisciplinary	e-Learning for Healthcare (UK)	www.e-lfh.org.uk
Pharmacists	Centre for Pharmacy Postgraduate Education (UK)	www.cppe.manchester.ac.uk
General practitioners	UKRCGP	www.rcgp.org.uk
Conference and trial updates	Clinical Care Options HIV Also see relevant association web sites	www.clinicaloptions.com/hiv

Table 23.4 Sexual health professional body web sites.

Target professional group	Organisation	Web address
Multidisciplinary	American Sexually Transmitted Diseases Association (ASTDA)	www.depts.washington.edu/astda
	British Association for Sexual Health and HIV (BASHH)	www.bashh.org
	British HIV Association (BHIVA)	www.bhiva.org
	Faculty of Sexual and Reproductive Healthcare (FSRH)	www.ffprhc.org.uk
Doctors	Australasian Chapter of Sexual Health Medicine	www.racp.edu.au
Pharmacists	Royal Pharmaceutical Society of Great Britain (RPSGB)	www.rpsgb.org.uk
Sexual health advisors	Society of Sexual Health Advisors (SSHA)	www.ssha.info
Nurses	Genito-Urinary Nurses Association (GUNA)	www.guna.org.uk

Centre for Postgraduate Pharmacy Education (CPPE). For general practitioners, the UK Royal College of General Practitioners (UKRCGP) has developed a basic online educational programme aimed to provide the minimum sexual health knowledge required by all GPs (Table 23.3). The National Network of STD/HIV Prevention Training Centers (NNPTC) web site provides links to online training for health care professionals as well as information of non-web-based courses. Details of non-web-based training courses in sexual health and HIV can also be found through relevant professional body web sites (Table 23.4).

Conference web sites often publish submitted abstracts and upload videos and commentaries of plenary sessions. Several web sites also summarise key messages from conferences and published trial data (Table 23.3).

In conclusion, we believe that the internet can and should have a key role in providing information and education about STIs and HIV to both patients and professionals. The very nature of the infections we manage means that patients may be much more likely to access health information this way. Professionals have a responsibility to be familiar with high quality sites and guide patients to these appropriately. Advances in online education provision in this speciality are likely to lead to a great expansion in online provision in the next few years.

Further reading

Andreassen HK, Bujnowska-Fedak MM, Chronaki CE, Dumitru RC, Pudule I, Santana S, *et al.* European citizens' use of E-health services: a study of seven countries. *BMC Public Health* 2007;**7**:53.

Dickerson S, Reinhart AM, Freely TH, Bidani R, Rich E, Garg VK, *et al.* Patient Internet use for health information at three urban primary care clinics. *J Am Med Inform Assoc* 2004;**11**(6):499–504.

Pew Internet and American life project. Online health search 2006. Available at http://www.pewinternet.org/pdfs/PIP_Online_Health_2006.pdf.

Purcell GP, Wilson P, Delamothe T. The quality of health information on the internet. *Br Med J* 2002;**324**(7337):557–8.

Schembri G, Schober P. The Internet as a diagnostic aid: the patients' perspective. *Int J STD AIDS* 2009;**20**(4):231–3.

APPENDICES

Proformas for Taking Sexual Histories

Appendix 1: Male sexual history proforma

MALE (New patient/episode)

PATIENT STICKER

DATE **SEEN BY (print/stamp)**

Presenting complaint

Last sexual contact	M/F Known	Reg/Cas/ and duration	Country	TYPE OF SEX				Condoms used?	Condom breaks/failure?
				Oral	Vaginal	Anal	Other		

Number of partners in last 3/12

Past history of STDs

Past medical history

Hepatitis A/B vaccination

Medication

Allergies

Recreational drugs (last 3/12)

Injecting drug use
Smoking
Alcohol

HIV TEST
Previous test
Blood donor

Risks
Male partners
HIV positive partner
From high prevalence area
High risk partner

Window period

Expectation of result

PN/support

Test today

EXAMINATION

LN

Testes

Penis

Perianal area

Tests (stick pathology form here)

Nursing notes

Diagnosis/Management Plan

Health promotion

Safer sex

Condoms

HIV

HAV/HBV vaccine

Contraception

Partner notification
Contact slips issued (number)

Treatment

Checked for drug interactions Yes/No

Referral to HA
Reason

Advice/information

KC60 Diagnosis codes
1.
2.
3.
4.

Orientation

Source of referral

GP letter required

Follow-up: Attend.......... Letter.......... Phone........

Doctor/SpN signature ....

Male proforma May 2003

Appendix 2: Female sexual history proforma

FEMALE (New patient/episode)

PATIENT STICKER

DATE **SEEN BY (print/stamp)**

Presenting complaint

Last sexual contact	M/F	Reg/Cas/ Known and duration	Country	TYPE OF SEX				Condoms used?	Condom breaks/failure?
				Oral	Vaginal	Anal	Other		

Number of partners in last 3/12

Past history of STDs

Past medical history

Medication

Current contraception

LMP Cycle

Pregnancies

Last Cytology Where taken

Result Ever abnormal

Allergies

Recreational drugs (last 3/12)

Injecting drug use

Smoking
Alcohol

Sex work

HIV TEST
Previous test
Blood donor

Risks
HIV positive partner
Bisexual partner
From high prevalence area
Other high risk partner

Window period

Expectation of result

PN/support

Test today

EXAMINA TION

LN

Vulva

Vagina
pH

Cervix

Bimanual

Tests (stick pathology form here)

Nursing notes

Diagnosis/Management Plan

Health promotion

Safer sex

Condoms

HIV

HBV vaccine

Contraception (including need for EC today)

Partner notification
Contact slips issued (number)

Treatment

Checked for drug interactions Yes/No

Referral to HA
Reason

Advice/information

KC60 Diagnosis codes
1.
2.
3.
4.

Orientation

Source of referral

GP letter required

Follow-up: Attend.......... Letter........... Phone...........

Doctor/SpN signature ....

Female proforma May 2003

Appendix 3: Assessment proforma for young people attending sexual health services

Name/ID: .... **Age:** ....

ESSENTIAL			ADDITIONAL INFORMATION
Age	Under 13	13-15	
Parental awareness of sexual activity	No	Yes	
Involuntary sexual activity			
Current	Yes	No	
Previous	Yes	No	
More than 1 partner	Yes	No	
Partners ages (specify)			
Partner in position of trust	Yes	No	
Alcohol use	Yes	No	
Drug abuse	Yes	No	
Pre-puberty	Yes	No	
Intellectual understanding	No	Yes	
Other young people/children at risk	Yes	No	
			ADDITIONAL
Involvement of other services	Yes	No	
Home circumstances of concern (e.g. in care/looked after)	Yes	No	
Out of school	Yes	No	
Aggression/coercion/bribery/grooming	Yes	No	
Mental health issues	Yes	No	
			FRASER COMPETENCY FOR TREATMENT
Understands advice given	No	Yes	
Cannot be persuaded to inform parent(s)	Yes	No	
Is likely to have intercourse	No	Yes	
Physical and/or mental health likely to suffer if care not given	No	Yes	
Best interest is care with or without parental consent	No	Yes	
			ACTION
Need to disclose	Yes	No	
Reasons			
Consent to disclose	Yes	No	
Discussed with/seen by senior doctor	Yes	No	
Action			
Referred to Health Adviser	Yes	No	
Follow up	Yes	No	
Name of Doctor/Nurse/HA			
Date:			

Index

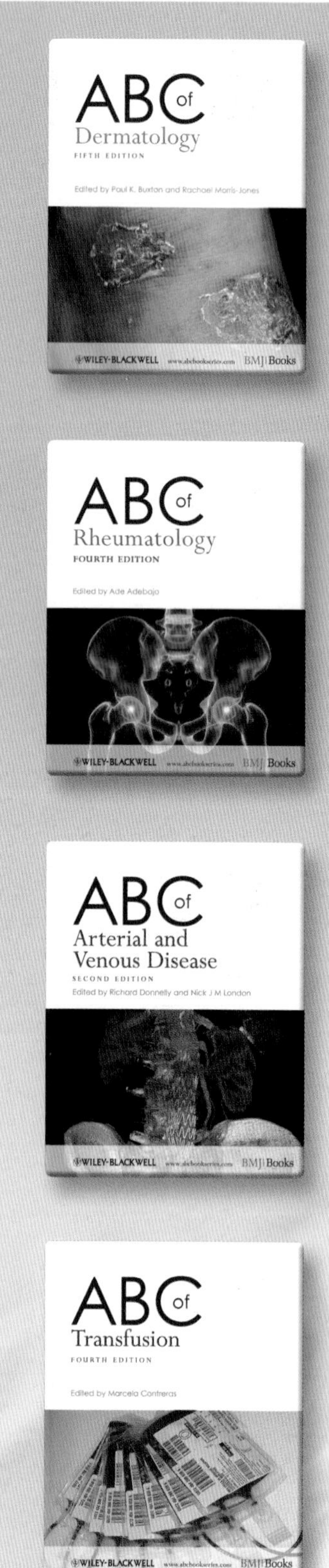

ABC of Dermatology

5TH EDITION

Edited by Paul K. Buxton & Rachael Morris-Jones
Consultant Dermatologist, Hampshire; King's College Hospital, London

- A new 20th anniversary edition of this bestselling *ABC* covering the diagnosis and treatment of skin conditions for the non-dermatologist
- Covers the core knowledge on therapy, management and diagnosis of common conditions and highlights the evidence base
- Provides clear learning outcomes and basic science boxes
- Includes a new chapter on the general principles of skin condition management for specialist nurses

March 2009 | 9781405170659 | 224 pages
£28.99/US$52.95/€35.90/AU$57.95

ABC of Rheumatology

4TH EDITION

Edited by Ade Adebajo
University of Sheffield

- A practical guide to the diagnosis and treatment of rheumatology for the non-specialist
- Fully revised and updated to include information on new treatments and therapies while covering the core knowledge on therapy, management and diagnosis
- A highly illustrated, informative and practical source of knowledge offering links to further information and resources
- This established *ABC* is an accessible reference for all primary care health professionals

October 2009 | 9781405170680 | 192 pages
£27.99/US$44.95/€34.90/AU$57.95

ABC of Arterial and Venous Disease

2ND EDITION

Edited by Richard Donnelly & Nick J.M. London
University of Nottingham; University of Leicester

- A practical guide to the diagnosis and treatment of arterial and venous disease for the non-specialist, focusing on the modern day management of patients
- Explains the different interventions for arterial and venous disease
- Covers the core knowledge on therapy, management and diagnosis and highlights the evidence base on varicose veins, diabetes, blood clots, stroke and TIA and use of stents
- This revised new edition now includes information on new treatments and therapies, antithrombotic therapy, and non-invasive techniques

April 2009 | 9781405178891 | 120 pages
£26.99/US$49.95/€33.90/AU$54.95

ABC of Transfusion

4TH EDITION

Edited by Marcela Contreras
Royal Free and University College Hospitals Medical School, London

- A comprehensive and highly regarded guide to all the practical aspects of blood transfusion
- This new edition is an established reference from a leading centre in transfusion
- Includes five new chapters on variant CJD, stem cell transplantation, immunotherapy, blood matching and appropriate use of transfusion
- Reflects the latest developments in blood transfusion management

March 2009 | 9781405156462 | 128 pages
£26.99/US$49.95/€33.90/AU$54.95

CURRENT TITLES

ABC of Mental Health
2ND EDITION

Edited by Teifion Davies & Tom Craig
Both King's College, London Institute of Psychiatry

- Provides clear practical advice on how to recognise, diagnose and manage mental disorders successfully and safely
- Includes sections on selecting drugs and psychological treatments, and improving compliance
- Contains information on the major categories of mental health disorders, the mental health needs of vulnerable groups (such as the elderly, children, homeless and ethnic minorities) and psychological treatments
- Covers the mental health needs of special groups: equips GPs and hospital doctors with all the information they need for the day to day management of patients with mental health problems

May 2009 | 9780727916396 | 128 pages
£27.99/US$47.95/€34.90/AU$57.95

ABC of Lung Cancer

Edited by Ian Hunt, Martin M. Muers & Tom Treasure
Guy's Hospital, London; Leeds General Infirmary; Guy's & St. Thomas' Hospital, London

- A practical guide for those involved in the care of the lung cancer patient
- An up-to-date evidence-based review of one of the most common cancers in the western world
- Written by the specialists involved in the launch of the NICE UK Lung Cancer Guidelines
- Looks at the epidemiology and diagnosis of lung cancer, focusing particularly on primary care issues

April 2009 | 9781405146524 | 64 pages
£21.99/US$37.95/€27.90/AU$44.95

ABC of Spinal Disorders

Edited by Andrew Clarke, Alwyn Jones, Michael O'Malley & Robert McLaren
Royal Devon and Exeter Hospital; University of Wales Hospital, Cardiff; Warrington Hospital; GP

- This brand new title addresses the causes and management of the different spinal conditions presenting in general practice
- Provides much needed practical guidance on the diagnosis, treatment and advice as back pain is one of the commonest causes for absence from work and is a chronic problem confronting general practitioners
- Includes guidance for the GP when they have to refer patients for more specialist treatment

December 2009 | 9781405170697 | 72 pages
£19.99/US$35.95/€24.90/AU$39.95

ABC of Medical Law

Lorraine Corfield, Ingrid Granne & William Latimer-Sayer
Guy's and St Thomas' NHS Trust, London; University of Oxford; Lawyer, Clinical Negligence and Personal Injury Specialist

- Fills the gap for a basic introduction to legal issues in health care that is easy to understand and act upon
- Provides up to date coverage of contentious issues such as withholding and withdrawing treatment and confidentiality
- Accessible to those without any legal knowledge, providing guidance without becoming embroiled in complicated legal discussion

June 2009 | 9781405176286 | 64 pages
£19.99/US$35.95/€24.90/AU$39.95

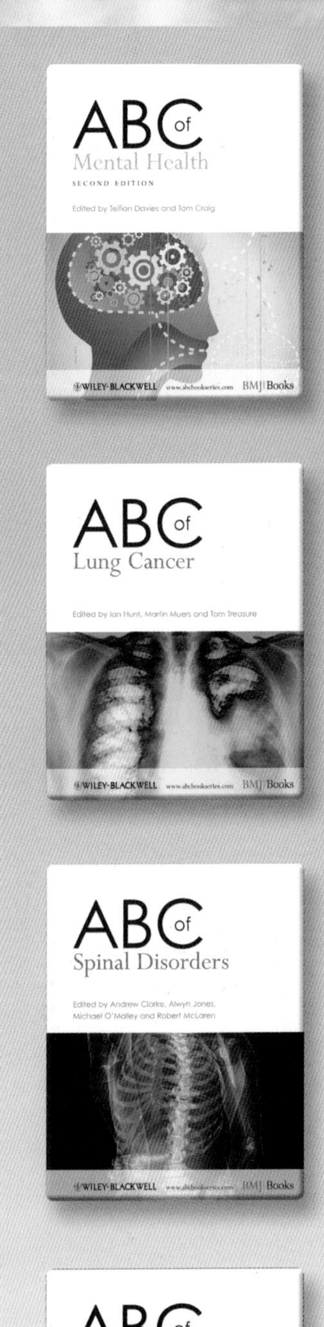

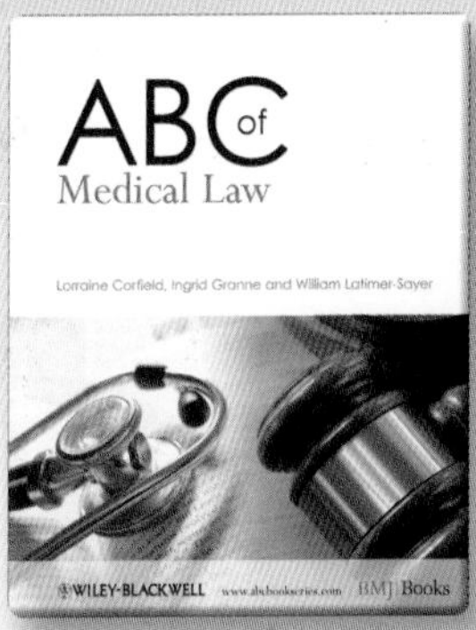